Dover
Gardner-Webb University
P.O. Box 836
Boiling Springs, N.C. 28017

HYPNOTISM
A HYPNOSIS TRAINING & TECHNIQUES MANUAL

"THE REAL QUESTIONS & ANSWERS"

ONE HUNDRED AND THIRTY QUESTIONS & ANSWERS OF HYPNOSIS
RAPID * INSTANT * SHOCK * HYPNOSIS INDUCTION METHODS
HYPNOTHERAPY SCRIPTS AND SUGGESTIONS FOR CLIENTS
SUBCONSCIOUS RECONDITIONED RESPONSE METHOD
INTERLINGUAL HYPNOTIC TRANCE INDUCTION
VISUAL IMAGERY SUGGESTION TECHNIQUES
EMOTION REPLACMENT THERAPY
REMOVING FEARS AND PHOBIAS
ENERGY VITALIZING HYPNOSIS
ACUPRESSURE HYPNOSIS
AND MORE

BY
TOM SILVER
ORMOND MCGILL
CLINICAL HYPNOTHERAPISTS

Forward by:
Ormond McGill
Dean Of American Hypnotists

SILVER HYPNOSIS INSTITUTE

Silver Institute Publishing Co.
Newbury Park * California

Published Copyright © 2003

Un-Published First Copyright © 1995
By
Tom Silver and Ormond McGill
(ISBN) 0-9678515-9-9

Library of Congress Catalog Card Number:
2002209867

All rights reserved. No part of this book may be reproduced in any form, electronic or mechanical, including photocopy, recording, or any information storage and retrieval system, without permission in writing from the publisher.

Printed in the United States of America

Published by:
The Silver Institute Publishing Co.
P.O. Box 189
Newbury Park, CA 91319-0189
www.tomsilver.com

In conjunction with:
Silver Hypnosis Institute
Training and Techniques Center

TABLE OF CONTENTS

NOTE TO THE READER xv

FORWARD BY ORMOND MCGILL xvii
(THE DEAN OF AMERICAN HYPNOTIST)

CHAPTER ONE
A BRIEF HISTORY OF HYPNOTISM 1

CHAPTER TWO
HYPNOSIS
 1. What Is Hypnosis? 5
  (a) What Is Mind?
  (b) What Is Hypnotic Suggestion?

CHAPTER THREE
CHARACTERISTICS OF HYPNOSIS
 2. What Is The Main Characteristics Of Hypnosis?
  A. Deep Relaxation Of The Body 11
  B. Absolute Fixation Of Attention 12
  C. Enhancement Of Senses Within The Field Of Attention 12
  D. Control Of Reflexes And Subconscious Nervous Activity
   Response to Post-hypnotic Suggestions 12

CHAPTER FOUR
QUESTIONS AND ANSWERS OF HYPNOTISM
 3. Are People Now Accepting Hypnotherapy? 14
 4. What Do Doctor's Think Of Hypnosis? 14
 5. How Does Hypnosis Change Brain Wave Activity? 15
 6. What Are The Different Stages Of hypnosis? 18
 7. Is Hypnotherapy Sessions Effective In All Hypnosis Depths? 18
 8. When Does Our Mind Start Operating? 20
 9. What Is Environmental Hypnosis? 22

CHAPTER FIVE
THE RELATIONSHIP BETWEEN HYPNOSIS AND SLEEP
10. Is Hypnosis And Sleep The Same Thing?   25

CHAPTER SIX
MORE QUESTIONS
11. Is There Any Danger Of A Subject Not Awakening?   27
12. How Long Does It Take To Hypnotize A Person?   29
13. Are Men Better Hypnotic Subjects Than Women?   30
14. Is It Difficult To Hypnotize A Strong Minded Person?   30
15. Can Animals Be Hypnotized?   30
16. Can Children Be Hypnotized?   31
17. Is Age A Factor In Hypnotizing?   31
18. Who Makes The Best Hypnotic Subject?   32
19. Who Can Become A Hypnotist Or Hypnotherapist?   32
20. How Can You Tell If A Person Is Hypnotized?   33
21. Is Willpower Important To Being Hypnotized?   33
22. Have I Ever Been Hypnotized Without Knowing It?   36
23. What Does It Feel Like To Be Hypnotized?   36
24. Can A Person Be Hypnotized With Their Eyes Open?   37
25. Can Hypnosis Program A Person?   37
26. Can Hypnosis Deprogram A Person?   37
27. What is The Hypnotic Trance?   38
28. What is The Best Time To Be Hypnotized?   39
29. What Technical Training Does One Need To Become A Hypnotist?   39
30. Can The Police Utilize Hypnosis?   40
31. Is Hypnosis Apposed By Any Religions?   40
32. Does Hypnosis Come From The Devil?   41
33. Is Hypnosis The Same Thing As Meditation?   41
34. What Is The Difference Between Western and Oriental Hypnotism?   41
35. What Is The Difference Between Mesmerism and Hypnotism?   42
36. What Is Stage Hypnotism?   42

CHAPTER SEVEN
PHENOMENA PRODUCED BY HYPNOTISM AND MORE
37. What Phenomena Will Hypnotism Produce?   46
38. Can A Person Be Too Eager To Be Hypnotized?   50
39. How Many Times Should A Person Be Hypnotized?   50

40. How Many Methods Of Hypnotizing Are There?	51
41. What's The Nancy School of Hypnotism?	51
42. What's The Salpetriere School of Hypnotism?	51
43. When Was Hypnotherapy Re-established Following its Decline After Charcot?	52
44. What Is Meant By The Body Rigidity Test?	52
45. Can A Person Resist Being Hypnotized?	54
46. What Is The Hypnotic Seal?	55
47. Are Some People Easier To Hypnotize Than Others?	55
48. What Type Of Things Can A Hypnotized Person Perform On Stage?	55
49. What Is The Role of A Hypnotherapist?	58
50. Is A Hypnotherapist Like A Parent To The Client?	58
51. What Is The Parent/Hypnotherapist Relationship?	58
52. What Is Meant By Ideo-Motor Response?	59
53. Is Proper Timing In Giving Suggestions Important In Hypnotizing?	59
54. Does Repetition Of A Suggestion Increase Its Influence?	60
55. Does The Combining Of Suggestions Help In Hypnotizing?	60
56. Can A Person Be Trained In Subconscious Conditioned Responsiveness?	61
57. Does Voluntary Actions Increase Hypnotic Suggestibility?	61
58. Does Deep Breathing Increase Suggestibility?	62
59. Are Non Verbal Suggestions Of Use In Hypnotizing?	
60. Does Personalizing Suggestions Add To There Influence?	62
61. What is Meant By Visualization And Visual Imagery?	63
62. Is Hypnotism Safe And Sane?	63
63. Can Hypnosis Be Used To Influence Or Even Commit A Crime?	64
64. What's Automatic Writing and Drawing?	65
65. Can A Person Stop Smoking Using Hypnosis?	66
66. Can A Person Lose Weight Using Hypnosis?	66
67. Can Hypnosis Help A Person Sleep?	67
68. What Is Meant By Hypnotic Relaxation?	67
69. What Is Hypno-Anesthesia?	69
70. Can Hypnosis Help Athletes In Sports?	69
71. Can Hypnosis Help Develop Talent?	69
72. What Is Meant By Age Regression Hypnosis?	70
73. Can Hypnosis Help Overcome Drug Addiction?	70
74. Does Alcohol Make A Person More Receptive To Hypnosis?	71

75. Can Hypnosis Stop A Headache? 71
76. Can Hypnosis Be Used In The Field Of Education? 71
77. Is There Any Value In Sleep Learning? 72
78. Do Subliminal Suggestion Tapes Have Value? 73
79. Do Hypnosis Audio Programs Really Work? 73
80. Can The Severally Mentally Challenged Be Hypnotized? 74
81. Can Drugs Be Used To Increase Hypnotic Receptivity? 74
82. Can A Person Hear Better Through Hypnosis? 75
83. Can Hypnosis Advance The ESP Powers Of The Mind? 75
84. Is It Possible To Hypnotize A Person Who is Sleeping? 75
85. Can A Person Learn Faster While Hypnotized? 76
86. What Psychological Disorders Can Hypnosis Helpfully Aid? 76
87. What Physical Disorders Can Hypnosis Helpfully Aid? 77

CHAPTER EIGHT
LINGUISTIC QUESTIONS AND ANSWERS
INTERLINGUAL HYPNOTIC TRANCE INDUCTION

88. Is It Possible To Hypnotize In Another Language? 81
89. What Is The Interlingual Hypnotic Trance Induction Method? 83
90. Can An Interpreter Hypnotize A Person? 83
91. How Effective Is Interlingual Hypnosis? 83
92. What Special Considerations Should Be Taken Into Consideration In Conducting The Interlingual Hypnosis? 84
93. How Deeply Hypnotized Can A Person Become With Interlingual Hypnosis? 84
94. What Hypnotic Demonstrations And Or Positive Changes Can Occur with Inter-lingual Hypnotism? 85
95. How Many People Can Be Hypnotized At Once With Translingual Hypnosis? 85
96. Can Children Be Hypnotized By Using This Method Translingual Hypnotism? 86
97. Who Makes The Best Interpreter? 86
98. Is It Possible To Hypnotize Over The Television Or Telephone? 90
99. Can Watching A Movie Hypnotize You? 90
100. Can Reading A Book Hypnotize You? 90
101. What Safety Considerations Should Be Taken When Conducting Group Hypnosis? 91
102. Can A Person Perform Super Feats While Hypnotized? 91

CHAPTER ONE

A HISTORY OF HYPNOTISM

Hypnotism in one form or another has been practiced for a very long time. For hundreds of years the Yogi have applied the practice in various ways. They would throw themselves and others into a trance state of mind through concentration on various mantras.

Hypnotic phenomena can be observed in the ancient practices of Egyptian priests used in Temples of Healing. Also, the Persian Magi and Chinese Mystics used it to alleviate suffering.

The psychic side of hypnotism, such as clairvoyance and mental telepathy (which today is referred to as ESP) were also recorded among the old forms of hypnotism. We read of such references in relation to the Hebrew prophecies and the Oracles of Greece. The ancients held those who practiced such strange and secret powers in awe. Little wonder, as the secrets were kept closely guarded and were passed on by word of mouth only among the elect. That is to say, handed on from father to son as a precious heritage.

With the advent of Jesus Christ, an avenue of enlightenment was opened. He told of such truths about the wonderful inner nature of man. This Master performed miracles through the power of the mind. He explained that they were miracles that all could perform. He willingly revealed these divine secrets, which cured people of many ailments. He even resurrected the dead by His hypnotic and occult power, which was manifested by suggestion and the laying on of hands. The masses, with few exceptions, were not ready to mentally grasp the principles of His teachings and preferred to stay in ignorance and superstition. However, the seed was sown, and it could not entirely be destroyed even by His death. His twelve Apostles carried on His work and spread His teachings among many nations. Today His doctrines and followers number in the billions.

We find a large number of mental healers among the early Christians who applied Christ's methods of curing the sick. They were persecuted by the Romans and then put to death. The result was that after a time, in that period of early history, such methods of healing (the laying on of hands and prayer mantras of suggestive therapy) almost became obliterated.

However, with the later rise of Christian Churches, numerous priests and monks returned to faith healing and the suggestive power of prayer.

In the later part of the 18th Century, a Jesuit Priest by the name of Father Gassner created a sensation in Germany. He would induce the hypnotic condition by suddenly entering a room where a person was waiting and, with an uplifted crucifix in one hand, walk towards the person to call out in a stentorian voice the word "sleep" in Latin.

Invariably he would thus induce a state of hypnosis. He performed some remarkable experiments. In one of his "sensitives" he suspended the heartbeat for several minutes and then called the person back to life after an apparent death.

Another 18th Century man who was instrumental in renewed interest in this subject was the Viennese physician, Dr. Frederick Anton Mesmer, who is credited with being the "father" of mental medicine in relatively modern times.

Mesmer came to Paris in the spring of 1778 from Vienna, Austria where he had obtained his original degree. From working with physical magnets, (which was popular with doctors of the period) he developed a theory of using his hands for curing, stating that they exuded the same magnetic influence as a physical magnet. As this influence was organic in nature, he called it "Animal Magnetism". He claimed that this magnetism was in the human body and could be communicated from doctor to patient. He performed remarkable cures and his process became known as "Mesmerism".

Paris received Mesmer and his doctrines with open arms. He soon opened one of the finest salons imaginable where he treated and cured hundreds of people, rich and poor alike. The demand for his treatments became so great that he conceived the idea of treating his patients "en masse". He installed a sort of fountain in the center of his treatment room, which was called the "baquet". It was filled with water, which had been previously "magnetized". The "baquet" was then covered with a lid that had holes in it and through these holes, iron rods protruded (one for each patient). Thirty or so patients could be treated simultaneously while seated around the contrivance. Mesmer was dressed in a lilac robe while music played in the background. He would walk around and touch each patient's troubled part of the body, while the patients held the energy rod from the baquet. Also, the patients were tied together by a silver cord. Hundreds of cures are on record, which he accomplished by this procedure.

It is recorded that he treated over 8,000 patients during the year of 1784. It has been said that he charged exorbitant fees for his services and that he made a fortune for himself. This is true in regards to his rich patrons, but it is equally true that the poor were treated similarly yet free of charge.

His success aroused the jealous antagonism of other French physicians who discredited his work. Mesmer returned to his native country where he died in 1815. Following Mesmer, the next historic figure that was prominent in the advancement of hypnotherapeutics was Dr. James Braid of England.

Dr. Braid was born in 1795 in Edinburgh. He graduated there as a physician and surgeon. He settled in Manchester after practicing medicine in Scotland for a number of years and remained there until his death in 1860.

Dr. Braid is regarded as the real rediscoverer of what is today called "hypnotism". In fact, it was he who coined that name. He took it from the Greek word "Hypnos", which means the god of sleep. Thus, "hypnotism", as we know it today, was born.

After having witnessed an exhibition on mesmerism and animal magnetism presented by a French mesmerist in the city of Manchester, England, Dr. Braid started a series of experiments on his own. He soon found that the same phenomena could be produced without using passes and without need for a belief in a so-called "magnetic fluid". He developed a method of having his subjects gaze intently at a bright object held some inches in front of and above the eyes that seemed to produce a state analogous to natural sleep. His method seeded to produce results similar to those claimed by the mesmerists. Braid concluded that "animal magnetism" had nothing to do with the production of the phenomena. In his opinion, it was a matter of the concentration of the subject upon the object held in front of his eyes. In his early work he used no verbal suggestions to amplify the trance state. In later years, Dr. Braid added suggestions to his technique. As was mentioned, he called the mental condition he induced "hypnotism" and the termination of the condition he called "dehypnotizing".

His conscientious work in the field led other prominent men of his times to study the phenomena, which advanced an understanding of its psychological nature. Among these was Dr. A.A. Liebault of France.

In 1864 Dr. Liebault settled in Nancy, France to practice medicine and hypnotism. His hypnotic patients grew so numerous that he was forced to enlarge his quarters.

His successful work with hypnotism soon attracted attention throughout France. Subsequently he joined forces with his esteemed physician friend, Dr. Bernheim, and together the Nancy School of Hypnotherapy was formed.

Liebault used Braid's method of inducing hypnotic sleep using verbal suggestions along with it at all times. Himself and Bernheim recognized the value of suggestions. They published an acclaimed work titled "Suggestive Therapeutics" some years later that was based on case histories of cures performed at their "Nancy Clinic."

At this same historic period, Dr. Charcot in the Sapetriere of Paris drew attention to the subject and attracted many followers.

The Sapetriere and the Nancy School held many differences of opinions about the causation of hypnotic phenomena. Charcot asserted that only neurotic and hysterical people could be hypnotized.

The Nancy School held that induced somnambulism (hypnosis) is universal to all humanity and healthy people actually made the best subjects. After the death of these pioneers in modern hypnotism, the therapeutic use of hypnosis fell in decline as Freud's work in psychoanalysis came to the forefront.

During that period it was stage hypnotists touring countries who kept hypnotism publicly alive.

It was during World War II that hypnosis again became revived for therapeutic use as an aid to help shell shocked soldiers. In that period hypnotism became officially recognized by the American Medical Association as having definite value as a form of healing art.

Since that recognition by the medical profession the advancement of hypnotherapy has been phenomenal. Today, a belief in the physiological transfer of human energy from doctor to patient (as Mesmer suggested) is given respect along with the psychological aspect of the psychology of suggestion.

In our opinion both aspects of the science have a place, while the association with hypnotism to programming the biocomputer of the human brain has had astronomical influence.

CHAPTER TWO

WHAT IS HYPNOSIS?

Question No. 1 ...
WHAT IS HYPNOSIS?

This the most frequently asked and the very first question that we have to answer is the same.

So for the first question ... What Is Hypnosis?

We have to look at this question from two sub-questions:
  a. What is mind?
  b. What is Hypnotic Suggestion?

(a) WHAT IS MIND?

Mind is nothing tangible and has many various names. Mind is a process for producing thoughts. Thoughts are forms of energy. Thoughts are what we think. What we think is how we are. What we are is in accordance to our behavior. This classic quotation expresses it well: As a man thinketh in his heart so is he.

There are five levels of conduct within us from which all behavior springs: instinct, reflex, habit, conscious thought, and the subconscious.

The first level, that of instinct, is located in the visceral region of the body where the impulses that drive us are felt. Here in our midsection is where we feel most strongly; it is the seat of emotions, even ambitions and the lure to drive on to an enticing future are felt in the torso.

Both the spinal cord and the lower brain control the reflex level. Within its scope are the numerous reflexes with which we are all familiar, such as blinking our eyes, dodging from danger, reaching with the hands to explore, and many others.

The third level that of habit behavior, probably located in the lower brain, works mechanically. As the reflex system does, but permeates the whole field of human endeavor.

The fourth level of behavior, which is that of conscious thought, is the crowning achievement of human performance.

It is designed to work through, and control, the lower levels of response and to stand as the progressive and civilizing force of mankind.

The fifth level of behavior, that of the subconscious, is that part of us that permeates all of the four levels of conduct here listed. An impulse may have a subconscious origin. A reflex is generally subconscious. Habit, in its last stage, is controlled subconsciously. Conscious thought, itself, may be colored by sub-conscious control.

Such is an anatomical presentation of human behavior, in the body via the brain and nervous system. The psychological presentation is to look upon mind in two aspects (phases); one involving what is referred to as conscious mind (10%), and the other as subconscious mind (90%). Each phase has it range of mental activities, i.e., conscious mind activity is induction, it can be critical of what it accepts or rejects. It is analytical utilizing logic & reason. Subconscious mind activity is deductive in that it accepts uncritically what it accepts, and acts upon such in spontaneous and automatic behavior.

The subconscious is the storehouse of memory. In it, every experience that happens to use from earliest infancy to the last hour of life is filed, and many people believe that memories of past lifetimes are therein also filed. These memories are not passive; they are vitally active, each one forming a thread in the texture of our personality. The total of all these impressions is the person himself. The latest scientific facts show that memories are formed with actual physiological changes of human nerve systems. Neuron connections are made according to various external stimuli.

The subconscious is also a dynamo. It is dominated by emotion, and emotion is the driving force of life. It is the energy source of creativity, motivation, and for the performance of the vital functions of the body.

The subconscious plays the role of supervisor over our body's physical processes. Digestion, assimilation, the circulation of the blood, the action of the lungs, the kidneys, and all the vital organs are controlled by its agency.

The subconscious never sleeps, indeed, during sleep it seems to be more alert and active than it is during waking hours, as evidence by the dreams we have. And it is protective.

The two aspects of mind, conscious and subconscious, in daily activity, are in perpetual interaction. If we consciously think a thought (idea), and cause it to be accepted by the subconscious, the idea will spontaneously go into action in producing the effect.

If it is a healthful thought we are so much the better: if it is a diseased one, we are so much the worse. For unlike consciousness, as has been mentioned, the subconscious has no selective power; whatever is presented to it is accepted and automatically acted upon. It is in the process of this transformation of a thought into an element of our life that we make use of the power of suggestion. And hypnosis places the mind in a mental state, which is hypersuggestible. In the hypnotic state the critical qualities of conscious mind are bypassed and the spontaneous qualities of subconscious mind are activated, by the power of suggestions.

(b). What is a Hypnotic Suggestion?

Suggestion in relation to hypnosis provides communication with the subconscious. A definition of suggestion is being a subconscious realization of an idea. What is interesting is that suggestion is used to induce the state of hypnosis and then is used to control the state it induces. This had lead some to say, Hypnosis and suggestion are one and the same. However, this cannot be true, as hypnosis is a state of mind which suggestion produces.

Examples of the power of suggestion are all around us. Examples of spontaneously aroused suggestions motivating our subconscious to action may be observed at every turn.

We listen to the description of some dread disease, and soon find ourselves developing the symptoms. We read a ghost story and while out walking that night every shadow seems a haunted spot. We meet acquaintances on the street and they with grave concern tell us that we are not looking well, and before long we find ourselves back at home sick in bed. The cause, in each case, is nothing more tangible than an idea that has become realized in the subconscious. If you wish, you could say hypnotized into the subconscious. Recognizing this truth, you will commence to gain an answer to the basic question:
WHAT IS HYPNOSIS?

It is obvious that the power of suggestion affects us physically as well as mentally.

The fact that suggestion can produce physical responses in our body can be easily proved by simply thinking of a juicy, sour, bitter lemon ... feel how the thought spontaneously starts the flow of saliva within your mouth. Or think of an itchy sensation about your body, and feel those itches commence.

But surely, you will comment that not every person would become ill because his friends told him he was sick. And right here, we come to a basic law in the operation of the Power of Suggestion:

Every suggestive idea that enters the conscious if it is accepted by the subconscious is automatically transferred by it into a reality and becomes an element in our life.

It will be appreciated from the examples cited, that the thoughts we think, determine our mental states, our sentiments and emotions, but also the delicate actions and adjustments of our physical body. Trembling, palpitation, stammering, blushing, the variety of pathological states which occur in neurosis are all due to modifications and changes in the blood-flow, in muscular action, and in the operation of the vital organs. These changes are not voluntary and conscious ones – they are determined by the capacities invested in the subconscious aspects of our mind, and come to us often with a shock of surprise.

Witness the remarkable change when we received a bit of good news, like the winning of a lottery, for example.

Our body seems to have lost all it weight, pain, and cumbersomeness. We appear to be walking on air. This is an interesting observation, for when the body is functioning at its best, we seem not to have a body. This is as it should be, for too much worry and concern over our physical condition frequently makes our body too much for us. Happy suggestion takes our mind off our body, and it functions more perfectly.

A study of suggestion and hypnosis reveal to us that when poor thinking is engaged in, meaning when a person experiences negative emotions, the body becomes a problem, and when a person thinks good positive, optimistic thoughts which activate positive emotions, the body is no longer a problem, but an asset. A happy state of mind is important to good health.

Where does hypnosis fit into the picture? The laws of applied suggestion impose first the acceptance of the idea (suggestion),and secondly its transformation into a reality. The subconscious aspect of mind performs both of these operations automatically – if the idea carries enough "Desire" to drive it home into the subconscious.

What is hypnosis? Hypnosis is the state of mind that gives every idea emotional wallop, and directs the power in a purposeful manner. Hypnosis is a technique that eliminates the possibility of the potent power of suggestion being merely a hit and miss proposition. Through the application of hypnosis we can select and use those suggestions we especially desire, and then deliberately start them to action to benefit our life.

Whether the idea is self-induced, as in the case of using Self-Hypnosis, or originates from an outside source is a matter of complete inconsequence. In both cases, it undergoes precisely the same process it is submitted (via suggestion) to the subconscious, accepted or rejected, and so either realized or ignored. Suggestions presented to a person by an outside hypnotist can sometimes be a great help in entering the state, as such becomes a dynamic situation between two persons working together to achieve a given end.

Of such is the answer to Question No. One: WHAT IS HYPNOSIS? Now that you have this understanding our answers to the various questions about hypnotism will have instant meaning to you. But first before we get into tackling detailed questions about hypnosis, let us give you a general consideration of the characteristics of hypnosis and phenomena. Such will make our submitted answers to your questions have even more meaning, and add comprehension of this fascinating subject.

Perhaps the simplest way to answer this question is to say that hypnosis is a state of mind produced through the use of suggestions, amplified by the energy of the hypnotist causing a mental condition of hypersuggestibility.

Outwardly hypnosis appears much like a state of sleep. However, internally it is quite different. In normal sleep, the attention of the sleeper is diffused, while in hypnotic sleep the attention of the sleeper is concentrated towards the suggestions presented by the hypnotist. A person may be awake and still be hypnotized. It may also by self-induced. What is of special interest is that the power of suggestion is both used to induce the state and to control the state it induces.

To understand hypnosis, it must be understood that mind functions on two levels: one, our normal waking state which we call conscious mind, and two, on an inner level which we call subconscious mind. Hypnosis brings into action the subconscious phase of mind in which the subject (often called the hypnotic) responds spontaneously and uncritically to the suggestions of the hypnotist. While in that state, the hypnotized person is not capable of inductive reasoning and cannot analyze, so to speak, what is real from the unreal.

Our subconscious mind does not distinguish between reality and imagination; our conscious logical part of our mind does that.

You will find there is a considerable difference in the actions of different people being hypnotically influenced. Some become entranced quickly (falling into a sleep-like state), and have no memory of the experience (or what occurred while in it) on being aroused. Some at first respond only to waking hypnosis tests. Others will on a first or second trial go into a light trance without complete amnesia. The memory recall is of a hazy nature, much like recalling an almost forgotten dream. As the induction is repeated several times, often the subject will drop down to deeper levels.

The more times you hypnotize a person the more responsive and deeper into hypnosis they will go. The deeper hypnotized they become, the quieter and less resistant the conscious mind or critical mind is and the more successful is the hypnosis or hypnotherapy session. Once hypnosis has been induced in a subject who has amnesia on awakening from trance, he can be quickly returned to profound hypnosis by giving him a post hypnotic suggestion to instantly re-enter hypnosis after you awaken him.

After you awaken the subject, simply look him straight in the eyes and say in a positive voice, SLEEP!

If the subject is receptive to hypnosis, they will instantly enter back into the hypnotic sleep.

CHAPTER THREE

CHARACTERISTICS OF HYPNOSIS

Question No. 2 ...
WHAT IS THE MAIN CHARACTERISTICS OF HYPNOSIS?
We consider that there are five main characteristics of the hypnotic state of mind
(Often referred to as Trance),

A. Deep Relaxation of The Body

The induction of hypnosis involves concentration on physical relaxation of the body. As the body relaxes so does the mind, in turn, relax. Concerns tend to disappear along with relaxation. Relaxation tends to cause the critical faculties of the conscious phase of our mind to submerge and allows the subconscious mind or bio computer to emerge. The scientific terms for these brain wave activities are Beta, Alpha, Theta and Delta. This is brain wave activity that can be scientifically documented with an E.E.G. machine, which is a brain-scanning device that measures brain wave frequency which is called "Hz" or (sounds like hurtz). The medical term is called an Electroencephalogram Machine.

The relaxation that hypnosis brings to the body is a most valuable asset. We live in a high-pressure world these days, and stress has become a major cause of illness and even death in some cases. Stress and body tension go hand-in-hand, and the deep relaxation hypnosis brings to the individual, removes tensions from the body, which in turn removes stress from the mind. Various mind chemicals are produced under the hypnosis sleep that can increase our body health and vitality. Sixty percent of our physical problems are caused by emotional anxiety. Stress, tension, worry, anger, depression can also lower our immune system thereby opening us to more frequent physical illness's.

If hypnosis offered no other characteristic than the deep therapeutic relaxation it provides, that alone would give proof of its invaluable nature. Some people say that twenty minutes of a hypnosis sleep, is equal to about five hours of a natural sleep.

B. Absolute Fixation of Attention

Entering the state of hypnosis consists in gradually limiting the field of attention until a perfectly concentrated and unvarying focus is reached. Attention in our waking state of mind is a bombardment of stimuli coming in via our fives senses of seeing, hearing, feeling, smelling, and tasting (varying in degree, of course, dependent on how the senses are activated at any particular moment). Entering hypnosis reduces this variety of incoming stimuli, and concentrates the full attention upon one in particular. That is to say, entering hypnosis has resulted in narrowing the field of attention so that only a very small range of stimuli is perceived, and this range is determined by the suggestions of the hypnotist. Hypnotic suggestions are nine times stronger than a waking conscious suggestion.

C. Enhancement of Senses Within the Field of Attention

Experiments in hypnosis indicate that the senses may be caused to function with much more accuracy when attention is directed to them by suggestion in the hypnotic state. The logical powers of the mind are greatly enhanced, and deductions may be performed with remarkable accuracy. The sense of smell and taste can be intensified under hypnosis. Some accounts of increased eyesight have been reported under hypnosis. The comparison between the waking and hypnotic state is much the same as the comparison between a shotgun and a rifle. Hypnosis hits the bull's eye with positive suggestions getting in with accuracy and even sometimes bypassing conscious resistance.

D. Control of Reflexes and Subconscious Nervous Activity

When a person is hypnotized, the pulse rate may be altered, areas of the body my become numb, menstrual periods may be regulated, blood circulation increased or reduced, breathing and oxygen intake reduced, body temperature changed, and other such automatic bodily functions controlled or altered under hypnotic suggestion by directly affecting "the autonomic nervous system", which regulates our respiratory and circulatory system.

E. Response to Posthypnotic Influences

Suggestions given under hypnosis for actions to be performed after the arousing from the trance will be performed provided these suggestions are not counter to powerful tendencies or the moral nature of the person that they are given to. When such suggestions are presented, the subject either refuses to accept them or may arouse spontaneously from the hypnosis relaxation. Post Hypnotic suggestions which are positive and healthy suggestions to help a person reach their goals in life and which the subject or client really wants in their life, will be more easily accepted than suggestions which are negative or contrary to the clients well-being.

More details of these basic characteristics of hypnosis will be considered in the following chapter dealing with the producible phenomena of hypnotism.

CHAPTER FOUR

QUESTIONS AND ANSWERS OF HYPNOTISM

Question No. 3 ...
ARE PEOPLE NOW ACCEPTING HYPNOTHERAPY?

We think that hypnotherapy is gaining international acceptance and is being utilized by thousands of medical practitioners, psychotherapists, psychologists, and psychiatrists because hypnosis is a science of the mind, and it works.

In the 1700s and 1800s, hypnosis was practiced by some of the top medical Doctors in Europe. Thousands of people were helped and even cured from emotional and physical ailments through the practice of hypnotherapy. Back in those days, the science was called magnetism and mesmerism. Since the mind is now being proven to be a haven of revitalizing chemicals produced in the brain, hypnosis is being used to activate these chemicals in the brain and the positive emotions in the subconscious to help heal and help people to enjoy living life more to the fullest. Hypnosis is not a cure for everything but it sure can help enhance the quality of life, health and happiness.

Hypnosis is becoming the number one form of mental health therapy and is helpful in healing the physical body pains that are created by emotional manifestations in the mind. A physical manifestation of an emotional anxiety is what hypnosis can help relieve. Hypnosis can also produce a chemical balance in the mind by creating and activating chemicals such as saratonin. We will see the science of hypnotism being used more and more every day.

Question No. 4 ...
WHAT DO DOCTORS THINK OF HYPNOSIS?

Medical Doctors are now really starting to accept hypnosis and hypnotherapy as a therapeutic tool, which can be utilized in combination with traditional medicine. Medical Doctors say that over 60% of our physical problems stem from our mind. Medical Doctors also say that stress, tension, anxiety, and worry are the biggest factors in the increase of heart attacks and even death in our American culture.

These are all emotions, and negative emotions can affect our health, our body and our life. All emotions come from the subconscious mind and can be altered, neutralized or changed through the practice and use of hypnotherapy. In the mid-1950s, the A.M.A. officially recognized the science of hypnotism and even recommended that students of medicine also should learn and study hypnosis.

Question No. 5 ...
HOW DOES HYPNOSIS CHANGE BRAIN WAVE ACTIVITY?

Yes indeed, our conscious brain wave activity, which is also called by wave frequencies do change from our waking state on into the different hypnotic states. The brain wave frequencies change as the different depths of hypnotic relaxation occurs. As a person goes deeper into hypnosis, the cycles of brain wave activity get slower and conscious brain wave activity is reduced. The conscious brain frequencies diminish and reduce.

In our waking state of brain wave activity that we call Beta, our conscious brain wave pattern frequencies might range in depth from about 14Hz up to 30 Hz (hertz are wave frequencies equal to one cycle per second which can be monitored by a EEG machine). At that stage of conscious brain activity, our conscious or cognitive mind, or what we might call, our waking state of mind is very active and alert. This state of consciousness occurs usually during the day.

The second stage of brain wave frequency activity is called Alpha. In Alpha, which is a state of light hypnosis or physical relaxation and restfulness, our brain wave frequencies, patterns or cycles slow down to about 7Hz to 13Hz brain frequency activity. Light relaxation might be considered Alpha.

The next deeper level or stage of hypnosis depth is called Theta. In the state of Theta, our conscious brain wave frequency activity slows down even more, and would register on a brain wave scanning device at about 4Hz to about 6Hz or cycles per second. When a person falls into a nice natural sleep at night, they are probably in the state of "Theta" drifting in and out of Delta.

The deepest depth of hypnosis is called Delta, or Somnambulism. In Delta, our conscious brain wave activity is reduced to only about 0.1Hz to about 4Hz. The deeper the level of hypnotic depth, the more unconscious the conscious mind becomes.

"BRAIN WAVE" TECHNOLOGY IS THE FUTURE
TOM SILVER AND TIMOTHY HUANG GIVING A LECTURE ON INTERLINGUAL HYPNOTIC TRANCE INDUCTION AND SOLVING CRIMES WITH HYPNOSIS AT THE NATIONAL GUILD OF HYPNOTISTS CONFERENCE IN NEW HAMPSHIRE *AUGUST 2002

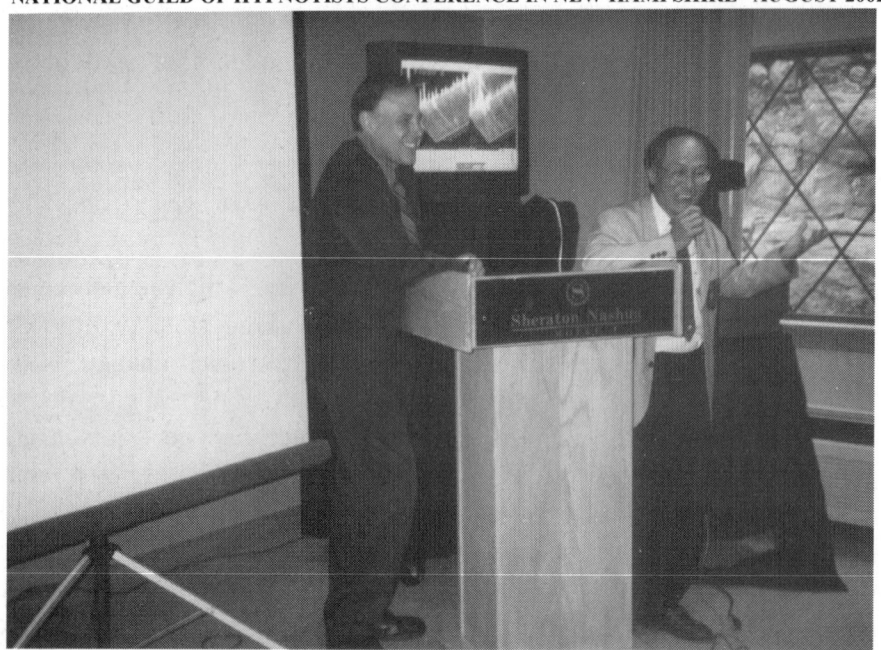

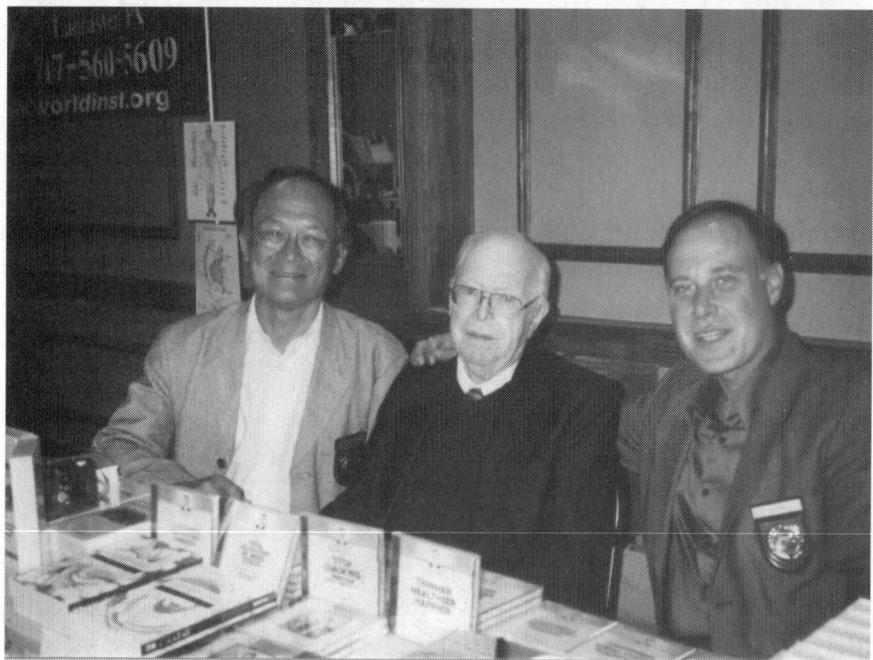

TIMOTHY HUANG * ORMOND MCGILL * TOM SILVER
SITTING AT TOM'S SELF HELP PROGRAMS BOOTH AT THE N.G.H. CONFERENCE 2002

EEG BRAIN WAVE SCAN OF SUBJECT WHO IS "NOT" HYPNOTIZED
CONSCIOUS BRAIN WAVE FREQUENCY ACTIVITY OF "BETA" (30Hz)

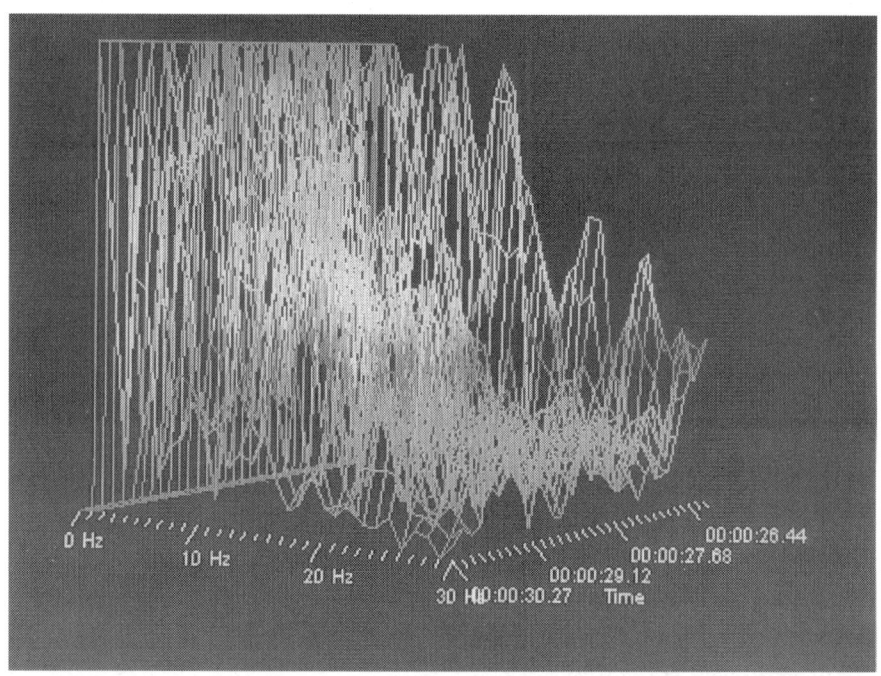

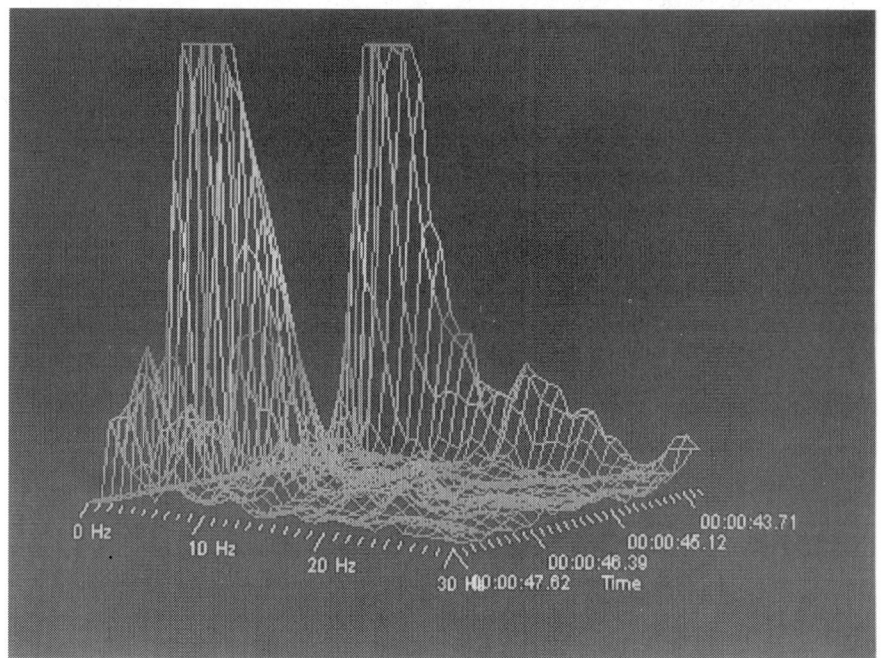

EEG BRAIN WAVE SCAN OF SUBJECT WHO IS DEEPLY HYPNOTIZED
SUBCONSCIOUS BRAIN WAVE FREQUENCY ACTIVITY OF "DELTA" (5Hz)

It is important to realize that there is indeed a way of monitoring levels of hypnosis using scientific medical devices such as the EEG machine. This type of monitoring levels of hypnosis is factual science and validates the true reality of hypnotic trance. EEG will be the physical tool to help cross hypnosis into full acceptance and usage in combination with all other mental and medical methods of healing.
In the future most clinical hypnotherapists be utilizing this technology.

Question No. 6
WHAT ARE THE DIFFERENT STAGES OF HYPNOSIS?

In modern hypnosis most theorists believe that there are three major stages of hypnosis. Some terms used to describe these stages are the hypnoidal, or light stage, cataleptic, which could also be called the medium or middle stage of hypnosis, and somnambulistic, which is considered the deepest stage of hypnosis.

Some hypnotists believe that there is also a fourth level or depth of hypnosis which they consider the psychic or medium state. In this deep hypnotic depth, E.S.P. and other psychic phenomena might occur. Maybe past life regression also occurs in this deeper level of hypnosis. More research is needed.

Relating to brain wave science. The hypnoidal or light depth of hypnosis could be considered the state of Alpha. The cataleptic depth of hypnosis could be considered the state of theta, and deepest stage of hypnosis, which we call somnambulism, could also be called the state of delta.

Question No. 7
IS HYPNOTHERAPY SUGGESTIONS EFFECTIVE IN ALL DEPTHS OF HYPNOSIS?

Hypnotherapy sessions to help people overcome negative emotions and health issues can be just as effective on a person who might be in a light stage of hypnosis, as it might be on a person who is deeply hypnotized. While a person is under light, medium, and deep hypnosis, positive suggestions, can be effectively transmitted by the hypnotherapist to the client. Only fifteen to twenty percent of the population will go into the deeper stages of hypnosis on their first time being hypnotized. When I (Tom Silver) perform hypnosis demonstrations on national television shows such as NBC's show called "The Other Half" with Dick Clark, or The "Beyond" Show on WB network with renowned physic James Van Praagh, I usually will pre-hypnotize the subjects before the taping of the television show to make sure that I can get them into delta so that I will able to show the power of hypnosis in just a few minutes. Under deep hypnosis, a therapist can create some very profound changes in a person's life. Sometimes a person can enter right into deep hypnosis on their first time being hypnotized, but for most people, it takes a few sessions to condition the conscious mind to relax and to let go. Most people tend to go deeper into hypnosis, the more times that they are hypnotized.

Our brain also produces certain mind chemicals under hypnosis or deep physical relaxation that can help to heal our mind and body. Serotonin, melotonin, dopamine, endorphins, and more. These mind chemicals in the brain are stimulated and produced naturally while a person is relaxing under hypnosis. That is why so many people feel so refreshed and energized after they awaken from a hypnotherapy session.

These "mind chemicals" can create a chemical balance in your mind and body as well as help to heal some physical pains that can occur from negative subconscious emotions. These are called body syndromes, which are physical manifestations of an emotional anxiety. These emotions are negative emotions and all emotions are located in our subconscious mind.

Hypnotherapy can be beneficial in all stages or depths of hypnosis. In deep hypnosis, somnambulism or delta, regression therapy can occur, where you can regress a person back to anytime period in their current life to help them overcome an event that has created ill health or mental disturbance. Past life regression therapy can also be achieved under the deepest stage of hypnosis.

For entertainment purposes with hypnotism, this depth of conscious silence can bring about illusion and even hallucinations in hypnotized subjects for the purposes of conducting stage hypnotism demonstrations.

We believe that only clinically trained and certified hypnotherapists should conduct stage hypnosis demonstrations. Some people believe that E.S.P. abilities might also become active in a person while under the deepest stage of hypnosis, but that is just an opinion and of course not a fact.

Question No. 8 ...
WHEN DOES OUR MIND START OPERATING?

The subconscious mind is formed and starts developing right after birth and some people think even in the womb before birth. It is located in the medulla oblongata or what is called the inner part of our brain.

From birth to about 3 years of age, everything that goes into a child's life goes directly into their subconscious mind or bio computer. The subconscious absorbs pictures, words, actions, tones and frequencies of the human voice and occurrences in the environment. It is like a sponge absorbs water. The most penetrating experiences are the emotions that are programmed or recorded into the subconscious mind. We are largely influenced and programmed subconsciously by our parents or primary caregivers.

Children record subconsciously from birth "positive and negatives" emotions into their bio computer from their parents, from other children, from the environment and from animals, like a small child or baby frightened by a dog.

Some children are filled with positive emotions such as love, trust, security, confidence, understanding, happiness and so fourth. Some children are given negative emotions, words and pictures from their primary care givers or parents of anger, fear, confusion, self-doubt, loneliness, pain, gilt, and other negative emotions, which will become deeply recorded into that child's subconscious mind.

Most people are programmed with a combination of both positive and negative emotions. Negative emotions might create really bad problems in your adult life, because once they are recorded in your subconscious mind, they will always haunt you, and they will be with you for the rest of your life, unless your subconscious mind let's go of them, and releases them through hypnotherapy, or by utilizing some other type of subconscious therapeutic procedure.

Positive emotions if programmed into your subconscious mind, will help you to enjoy life more, to be healthy, and to have success in your life. Most of us have a limited life script because of the negative emotions that are programmed into our subconscious bio-computer.

At about 3 years old, a child's conscious mind begins to become activated. That is our logic and reason part of our brain and is only about 10% of our total brainpower. It is actually our tiny bio-computer.

The conscious mind is located in the cortex of our brain or the outer part of the brain. The conscious mind is our cognitive or intellectual part of our mental power. Most people relay only on that part of their brain to succeed without realizing that to have 100 percent of total mental power, both of your minds need to be working together.

When our conscious mind is formed, we create a barrier between our conscious and subconscious mind, which can be called a critical factor or critical area of mind. When you are in a hypnotized state by a hypnotherapist, or by the environment, such as by watching movies or television, the critical factor or barrier between your conscious mind, and subconscious mind, opens up, and you are then in a hypnotic receptive state which can then record or activate positive or negative emotions. The movie "Jaws" hypnotized the viewers in the movie theaters and thousands of people all over the world had fears of the ocean and of sharks. Hypnosis is all around us in the environment.

Driving a car on automatic pilot and thinking thoughts of the day. You are hypnotized, because driving while daydreaming and then wondering how did I arrive at my destination, or was I going the right speed is what is called waking hypnosis. When you first learned how to drive, the pattern and program of driving an automobile had been recorded or embedded into your subconscious mind. The suggestions and patterns of driving were stimulated by your desire and emotions of wanting to drive. Therefore you can for the most part drive and think thoughts because the pattern of driving has been recorded into your strong bio-computer, your subconscious mind. When your conscious mind becomes active is usually when children our taught logical information in the schools. In America it is around the first grade.

Now our subconscious continuously operates with our conscious mind. When our conscious mind is operating, so is our subconscious mind operating by identifying and associating with our conscious thoughts. The subconscious, mind "Identifies and Associates" with the conscious mind thoughts. We are consciously bringing up thoughts, pictures, words and emotions from our subconscious mind. Those emotions and pictures and words are either helping us or hurting us.

If you have ever overreacted to a situation and looked back and wondered to yourself, why did you get so upset, it was because your subconscious mind identified that situation that was making you angry with a past experience and emotion of anger. The subconscious instantly related your conscious mind thoughts to the subconscious mind emotions.

Both of your minds are interacting during your waking state of life activity. We are not talking about the theory of right or left-brain, since this author's hypnotic opinion is that we have an outer and inner brain function. Your two mental bio- computers are either working together in harmony, or they are in discord, and in a dysfunctional state of limitation.

Our subconscious mind never sleeps. In a receptive hypnotic state, the subconscious records, retains, and freely accepts emotions, pictures, words and thoughts. It is receiving or imputing data. In a natural sleep like the one each and every one of us does every night. The subconscious in transmitting thoughts, emotions, pictures, words in the form of dreams.

Question No. 9
WHAT IS ENVIRONMENTAL HYPNOTISM?

Environmental hypnosis is the process of being hypnotized by the environment. Like I had mentioned earlier, driving your car and day dreaming you are hypnotized.

When you learned how to drive a car, the pattern of driving got accepted and recorded into your subconscious mind and when you daydream and drive, your subconscious mind is doing the driving for you. At that time, your subconscious is working for you.

Watching a movie we become hypnotized into the movie and feel the effects of the movie. As you start to watch a movie, you start to focus and concentrate on the movie, and after a few moments you become hypnotized into the movie and start to kind of live and feel the emotions of the movie. If the movie is sad, people cry, if it s happy or exciting people are going through a roller coaster of emotions. As I had also mentioned earlier, about the movie that showed sharks killing and eating people.

That movie created lots of fear in people after watching it, because it activated a fearful emotion in the subconscious mind. The horror movies depicting violence have helped create more insensitivity to human life, and people are now committing more crimes than ever before. Negative movies do affect your life and for some people are very harmful. Some people can watch a movie and simply just feel nothing except for the share enjoyment of the movie, like someone who enjoys going on a roller coaster at an amusement park.

Movies can put you into a hypnotized state of mind, and movies can produce good happy feelings or thoughts, or movies can activate fear, hatred, violence and other negative images and patterns. Be careful what movies you let your children watch and be careful what movies you watch.

You can be hypnotized many different times a day. Listening to music, watching a soap opera, watching a sports event, working, shopping in a super market, smelling a good smell to name a few. We go into hypnosis and magnified concentration all the time and each and every day. We are all hypnotized at times during the day by the environment.

TOM SILVER & ORMOND MCGILL

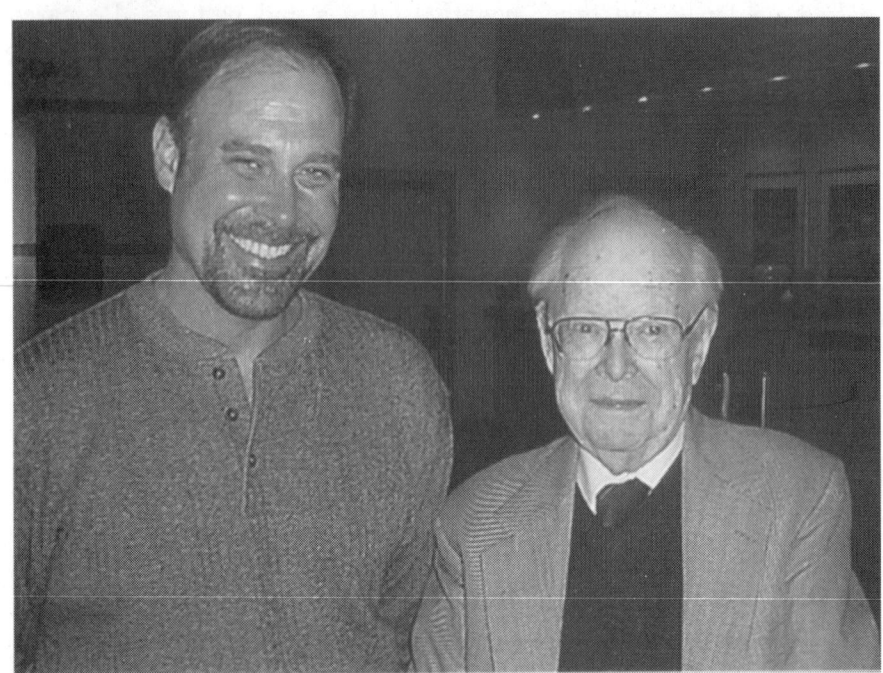

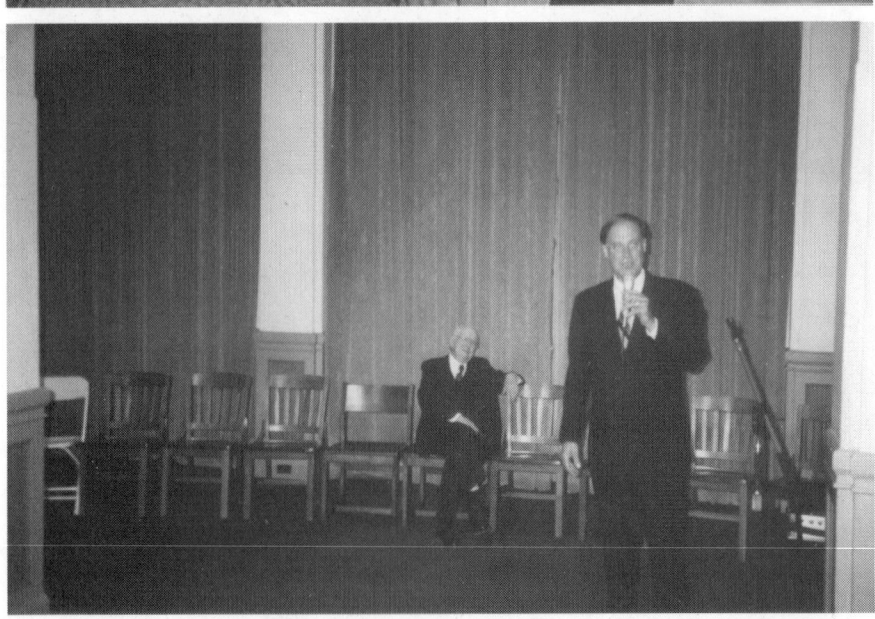

**ORMOND MCGILL AND TOM SILVER
APPEARING LIVE AT STANDFORD UNIVERSITY
TWO HYPNOTISTS PERFORMING TWO SHOWS**

CHAPTER FIVE

THE RELATIONSHIP BETWEEN HYPNOSIS AND SLEEP

Question No. 10 ...
IS HYPNOSIS AND SLEEP THE SAME THING?

Psychologically speaking, sleep and hypnosis represent directly opposite states of mind. In sleep, the attention of the sleeper is diffused, while in hypnosis it is concentrated. Yet, so closely has the state of sleep and hypnosis been associated throughout years of history, (indeed, the very word, hypnotism, coined by Braid, is derived from the Greek word, "Hypnos" meaning sleep or to sleep) those suggestions of sleep in relation to hypnotizing are almost invariably given, and from the practical standpoint of hypnotizing, the subject being asleep is almost synonymous with being hypnotized. Thus, from the standpoint of the subject's association of what being put to sleep means as well as from the audience's reaction in observing the phenomena, the suggestion of SLEEP is most important. So much is this the case that most methods of hypnotizing incorporate suggestions of sleep and or going to sleep in the induction formula.

Despite outward appearances, the internal mechanism of sleep and of hypnosis, are completely different. In truth, hypnosis does not produce a sleep state but produces a very heightened state of super awareness or super awake-fullness so much and to limit the awareness or awake-fullness to concentrated points of attention. Concentrated points of attention produces a unique alteration in consciousness – so much so that hypnosis can well be regarded as a unique state of mind in its own right. Further, this narrowing of this field of attention frequently produces an amnesia effect when the state is removed. Amnesia being a loss of memory as to what occurred while in hypnosis. This only occurs on a small percent of the population the first time they are hypnotized.

Amnesia is a form of conscious absent mindedness with which we are all familiar with, as for instance, when our mind has been diverted that when we return to full attention we find we have sped some miles down the freeway, even missing the turnoff we wanted, and return to our normal stream of consciousness bewildered as to knowing exactly where we are.

In some cases, we do not even recall having driven those vanished miles. Or an even simpler experience is how many times have you misplaced a familiar object? You know that you had it, but you can't remember where you placed it.

Have you ever misplaced the keys to your car or house? The suggestion of SLEEP is found to be productive of an automatic amnesia effect on the client in hypnosis, as not recalling what happens when one sleeps is an expected occurrence. Remember that the conscious mind goes to sleep under hypnosis, and the subconscious mind or unconscious mind wakes up under hypnosis. Since, we have all seen people hypnotized on television who look like they are sleeping in their chairs, we think that hypnosis sleep and natural sleep are the same, but they are not.

The similarity lies in the physical body appearing relaxed and resting with the person's eyes closed. The truth is that in both the natural sleep and the hypnosis induced sleep, the conscious mind becomes relaxed, quiet or silent, but in natural sleep, the subconscious mind transmits information in the form of dreams and in the hypnotic sleep, the subconscious mind can receive position information, visual imagery, and suggestions.

Accordingly, when a client goes into a hypnosis sleep, the factor of having no memory while asleep often does occur in hypnosis because of our long associations with normal sleeping habits. When conducting hypnotherapy sessions, sometimes it is better to maintain a medium depth of hypnosis where both the conscious and the subconscious minds can hear and remember the positive suggestions or changes.

Despite the fact that GOING TO SLEEP is a strong suggestion for inducing hypnosis, it is not actually essential to the phenomena. Subjects can be hypnotized without mentioning the word sleep at all. Some hypnotherapists prefer to substitute the suggestion of relaxation for that of sleep, however beyond question, the suggestion of sleep is far more powerful a suggestion then is that of relaxation.

Brainwaves in sleep and in trance clearly show the inner differences. While a person is in sleep, his/her brainwaves show very low activities in all brainwave ranges. But, while in hypnotic trance, although the beta waves are very similar to that of in sleep (low), the theta and delta waves are very strong. In this book, you will actually see real brain wave graphs of subjects and clients who were hypnotized. These graphs will show actual conscious and subconscious brain wave activity from high beta down to delta.

I (Tom Silver) believe that the only way for hypnosis to become truly accepted in the scientific community, it has to utilize scientific applications such as the EEG device to monitor brain wave frequencies and activities. With this type of medical/scientific device, a therapist can actually see the client has entered into hypnosis as well as the depth of hypnosis. Brain wave utilization will be discussed later on is this book.

Question No. 11 ...
IS THERE ANY DANGER OF A SUBJECT NOT AWAKENING FROM HYPNOSIS?

The term awakening from hypnosis is what's most generally used, but actually the term arousing from hypnosis is more accurate.

There is no danger whatsoever of a person not arousing or awakening from hypnosis, even if in the very deepest trance levels of somnambulism. Occasionally a subject will take a little time to come back from trance, as the experience of being in hypnosis can be so pleasant that one almost doesn't want to leave it, and return again to the high paced world of today. However the subject will always arouse or awaken from hypnosis even if left entirely alone. Now if you hypnotize a person and leave them in hypnosis, they will naturally convert to from hypnosis to natural sleep and awaken feel peaceful and refreshed.

Since hypnosis is induced by a process of suggestions affirming ideas of going to sleep it stands to reason that the reverse of that process presenting suggestions for the removal of sleep and the awakening from trance are bound to arouse the subject. If you leave a person in a hypnotic sleep, they will convert to natural sleep and awaken when ready from natural sleep.

We have only one thought to add in relation to awakening the subject after they are hypnotized, and that is to do so in a pleasant and gentle manner while giving suggestions of well being. Consider this observation. A hypnotisterpist puts his or her subject/client to sleep by a soothing process, and then, suppose, that when the hypnotherapist is ready to awaken the client, instead of being soothing he suddenly claps his hands and shouted in the client's ear, WAKE Up! Under such a stimulus some sensitive people will almost jump out of their skins. Such a startling arousing from hypnosis, is a very unprofessional way to waken a person up from hypnosis.

Hypnotism is a dynamic situation between two people who willingly place themselves in close rapport. Each must respect the other in everyway. The hypnotist must keep in mind that the hypnotic state of mind was induced in a soothing way and the same gentle and soothing approach must always be maintained in the perfect arousal from hypnosis. Now some hypnosis inductions may not always be a soothing induction, such in rapid and physical inductions which we will get into later in this book, but the awakening from hypnosis should be conducted in a very maternal nurturing way and should include positive suggestions before they awaken.

<u>The hypnotherapist has a moral obligation to the subject that the person coming out of hypnosis feels better than he or she ever did when they went into hypnosis.</u>

CHAPTER SIX

GENERAL HYPNOTISM QUESTIONS

In the foregoing chapters, we have carefully gone into answering in some detail the questions related to the entire field of hypnosis. With the understanding you now have, it will be possible for us to answer in a condensed manner, a full one hundred and thirty question about hypnotism that we are most frequently asked. There is no particular sequence to these questions. We have simply jotted them down as we wrote this book, and have answered them, each in turn, as directly as we can. Let's start this chapter now by answering question number twelve. How long does it take to hypnotize a person?

Question No. 12 ...
HOW LONG DOES IT TAKE TO HYPNOTIZE A PERSON?

The potential to enter hypnosis lies within the mind of every person. Mind operates like a computer, so hypnosis can occur in an instant with some subjects. The length of time it takes to hypnotize rather depends on the situation. In my (Tom Silver) television shows and stage show demonstrations, I induce hypnosis on a subject or in an entire group inside a few minutes. In some occasions we accomplished the induction to a very deep trance in less than 10 seconds.

In your private office work as a clinical hypnotherapist the situation is very different. There is no need to use a rapid induction except for certain situations, and indeed many clients seem to prefer a longer procedure of being hypnotized which may include what we call a physical relaxation. When working with your client, you might want to devote a half hour or less to the hypnotherapy part of the session. Hypnotherapy sessions also should include conscious discussions with your client, prior to hypnotizing them.

You might devote a full half hour to just conscious discussion with your client before you hypnotize them. As a hypnotherapist you want to get to know your client and find out from your client what there goals are and what they would like to accomplish by being hypnotized. I (Tom Silver) write a "mental prescription" for each of my clients during the discussion part of my hypnotherapy session. I will talk about my method I call a "mental prescription" that later on in this book.

Question No. 13 ...
ARE MEN BETTER HYPNOTIC SUBJECTS THAN WOMEN?

Sex does not seem to be a factor. Men and woman appear to be equally hypnotizable. The individual them-self is the factor depending if they are resistant to allowing themselves to get hypnotized, and on how effectively they can learn the skill of entering the hypnotic state of mind. Being able to be hypnotized and using the power of mind is truly a learned skill. Some people both male and female seem to have a natural aptitude for it. Others take longer to learn, but both men and woman are equal when it comes to being hypnotized. Focus and concentration can also be a factor in person entering into hypnosis.

Question No. 14 ...
IS IT DIFFICULT TO HYPNOTIZE A STRONG MINDED PERSON?

Actually we prefer to work with a strong-minded person, as a strong-minded person is someone who achieves the goals they set out to achieve. We would say that being strong-minded is really an asset to being hypnotizable. A strong-minded person can concentrate better and can focus better on the suggestions of the hypnotherapist, and are sometimes the best clients in hypnotherapy. Lawyers, doctors, teachers and even military personal can make great subjects for deep hypnosis and hypnotherapy sessions. Remember a stubborn person is not a strong-minded person. Stubborn people may be difficult to hypnotize. A strong minded person who is an open minded person, willing to allow themselves to be hypnotized, may be some of the most receptive types of people for hypnotherapy.

Question No. 15 ...
CAN ANIMALS BE HYPNOTIZED?

Animals can be place into a catatonic state resembling hypnosis in that the eyes become glazed and fixed and the body immobile, such as when a rabbit is stretched out on its back and held motionless for some moments, or when a chicken has its bill placed with eyes starring at an extended chalk line, however the state induced cannot be said to be true hypnosis for sure. Turning a shark in the ocean belly up will put it into a calm state as if it's been hypnotized.

However is this a trance states? We don't know. True hypnosis appears to require the higher mental faculties of man. Animals as we know it cannot be hypnotized. Animals can be taught behavior modification through conditioning. Animals work also on a primitive type of mind where as during what the animal might perceive as danger, it might appear of look lifeless or even dead to instinctively protect itself. A kind of flight mechanism of shutting itself down physically for the animal's survival.

Question No. 16 ...
CAN CHILDREN BE HYPNOTIZED?

Indeed they can, and wonderfully so. Children go in and out of hypnotic mental states often in the games they play. In our clinical work with children, we employ a let's pretend or make believe we are hypnotized technique which provides an exceedingly rapid method of hypnotizing children, as they make a game of it. When you watch children playing you can see that they are hypnotized almost naturally by pretending they are cowboys or pirates or playing with pretend friends. Children understand simple suggestions the best.

Children tend to stay in hypnosis shorter periods of time, but they seem to also go in and out of hypnosis a number of times during a hypnotherapy session.

Question No. 17 ...
IS AGE A FACTOR IN HYPNOTIZING?

It would be rather difficult to classify any particular age as being hypnotizable in such an individual matter. Every person is hypnotizable to some degree, however we have had the opportunity of working with different age groups ranging from children to senior citizens, and if we were to vote our choice, we would say we prefer to work with young adults because they seem to be a little more willing to allow themselves to be hypnotized. We think that misconception's and misinformation of what hypnosis is and is not can be a major factor in a person's resistance to allowing themselves to be hypnotized. Some people might have a fear of losing control and prevent hypnosis. Our belief is that people are hypnotizable at any age.

Question No. 18 ...
WHO MAKES THE BEST HYPNOTIC SUBJECT?

To answer this question we would say that people who are willing to allow themselves to be hypnotized make the best subjects. A person who has an intelligent interest in hypnosis and has an understanding of what hypnosis is will let himself or herself experience it and usually make the best, deepest and receptive hypnotic subjects. People who do not think too much about the process of hypnosis but instead just "go" with the flow of the process tend to make the best hypnotic subjects. Hypnosis also depends on a person's willingness to be hypnotized. All hypnosis can be considered "self hypnosis". A person's willing desire to be hypnotized will make them the best candidates for hypnosis.

Question No. 19 ...
WHO CAN BECOME A HYPNOTIST OR HYPNOTHERAPIST?

There is no special mystical power in being a hypnotist or a clinical hypnotherapist. Anybody can learn about hypnosis and how to hypnotize a person but how good of a hypnotist you will be is quite another matter. Becoming a hypnotist is a developed skill that takes time and patience. It also takes a lot of practice and experience.

Ask yourself a question: can you be a singer? Yes, you can if you have some talent in that direction, but that does not mean you are going to become Elvis Presley.

Generally speaking the more skilled you are in dealing with people and in influencing people the better hypnotist you will be. There are many schools of training in hypnotherapy around the world. We have personally trained hundreds of people to be clinical hypnotherapist in America and in Asia. Personal one on one training with a practicing hypnotherapist who has had years of experience in hypnotism is also recommended. I (Tom Silver) am fortunate to have as my close friend Ormond McGill.

An educational training through a clinical hypnotherapy institute is highly recommended as well as continued follow up education is also recommended. Anybody can learn how to become a hypnotherapist and how to hypnotize, but to develop a real skill in it takes time and practice.

Question No. 20 ...
HOW CAN YOU TELL IF A PERSON IS HYPNOTIZED?

There are certain physical and brainwave characteristics, which occur when a person is in hypnosis. Sometimes a fluttering of the eyelids called "rapid eye movement" can be seen, and the eyes may also to appear to roll upward under the upper lids. A certain letting go will be noted in the individual as well as all tension leaves the body and face and a sort of deep relaxation sets in. The breathing will appear to become slower and lighter. You might notice a relaxed jaw with the mouth open a little.

The more experience one has with working with the state, the more instinctively one becomes to recognizing the state. There are also medical devices as mentioned previously such as the EEG device that measures brain wave activity. This EEG brain frequency device called an Electroencephalogram, measure conscious and subconscious brain wave activity scientifically proving a person is in a hypnotic receptive state. With this type of device, a hypnotherapist can actually see when a person has entered the state of "theta" or "delta" which is of course somnambulism or deep hypnosis.

Question No. 21 ...
IS WILL POWER IMPORTANT TO BEING HYPNOTIZED?

We had better go into some detail in answering this question, as it is important to your hypnotic knowledge.

Will Power has little to do with hypnosis. For a suggestion to carry power it must be accepted by the subconscious, and no amount of willing will bring about the desired results, for willing only makes the conscious aspect of mind more active and submerges deeper the subconscious.

A person trying to use his Will to implant ideas in his subconscious is attempting the impossible. A sick man tries thinking over and over ideas of good health in order to will himself back to health. Instead of feeling better he feels worse, as such ideas only serve to bring him to an increased realization that he is sick. Consequently he finds himself contemplating the exact opposite of what he desires. He battled with his Will to repress the aroused thoughts of illness, but it seems that the more he struggles to hold in check the unwanted ideas the more fully opposing thoughts obsesses him.

How many times have you had trouble willing yourself to sleep at night because you were going to have a busy day, but instead of falling instantly deep asleep, you stayed up half the night trying to fall asleep?

This brings us directly to another important law in the operation of suggestion:

Whenever the "Will" is in conflict with an "Idea" The "Idea" invariably wins the struggle

The idea is stimulated and colored with emotion and thus the idea is the subconscious and the will is actually the conscious mind. The will part of our mind is 10% mind power and the idea part of our mind power is 90% of our mind power operation.

You can prove this to yourself with a little experiment.

Take a plank of wood about six inches wide and twelve feet long and place it on the floor of your room. Now try walking along that plank from one end to the other. Narrow as it is you can do it easily. Next, take that very same plank of wood and suspend it over the canyon or between two high buildings and try walking over it. You take a few timid steps out upon it, and unless you make a hasty retreat your life is in danger as you would soon lose your balance and fall into the depths below.

Do You Want To Know Why?

The new position of the plank has aroused in your mind the suggestion of the idea of falling, in which this idea is colored with the emotion accompanying such possibility. Immediately your subconscious goes into action and accepts the idea of possibly falling.

With your will Power you try to overcome the impulse to fall after-all your logic tells you that you have just proved you can walk along that plank without falling. But reason about it as you will, the more you think about not falling, the more the counter-idea that you will fall is aroused until were you to stubbornly persist in taking the risk, you would lose your balance and fall off the plank of wood down to the ground. The operation here is that the more you try not to think of falling the more you will feel that you will fall. The harder the will force not to fall the greater the anxiety and fear of falling.

This is what we call "<u>The Law of Opposite Operation</u>", which is basic to the use of suggestion, viz.:

When the "Imagination" and the "Will are in conflict the "Imagination" will always WIN

In the conflict between the will and the imagination, the force of the imagination is in direct ratio to the square of the will. The more you try, the more difficult it will be.

Thus willpower turns out not to be the commanding monarch of life as many people would have it but instead is a blind Samson capable either of turning the mill or pulling down the pillars. Willpower should be used as a conscious motivational tool to stimulate positive emotional responses so that both of your minds are working together, instead of challenging each other.

A person who comes into your office for hypnotherapy needs to be taught how to operate their conscious mind instead of their mind operating them. Learning how to operate your will power to direct subconscious positive response in really the key to being a successful hypnotherapist. Subconscious reprogramming through hypnotherapy, and exercising your conscious mind to think the thoughts that you want it to think is what we could call having total mental or mind power.

Hypnotizing is not a question of a weak mind verses a strong mind. It is not a question of willpower. Becoming an expert hypnotist comes from learning how to effectively influence subconscious mind activity while bypassing conscious mind non-acceptance. Willpower comes solely as the directive aim of the hypnotist. Directive aim of the mind to accomplish anything in life is the key to success. In such regard, learning the art of hypnotizing is a key factor to success in accomplishing whatever you will yourself to accomplish. In relation to hypnosis, such can almost be likened to a direct telepathic influence of mind upon mind, while the verbalized suggestions affirm the inner mental purpose of the hypnotist is to effectively influence the subject. In a nutshell, effective hypnotizing of others comes via the hypnotist knowing with positive assurance that what he suggests to the hypnotized subject/client will be performed by the subject/client in the hypnotherapy session. Learning how to hypnotize automatically increases one's willpower, and willpower properly directed will cause things to come one's way with half the difficulty compared to one who does not use this remarkable mental gift.

Of course, do not expect to influence everybody because there are some people who for some reason may be resistant to you hypnotizing them, but you will be able to influence a full seventy-five percent of those you try to hypnotize. You can hardly call that percentage bad. Learning how to hypnotize is like everything else in life. Hypnotizing your first subject is the first hurdle you must pass. Once you have had your first success, you will advance by leaps and bounds.

Question No. 22 ...
HAVE I EVER BEEN HYPNOTIZED WITHOUT KNOWING IT?

Assuredly you have been environmentally hypnotized. Every time you become completely absorbed in anything you enter a hypnotic state of mind. You go to a movie and become absorbed in the drama and the movie makes you cry or it makes you laugh, and yet it is only a motion picture and you know it is. But the movie has stimulated your emotions and you automatically respond to the way the story suggested. Even advertising campaigns and slogans can emotionally move you in certain directions to make purchases. Remember the slogan that went like this: "Things go better with _____. You can fill the blank.

Question No. 23 ...
WHAT DOES IT FEEL LIKE TO BE HYPNOTIZED?

When you are hypnotized, you feel very calm and relaxed as though nothing else matters but being in this deep peaceful relaxation. Your entire body becomes lose, limp and relaxed also. You can be aware of everything around you, yet you are very peaceful and receptive to subconscious suggestions without resistance from the conscious critical facility of mind. It may feel like you are having a wonderful dream also. If you have ever been caught up in a vivid dream you will know what it feels like to be hypnotized. Even when you know the dream is a dream, it still powerfully affects you. Dreams are very real to the dreamer. Hypnosis is very real to the hypnotized. And being hypnotized like I had mentioned earlier for about 15 minutes, is equal to about 5 hours a deep natural sleep. Some people when they awaken from hypnosis may not remember what took place during the session and other will remember everything. When you awaken from hypnosis, you feel very calm and peaceful.

Question No. 24 ...
CAN A PERSON BE HYPNOTIZED WITH THEIR EYES OPEN?

Yes, a person can be hypnotized with their eyes open, but usually, when inducing the state for hypnotherapy purposes the eyes are usually closed. Closed eyes tend to take one more into their private world free from outside distraction. Once the person is in a deep state of hypnosis, open or closed eyes makes little difference. When you see a hypnosis stage show demonstration, those people hypnotized may have their eyes open, but they are still in complete focused concentration and are very hypnotized. Conscious hallucinations can occur on some people who are hypnotized for stage show demonstrations.

Most hypnotherapy sessions take place in a quiet room, with the client sitting or reclining on a recliner, with their hands resting on their lap and their eyes closed and relaxed.

Question No. 25 ...
CAN HYPNOSIS PROGRAM A PERSON?

Your brain functions much like your personal computer. Just as you can program the computer on your desk, so your personal computer can be programmed and using hypnosis is an effective way to reprogram yourself. Just remember to program yourself in helpful and positive ways.

Every experience one has in life has the effect of programming a person. If the programming is good, hypnosis can be used to amplify the programming. If the programming is harmful, hypnosis provides a means of deprogramming that, which is not wanted. Hypnosis provides a directed means of allowing you to become the person that you want to be. Hypnosis can reprogram your bio computer to work for you and for you be in control of your mind.

Question No. 26 ...
CAN HYPNOSIS DEPROGRAM A PERSON?

This question is just the reverse side of the foregoing. Your living of life is constantly programming your behavior (both mentally and physically). If the programming is good you benefit. If the programming is not good, it is harmful. Using hypnosis provides the means of being selective in your mental programming, and makes it possible for you to deprogram and remove unwanted program and habits. Lot's of people could benefit from some type of deprogramming through the usage of hypnotherapy.

In real life, there are cases when deprogramming is very valuable, such as for the victims of certain miss-guided cults. When the authority (usually, parent or relatives) pulls the victims (usually kids) out of such cult environment, the subject may still be under the influence of the cult. We may even say that the subject is still under the hypnotic influence of that cult.

To do the deprogramming, or in layman's term, to bring the person back to common sense is to hypnotize the subject even deeper and then give the subject the suggestions of removing the unwanted suggestions given by the cult environment. This hypnosis deprogramming technique is used all the time and can work well.

Question No. 27 ...
WHAT IS THE HYPNOTIC TRANCE?

The Hypnotic Trance is Hypnosis. Throughout the years, the word trance has taken on a connotation of something bad or controlling. All trance really means is "state" of hypnotic depth. It is a state of mind in which the "blossoming" or awakening of the subconscious mind activity is produced and becomes active and receptive. This "blossoming" or awakening of the subconscious occurs naturally twice daily in the morning just before you fully awaken, and at night just before you drift off to sleep. This is the NATURAL TRANCE STATE in which you can subconsciously influence your own actions, habits and behavior.

Through hypnotherapy you can bring forth this awakening of the subconscious mind of a client anytime that they come into your office day or night. You can even do it for yourself with your practice of "self-hypnosis".

Think of your subconscious and conscious minds as the oceans tide. When the tide is "high" and the water has risen on the sand, your subconscious mind is very active. At that point, your conscious mind is resting or quiet, and you are physically relaxed and hypnotized.

Positive suggestions, which are given to your subconscious mind by a hypnotherapist, will be easily accepted and recorded. Still imagining both of your minds as the ocean surf, when the tide is low on the beach you are wide a wake and your subconscious mind is simply just responding and relating to your conscious thoughts. In the waking state such as during the day, your subconscious mind identifies and associates with your conscious thoughts and you are continually bringing up various emotions that are colored with conscious thoughts.

That's why so many people walk around feeling bad, because they are giving themselves negative suggestions with their will or conscious mind, and activating negative emotions from their subconscious. There are many depths of the hypnotic trance and they will be discussed in this book. This manual will help to make you an expert in hypnotism.

Question No. 28 ...
WHAT IS THE BEST TIME TO BE HYPNOTIZED?

There is no absolute time set as to a best time to be hypnotized. Generally speaking, the best time to be hypnotized is when you can direct all your attention to it without being distracted by other things you have to do. We have successfully presented hypnotism stage shows and worked with hypnotherapy clients at all hours of day and night. Some hypnotherapists prefer seeing clients in the mornings because they feel that the clients are more alert and fresh. Some hypnotherapists feel that after a client with through with work can be a great time for a hypnotherapy session because it can allow your client time to relax and let go of the days stress and tensions.

Question No. 29 ...
WHAT TECHNICAL TRAINING DOES ONE NEED TO BECOME A HYPNOTIST?

The best training for becoming a hypnotist actually comes from gaining experience with hypnotizing. And being hypnotized yourself too, as you then gain an introspective understanding of the hypnotic state. In relation to technical training, college courses in psychology are valuable. Likewise there are numerous private schools and hypnosis institutes across the country that give courses in hypnotherapy like the courses that we teach at the Silver Hypnosis Institute in Southern California.

Training in hypnotherapy is very important and we feel that if you are serious in wanting to become a hypnotherapist, you should enroll in a hypnotherapy program and start taking as many different courses as you can. The more knowledge you have, the better you will be.

We also feel that the study of the science of hypnosis and techniques to hypnotize a person should be taught to every person studying medicine and psychology. Again remember the A.M.A. officially recognized hypnosis back in the fifties and also requested medical students to also study hypnotism.

Question No. 30 ...
CAN THE POLICE UTILIZE HYPNOSIS?

Some Police Departments in major cities have trained personnel in forensic Hypnosis. It has proved useful in activating memories about specific events and in tracing stolen articles by hypnotizing witnesses to remember license plate numbers on cars, recalling names and descriptions of suspects, etc. However as incriminating evidence, it is not legally accepted in court in most countries. However, it's found that hypno-Investigation is a very powerful and useful investigational tool to obtain leads and to sort out wrongful information. It's been widely used but not publicized by many legal agencies, such as the Police, FBI and CIA.

I (Tom Silver) used hypnosis in Taiwan to help the Taiwan Department of Defense get to some of the answers of a crime by hypnotizing the witness, victims, and even the accused criminals who might have been involved in the crime and murder. The Taiwan D.O.D. awarded me, and my assistant/interpreter Timothy Huang, "Gold Plates of Honor" in July of 1997. Timothy Huang and myself worked three separate times on the case between January 1997 and September 1999. The subconscious mind remembers everything that has taken place in your life and under deep hypnosis a person may be able to activate those memories.

In my book which is called "Solving Crimes With Hypnosis I give you the techniques and method formulas that Timothy Huang and myself created to help the Taiwan Military and Department of Defense.

Question No. 31 ...
IS HYPNOSIS OPPOSED BY ANY RELIGIONS?

Any religious opposition to hypnosis is purely based on superstitious ideas from the past. Hypnosis has nothing whatsoever to do with religion. Hypnotism today is recognized as a way to subconsciously motivate behavior. Remember this is the latter Twenty-First Century not middle ages. Let's not talk nonsense. If hypnosis is apposed by any religion, it is because of ignorance and misinformation. Maybe hypnosis is used more in religion, than we think.

Question No. 32 ...
DOES HYPNOSIS COME FROM THE DEVIL?

Here's a question related to the foregoing. Poor Devil, he gets blamed for so many things. Hypnosis is a state of mind you induce in yourself or someone induces in you. Some people say that all hypnosis is, is really a form of self-hypnosis and as you now know every one of us, have been hypnotized by the environment. Are you a Devil? If you are not, obviously hypnosis does not come from any imaginary devil. Honestly, it's about time people began taking responsibility for their own actions, and stop shifting the blame for what they do on some outside influence ala The Devil Made Me Do It! Many people felt that Jesus himself had hypnotic healing powers with his voice and his touch and he was not the devil. The more understanding and education that you have about the science of hypnotism, the more you can help to educate the general public and even the scientific community about it.

Question No. 33 ...
IS HYPNOSIS THE SAME THING AS MEDITATION?

Hypnotism and Meditation are opposites of the same. Hypnosis is motivated to achieve a given goal. Meditation is non-motivated and has no goal (unless you can conceive that just BEING is a goal). In hypnosis, a person is given positive suggestions or visual images, while in meditation the person is to have their mind become clear and free from thought.

To instantly understand this, appreciate that meditation is a state a BEING while hypnosis is a state of DOING.

Question No. 34 ...
WHAT IS THE DIFFERENCE BETWEEN WESTERN
HYPNOTISM AND ORIENTAL HYPNOTISM?

Western hypnotists, more or less, look upon being hypnotized as a self-induced process by the subject in himself. The operator functioning mainly as an instructor and assistant, as to how the subject is to think. Oriental hypnotist definitely believe in the transmission of thought premise, and that the operator is the director of the hypnotic influencing of the subject.

In other words, Oriental hypnotists feel that hypnosis is produced by the directed thought influence of the hypnotist upon the subject. Oriental hypnotists hold to what they call the threefold formula of visualization, affirmation, and projection. This method can apply also to hypnotherapists in the west and this is how the method is conducted.

The process starts with the hypnotist visualizing in his mind how the subject is going to respond to his influence. The hypnotist then affirms it is going to occur exactly as he affirms it to be. Finally, the thought forms generated are projected into the mind of the subject, producing hypnosis as the hypnotist gives the suggestions. We will get into this method later on in this book because we both feel it is a very valuable tool to use and should be considered.

Question No. 35 ...
WHAT IS THE DIFFERENCE BETWEEN MESMERISM AND HYPNOTISM?

Mesmerism was the original name given to the hypnotic state by Dr. Frederick Anton Mesmer. Dr. Mesmer believed in the invisible liquid energy projection idea from hypnotist to subject (as he was a physician, he regarded such as from doctor to patient). He called this projected energy animal magnetism.

Subsequently, later hypnotists renounced Mesmer's theory of an energy transference and came to regard much as entirely a psychological state produced in the subject via suggestion, and called it hypnotism. Hypnotism is a process of concentration, relaxation and can include positive suggestion and or visualization. Hypnotism involves the focus of concentration on a thought, object or idea.
What we call a "suggestive" state of mind based on concentration.

Question No. 36 ...
WHAT IS STAGE HYPNOTISM?

Stage Hypnotism is the demonstrating of hypnotic phenomena to an audience. It is presented upon a stage. While designed to be instructive, it is primarily produced in a manner to be entertaining and fun.

Many of us have seen a stage hypnosis show before at a school event, or on television. Actually, stage hypnotism is an excellent way to learn about hypnotism, as we learn best when things are entertaining. Dr. James Braid who was a Scottish medical doctor who created the name "Hypnosis" became interested in hypnosis after watching a stage demonstration from a 1800s stage hypnotist named La Fontaine.

In the long history of hypnotism, it was stage hypnotists with hypnotism shows touring the country that kept hypnotism alive in public interest. With the death of Charcot the serious use of hypnosis in therapy all but vanished. Sigmund Freud was there after that, but he turned his attention in the direction of developing his method of psychoanalysis. It has been speculated that Dr. Freud had trouble in being a proficient hypnosis technician and had trouble in hypnotizing people. Since both of us have performed stage hypnotism shows all around the world as well as on national television shows, we have been able to literally introduce millions of people to the science of hypnotism, and have helped to educate them, entertain them, and even enlighten them about the tremendous potential of our subconscious mind.

Friday, January 31, 1997

China News
World

Hypnotist assists inquiry into naval officer's death

An American hypnotist, who was invited to Taiwan to help investigate the murder of Navy Captain Yin Ching-feng, might have collected useful information about the case after questioning some witnesses under hypnosis, sources in the military said yesterday.

Yin's body was found floating off the northeastern coast of Taiwan in December 1993. An investigative report suggested that Yin was possibly murdered because of his plan to inform the authorities about a bribery case in the Navy concerning weapons procurements.

Hsu Ming, an artist who invited the American hypnotist to Taiwan, said he believed the military had made some breakthroughs in the case after questioning Navy Captain Kuo Li-heng, who is serving a life term in prison for his involvement in the arms scandal.

At least two witnesses told the hypnotist what they knew about Yin's murder, but neither of them could recall confessing after regaining consciousness, Hsu said.

Investigators had earlier suspected that Kuo may have taken part in Yin's murder, but they could not find any evidence to prove his involvement.

Hsu said Kuo might have named the people who planned Yin's murder. Hsu said he could not disclose their names because of a contract he had signed with the Ministry of National Defense to keep the investigation secret.

However, sources said that, according to Kuo's replies to some key questions, investigators were convinced that there was a ring behind Yin's murder because of the huge profits involved in the purchase of navy weapons.

The sources said the murderers appeared to have fled to other countries. The authorities were still wondering whether to deal with those who might have ordered Yin's murder because of their prominent positions in the military.

The sources also said authorities feel the case has adversely affected morale of Taiwan's armed forces.

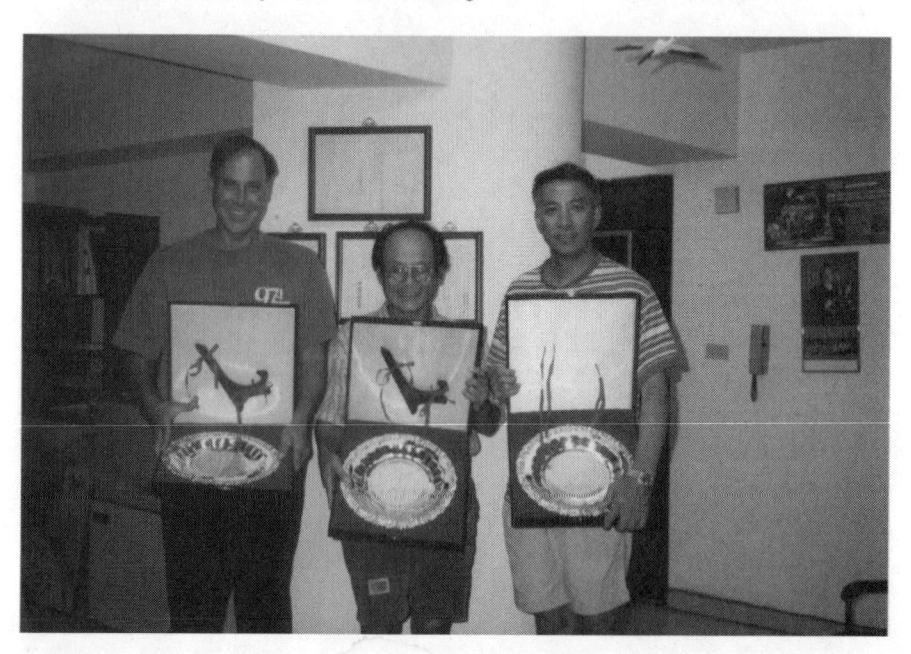

GOLD PLATE OF HONOR
TAIWAN DEPARTMENT OF DEFENSE
AWARDED TO DR. TOM SILVER
TAIWAN MINISTER OF DEFENSE *JULY 1999

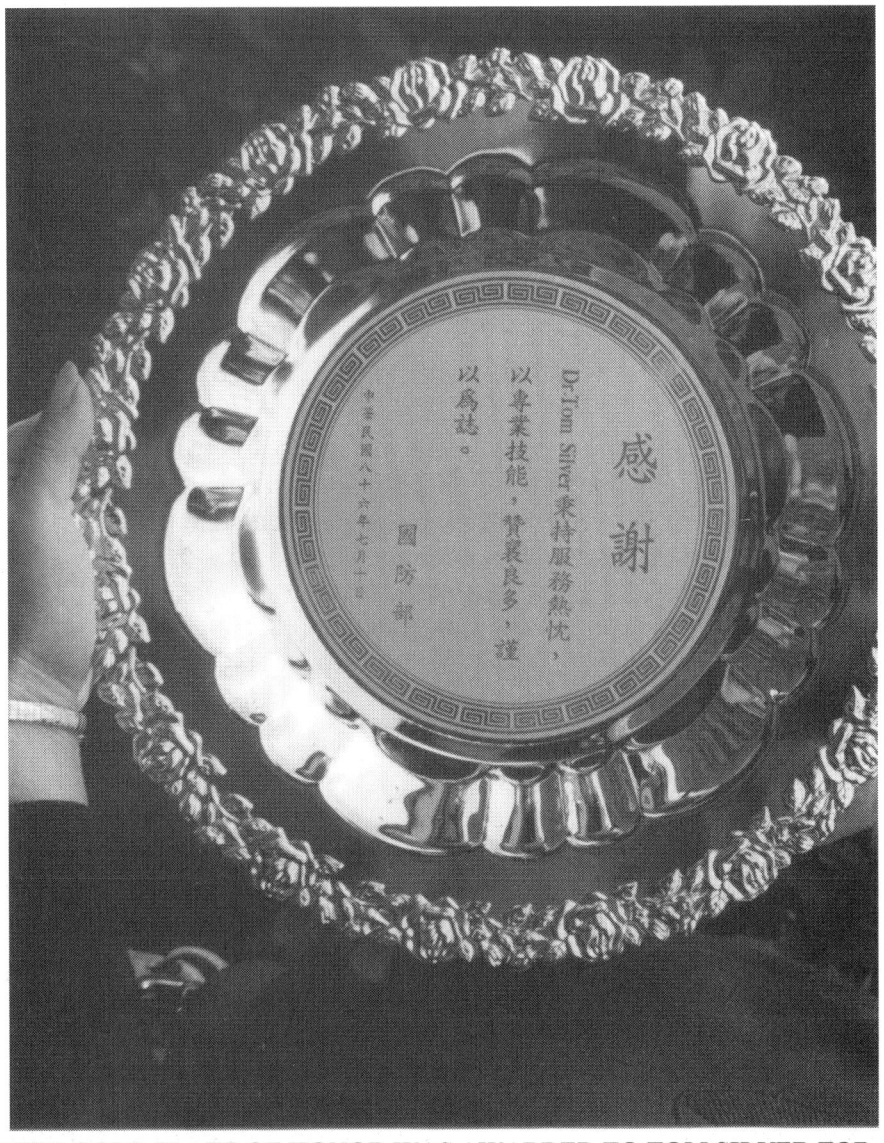

THIS GOLD PLATE OF HONOR WAS AWARDED TO TOM SILVER FOR HIS WORK WITH MEMORY ACTIVATION IN USING HYPNOSIS TO GATHER INFORMATION PERTAINING TO A WEAPONS PROCUREMENT SCANDLE AND THE MURDER OF NAVY CAPTIAN YIN CHING-FENG

CHAPTER SEVEN

PHENOMENA PRODUCED HY HYPNOTISM

Question No. 37 ...
WHAT PHENOMENA WILL HYPNOTISM PRODUCE?

Hypnosis is a state of mind in which suggestions exert their maximum influence. You might say hypnosis magnifies mind power receptors.

Suggestions are ideas, which produce active automatic responses in the mind and body, especially powerful when in hypnosis. A small organ within the lower part of our brain receives these suggestions. This organ is called "The Hypothalamus". The hypothalamus acts as a modulation or transceiver box between our mind and body. You will learn more about the hypothalamus later on in this book on the chapter of fear removal.

The effectiveness of suggestions in the waking state compared with suggestion in the hypnotic state differs only in the matter of degree of influence. Insofar as we consider hypnosis as that state of mind where the influence of suggestion can have its greatest effect. All suggestive efforts by the hypnotist are directed towards the hypnotic end of the scale, which appears to be more productive in producing the interesting, entertaining, instructive, and beneficial aspects of the phenomena of hypnosis.

PHENOMENA OF HYPNOSIS

In response to the direct and specific suggestions of the stage hypnotist, the subject may be rendered happy and joyous, sad, angry, bold, timid and be able to show many emotional changes in a creative way. The deeply hypnotized subject may be motivated to sing thinking she's Madonna or dance like a professional ballerina.

The expressions of the subject during these responses while in hypnosis, is most important, as its very earnestness is profound. The attitudes and gestures are equal to or surpassing the most accomplished actor although the hypnotized subject may be a person normally limited in such direction and show no particular talent for acting in the waking state.

The hypnotized subject is not acting a part in the ordinary sense of the word. He believes himself to be the actual personality suggested. The subject will impersonate to perfection any suggested character with which he or she is familiar with. Since our subconscious mind remembers everything that we have seen or experienced, under deep hypnosis you can bring up that memory and act upon it or convert it into a physical action such as when I (Tom Silver) have hypnotized a person into thinking that they were Michael Jackson and they imitated Michael's dance moves perfectly while hypnotized. I remember that after I had awoken the person who under hypnosis thought he was Michael Jackson, and asked him if he could dance like Michael Jackson, he said absolutely no. He said that he did not even know how to dance. He consciously did not remember what he had performed under hypnosis. His subconscious under deep hypnosis, gave him the ability to dance great without the fear. Fear stands in the way success.

One of the most striking abilities of the subconscious phase of mind as distinguished from the conscious phase of mind consists in its memory accessing abilities. In all degrees of hypnotic trance, memory is one of the most pronounced of the phenomena's.

One of the remarkable effects of hypnotism is this recollection of events, dates, memories and circumstances, and the revival of impressions long since past. The images of which have been completely lost to ordinary conscious memory and are not recoverable in the normal state of mind can be activated through hypnosis opening up these memories which are recorded in our subconscious mind. Memories recorded of our current lifetime (and some believe even those of past lifetimes) are there stored in the subconscious much as memories are stored in the memory-bank of a computer. Consider our subconscious mind as the "hard drive" on a computer. Our subconscious mind remembers and stores everything. Even blocked or repressed memories are stored memories. Hypnosis makes it possible to flash these memories upon our screen of mind, much as a computer likewise does upon its electronic monitor screen.

Everything learned in the course of life can be remembered in hypnosis, even when apparently it has long been forgotten consciously.

Equally, false memories can also be suggested as for example when it is suggested to the subject, you remember we visited Florida yesterday and we went to Disney World. Tell me about it and about all the different rides you went on. The suggestion will take effect, and he will at once if in a very deep depth of hypnosis (somnambulism) begin to relate all that he believes he did at Disney World. This is an example of what might be called retroactive hypnotic phenomena because the subject believes he experienced something in the past, which never really occurred. It is also considered an "imagined or false memory".

Memory may also be removed. The subject may be caused to forget whole periods of his life at the suggestion of the operator. We can show this demonstration in the "memory loss" test that we have performed at various events and shows. In a stage show performance, a person can be given the suggestion that they have forgot their name or that they cannot remember how to spell their name. Instant memory loss is a remarkable demonstration.

Sense delusions of both hallucinations and illusions can be induced through hypnosis. An illusion is the false interpretation of an existing external object, as, for instance, when a table is mistaken for a stack of books, a broomstick for a beautiful woman, a noise in the street for orchestral music, etc. An hallucination is the perception of an object which does not exist in fact, as for instance when the hypnotist suggests to the subject, Sit down in this armchair, where there is really no chair at all yet the hallucination is so perfect that the subject does put himself in the same positioning as if he were sitting in an actual chair. Only if you ask him, are you comfortable? He may reply, not particularly, and he asks for a chair that is more comfortable to sit on.

It seems incredible that a hallucination could be so real that a person would assume an attitude so strained, but it is so.

Hallucinations of all the senses and delusions of every conceivable kind can be suggested to a responsive subject. Just how real these effects are evidenced in experiments where the image of the hallucination has been caused to double by a prism or mirror, magnified by a lens, and in every way behave optically like a real object.

In suggestion a hallucination say that of a bird flying in, the suggested approach of the object causes contraction of the pupil and vice versa. At the same time, there is often convergence of the axis of the eyes, as if a real object were really perceived.

Various physiological effects can be produced in the state of hypnosis. A subject can be caused to weep and shed tears on his face. The heart can be quickened or retarded, respiration slowed or accelerated, and perspiration can be produced all by hypnotic suggestion. Even the temperature can be affected. Thus it has been observed that if a subject is told that the room he is in is very hot, his pulse will become rapid, his face flushed, and his recorded temperature increases. Or, if a person is told that he is standing on ice, he feels cold at once. He trembles, his teeth chatter, he wraps himself up in his coat. Goose bumps can be produced by the suggestion of a cold bath. Hunger and thirst can be created, and other bodily functions increased or retarded. This is due to a hypnosis suggestion activating and affecting a persons "Autonomic Nervous System".

The mind can be so concentrated upon a physiological process as to stimulate that process to normal activity, so as to produce curative effects, and even to superabundant activity, so as to produce a pathological positive effect. Blisters, warts, and burns have been annulled and even disappeared through the use of hypnotic suggestion.

Sense organs can be influenced by hypnotic suggestion at the same time. Tell the hypnotized subject, "here is a rose", and once the subject not only sees, but feels and also smells the rose. The suggestion here affecting the subject's sight, touch and smell simultaneously.

When the delusion is positive, the hypnotized subject believes he sees what does not exist; when it is negative, he fails to recognize the presence of an object really placed before him. An excellent demonstration of a negative illusion is to suggest to the subject he will not be able to see you, although you will remain in the room so he can feel and hear you. The suggested effect is strikingly performed. This is a negative illusion hallucination of sight. Similarly it may be suggested that the subject is deaf to certain words but not to others. An entire cessation of the functions of any sense organ can be induced in the same way, as a negative delusion. The sense organ affected is susceptible to hypnotic suggestion and hypnotic commands can remove the sense organ suggestion.

It is certain that the blindness and deafness produced in this way are of a mental nature, for the corresponding organ of sense performs its function, though the impressions do not reach the consciousness. In the same way, the sight on one eye can be negated, though the other can see as usual. Hypnosis has helped restored eyesight, use of limbs and even the human voice in some people who were hypnotized in the past. There are many documented recorded accounts of people regaining the use of limbs, eyesight after being blind, and even being able to regain speech through hypnosis.

ALL SUCH PHENOMENA OF HYPNOSIS CAN BE PRODUCED WHILE THE SUBJECT IS IN THE HYPNOTIC STATE AND ALSO POSTHYPNOTICALLY

THIS IS VERY IMPORTANT TO THE USE OF HYPNOSIS IN THE FIELD OF HYPNOTHERAPY. IF SUCH PHENOMENA WERE ONLY POSSIBLE TO PRODUCE WHILE THE SUBJECT WAS IN HYPNOSIS, ITS USAGE WOULD BE LIMITED. THE FACT THAT SUCH PHENOMENA CAN CARRY OVER INTO THE WAKING STATE MAKES ITS VALUE LIMITLESS.

Question No. 38 ...
CAN A PERSON BE TOO EAGER TO BE HYPNOTIZED?

Yes, we have found that people too eager to be hypnotized often defeat themselves from obtaining a deep level of hypnotic trance. The intensity of effort to be hypnotized brings in the objective mind, while hypnosis is a subjective mental state. Effort to do anything is fine, but the effort must be without effort. The obtaining of any real art is always that way. For example, a piano virtuoso has so mastered his art that he now plays without effort. So it is with being hypnotized. The subject simply has to let GO and that is all. Don't try and just let it happen. We also tell our clients to simply do everything that we ask them to do without thinking.

Question No. 39 ...
HOW MANY TIMES SHOULD A PERSON BE HYPNOTIZED?

The answer to this question depends entirely upon the individual. Being hypnotized is not harmful in itself, however one should not become addicted to anything.

Entering hypnosis is rather like a temporary escape from the hurly burly world for a time, so it can become sort of a retreat. Life is to be lived not escaped from, so using the repeated use of hypnosis should be kept in balance. Use hypnosis wisely on proper occasions and for proper purposes, but do not overdo it just to get away from things.

Hypnotherapy suggestions do need to be reinforced and most people need a number of repetitions of subconscious suggestions in order for them to create a new positive habit or change in is a person's life. We believe that hypnosis subconscious suggestions should to be reinforced at least 20 or times in a row to create a new change or positive habit. Some people may need reinforcement every once in a while for the rest of their life. Good mental health and physical health both need to be exercised on a regular basis.

Question No. 40 ...
HOW MANY METHODS OF HYPNOTIZING ARE THERE?

There are almost as many methods of hypnotizing as there are hypnotists as each hypnotist tends to develop an individuality of procedure unique to them self. However, if we are to get right down to basics, there are only two diverse forms of hypnotizing that have come to scientific attention throughout its history. Hypnotizing by the use of a transference of human energy such as Mesmer employed in his animal Magnetism inductions, and the psychological approach using suggestion as specialized in by the old masters of the Nancy School in France and Dr. James Braid of Scotland. Methods of hypnotizing are much like methods of painting. Paint and brushes are basics, but how they are applied is an individual matter. Ask yourself how many artists there are and you can name many. They all paint pictures, but each has their own artistic style.

In this book, we will discuss various methods of hypnosis inductions including progressive relaxation, physical induction, rapid induction and shock induction methods.

Question No. 41 ...
WHAT'S THE NANCY SCHOOL OF HYPNOTISM?

In the late 19th Century in France, Dr. Liebeault and Dr. Bernheim built the foundation of modern hypnotherapy based on the studies done by Abbe Faria and James Braid. They based their practice on the principles of hypnotic induction by suggestion, rather than by the doctrine of Jean-Martin Charcot's Paris Salpetriere School. The name of Nancy came from the location in the city of that name in eastern France. Current hypnotherapy practice is derived from the Nancy School of Hypnotism.

Question No. 42 ...
WHAT'S THE SALPETRIERE SCHOOL OF HYPNOTISM?

At the same time as Liebeault and Bernheim were founding the Nancy School, one of the most brilliant neurologist and anatomist, Dr. Jean-Martin Charcot of the Salpetriere hospital in Paris insisted that the hypnotic state was primarily an artificially induced nervous hysteria, a pathological phenomenon, and thus, it had little, if any, therapeutic function or merit. Charcot was a believer in the transparent magnetic fluid theory of Mezmer. Later on, it was proven that this is not the case on either front. There appears to be no magnetic fluid and hypnosis is not at all associated with hysteria.

Question No. 43 ...
WHEN WAS HYPNOTHERAPY RE-ESTABLISH FOLLOWING ITS DECLINE AFTER CHARCOT?

After World War I and through the depression in the 1920s hypnosis started to increase more in popularity. Work with shell-shocked soldiers in World War II caused a leap of renewed interest in hypnotherapy. Then the American Medical Association (AMA) gave acceptance to hypnosis as an adjunct to the healing arts in the 1950s. This was another big boost, and interest in the practice of hypnotherapy has advanced ever since. Hypnosis was used extensively in America after World War II and after the Korean War to reduce pain was injured military soldiers and for "post traumatic stress disorder" also called "shell shock". Medical documents show that hypnosis proved effective in pain control on some than morphine.

Question No. 44 ...
WHAT IS MEANT BY THE BODY RIGIDITY TEST?

This is a popular stage hypnotism demonstration, in which the hypnotized person it told to stand up straight. It is then suggested that that the muscles will become set and solid – the body becoming like steel and will not bend. Two assistants then help you take the rigid subject and stretch his body out between two chair, placing his shoulder on the back of one chair and his legs (just above the ankle) on the back of the other chair.

The subject will remain in that position supported between the chairs, with his body forming a human bridge. It becomes so rigid that a person can sit or stand in the center of the person's body without it even sagging under the weight. The test is not hard to do and is not dangerous, however two cautions are important:

Number one is to be sure you place the back of shoulders on the chair support at the head end (never place the support under the neck to prevent injury to the neck.

BODY RIGIDITY TEST

TOM SILVER HYPNOTIZES A SUBJECT TO MAKE HER BODY BECOME STIFF AND RIGID AS A STEEL BAR!

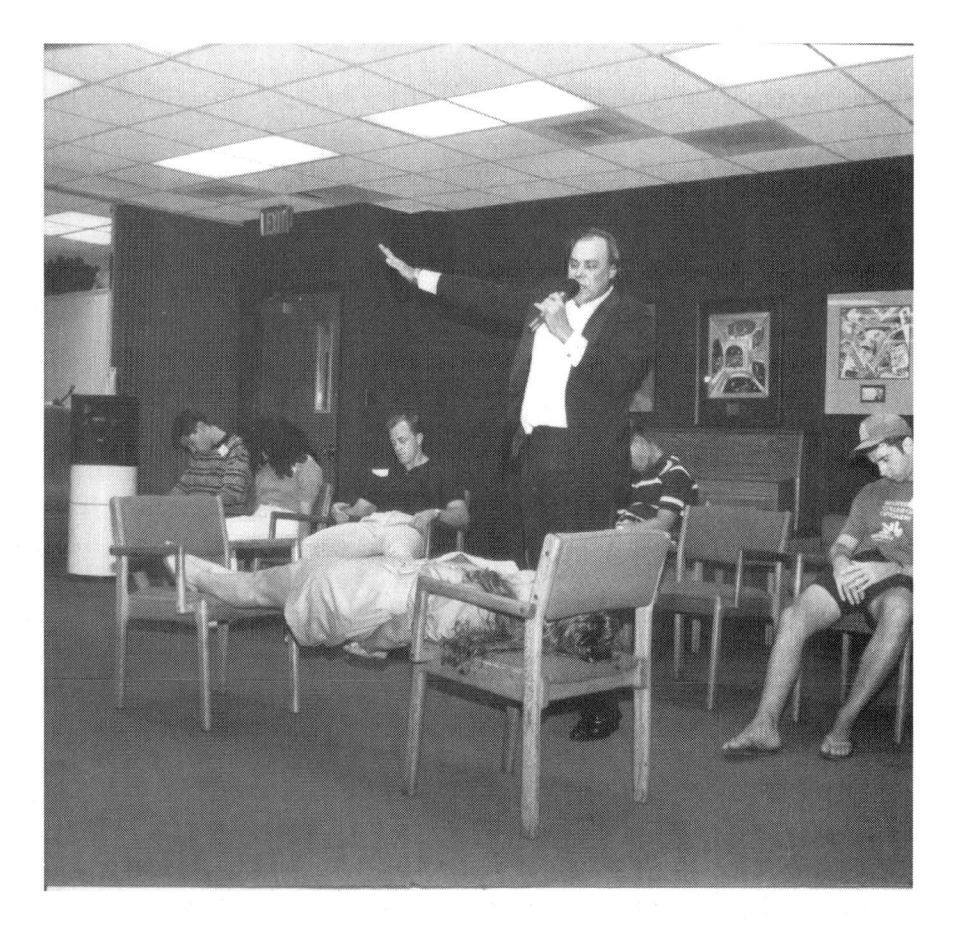

THE SUBJECT IS SUSPENDED BETWEEN TWO CHAIRS WITH HER BODY STIFF AND RIGID AS A STEEL BAR SHOWING A POWERFUL HYPNOTIC DEMONSTRATION OF A BODY CATALEPSY UNDER THE POWER OF HYPNOSIS!

Number two is to have assistants hold head and feet securely in position, so there is no possibility of the subject slipping and falling from the back of the chairs. This unusual feat is an effective stage demonstration but it is not recommended for demonstrational hypnosis.

When completed, assistants remove the subject's rigid body from the back-of-chair supports, and return it to an upright standing position. You suggest the person's muscles are now relaxing completely and are flexible in everyway. Subject is then aroused from the trance. The demonstration is usually shown to demonstrate catalepsy, and the advanced degree of muscle strength that can be produced in hypnosis. I (Tom Silver) once performed that demonstration on three people all at the same time, two thousand miles away from me live on a national American Television Special called "Powers of the Paranormal". We however really do not recommend the performance of the body rigidity because; a subject who has physical problems or a pregnant person might injure himself or herself. It is a specialized demonstration that should be conducted by only seasoned hypnotists and we do not recommend conducting this demonstration.

Question No. 45 ...
CAN A PERSON RESIST BEING HYPNOTIZED?

The induction of hypnosis is a <u>willingness</u> on the part of operator and subject to assist the latter to enter the hypnotic state of mind. The operator/subject with hypnotism is a dual role process, in which each has a specific role to play. The subject takes on the passive role of being receptive and concentrating on the suggestions, while the hypnotist takes on the active role to properly present the hypnotizing suggestions. Both devote their complete attention to the process. In this context, one school of hypnosis states the hypnosis as a form of social role-playing. In life, it is difficult to accomplish anything by resisting doing it. Hypnotizing is no exception to this general rule. Unless the subject is willing and agreeable to be hypnotized, the whole thing is a waste of time for both parties.

However, a great hypnosis master may have many techniques to overcome the subject's conscious resistance in a very subtle way, and bring these resistant subjects into a deep trance. It has been said by many that everyone is hypnotizable. Both of us teach physical and various what we call "Shock Induction" methods that sometimes can by pass a consciously resistant or analytical resistant person.

Question No. 46 ...
WHAT IS THE HYPNOTIC SEAL?

The Hypnotic Seal, so called, is a process some hypnotist employ in telling the deeply entranced person that no other hypnotist other than them-self, can hypnotize them. The subconscious mind may accept or reject such a suggestion and respond accordingly. It is certainly not a very a good thing to do because it limits the use of hypnosis to working with one particular person. A clever hypnotist can break the seal, but generally speaking such an ego-centered procedure on the part of the hypnotist is not to be tolerated.

Question No. 47 ...
ARE SOME PEOPLE EASIER TO HYPNOTIZE THAN OTHERS?

Of course, just as some people are easier to communicate with than others. Some people are able to enter the hypnotic state almost in the instant and go into deep trance. Others take longer to learn how to do it. Entering hypnosis is possible for everyone, but in a way it is a talent, and the degree of talent each person has varies with each individual.

Question No. 48 ...
WHAT TYPE OF THINGS CAN A HYPNOTIZED PERSON PERFORM ON STAGE?

A hypnotism show is mainly designed for entertainment, and subjects on stage have a natural freedom to perform. Being on stage is a suggestion in itself, and most who volunteer to come on stage have a natural enjoyment of it. For persons who like to entertain others, the hypnotic stage situation presents a wonderful opportunity. Even some persons who are normally shy about performing on stage while hypnotized on stage are able to let GO of such inhibitions and have a great time. Singing and dancing, playing a piano, watching a funny movie and other fun and amusing demonstrations can be conducted at a hypnosis show. If you conduct an educational and entertaining stage show, you may also find your private hypnotherapy business increasing. People are eager to learn how hypnosis can also create positive changes in their lives.

HYPNOSIS SHOW POSTER
ORMOND MCGILL AND TOM SILVER'S TWO MAN SHOW
HYPNOSIS PERFORMANCE POSTER CREATED FOR SHOW AT
STANFORD UNIVERSITY IN PALO ALTO CALIFORNIA IN 1998

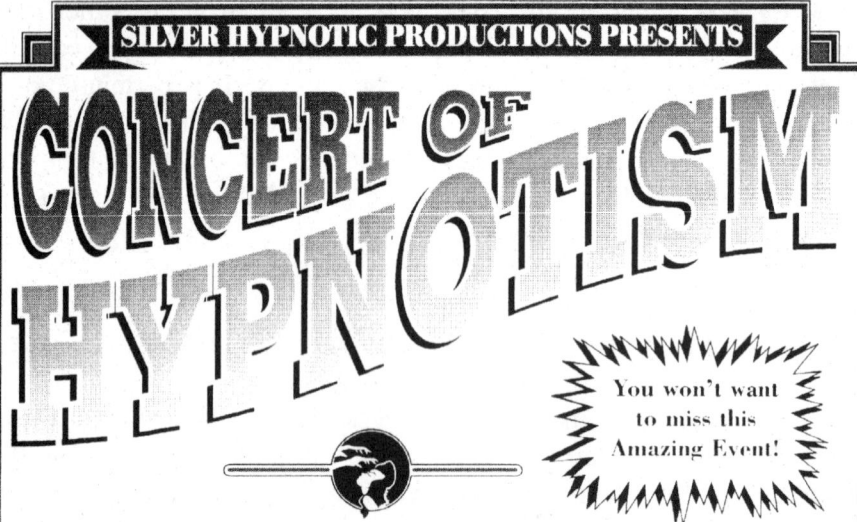

SILVER HYPNOTIC PRODUCTIONS PRESENTS

CONCERT OF HYPNOTISM

You won't want to miss this Amazing Event!

THE WORLD'S GREATEST HYPNOTISM SHOW WITH TWO GREAT MASTERS

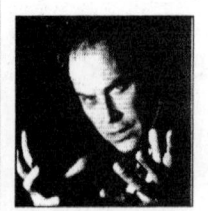

TOM SILVER
Star of CBS Special "Hypnotized"

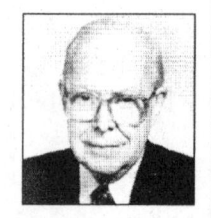

ORMOND McGILL
Dean of American Hypnotists

A GALACTIC HYPNOTIC EVENT

THE FORCE

Exclusive! The entire attending audience given the opportunity to participate in "Abundance Hypnotism"... concert hypnotism at its best.
How to use your creative mind to bring wealth, love, health and success into your life.
Plus...A new form of hypnotism "Psychology In Action"...
Startling Educational Superlearning

"CONCERT OF HYPNOTISM"
TWO GREAT HYPNOTISM SHOWS IN ONE PERFORMANCE!
POSTER CREATED BY DEAN OF HYPNOTISTS "ORMOND MCGILL"

THE N.B.A. HALFTIME SHOW HYPNOTIST TOM SILVER

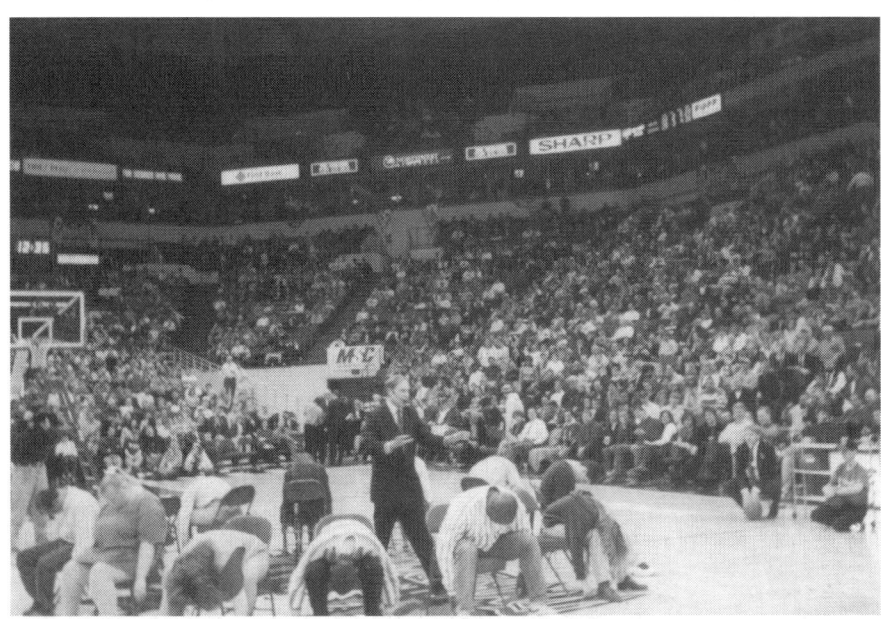

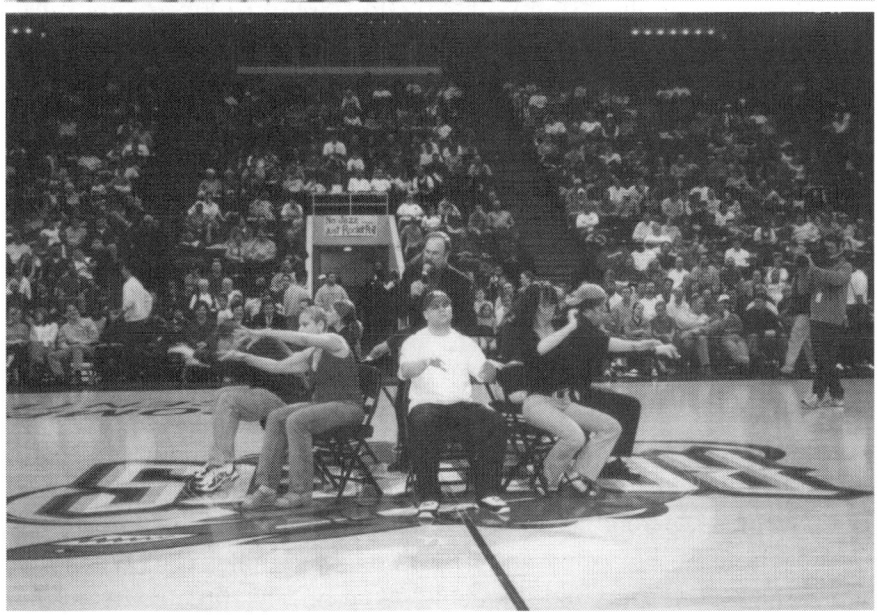

**AUDIENCE MEMBERS HYPNOTIZED TO BE "THE STARS OF THE SHOW"
"TAPPING INTO CREATIVE HIDDEN TALENTS INFRONT OF 20,000 FANS"**

As a clinical Hypnotherapist, I (Tom Silver) say during my stage show presentations that, "My motivation is in helping people change their lives, but I also love to show the creativity of our subconscious minds.

Question No. 49 ...
WHAT IS THE ROLE OF A HYPNOTHERAPIST?

The role of the hypnotherapist is not so much that of a physician (healer) as it is that of an educator (teacher), and his office is the school to which the student (client) goes. Actually the therapist role is more of a re-educator rather than educator as the student has already learned many things, some of which it would be better if they had not been learned. And so the hypnotherapist helps his clients unlearn things that are harmful, and learn, instead, things that are helpful and beneficial to the clients health and happiness.

Question No. 50 ...
IS A HYPNOTHERAPIST LIKE A PARENT TO THE CLIENT?

There is a definite analogy there. The Hypnotherapist is more like a friend creating a mutual agreement with the friend/client to help them. Mind can be likened to a family situation also. Conscious mind can be considered as the parent and subconscious mind can be considered as the child, a child with remarkable talents and mental abilities distinctively its own. For a while it can think deductively wonderfully, it cannot think inductively at all. So it needs directions to get it started. To instruct it correctly is the role of the hypnotherapist.

Question No. 51 ...
WHAT IS THE PARENT/HYPNOTHERAPIST RELATIONSHIP?

Okay. Let's say that some parents are wise and some are not so wise. An unwise parent teaches their child wrong and so the child performs poorly. Such a parent needs help. The hypnotherapist temporarily takes over the role of the parent and helps straighten things out. When things are straightened out and the child is properly directed to use it's personal talents, then things go along wonderfully. Hypnosis is the training medium the hypnotherapist uses, and the more profound the medium the more rapidly the student advances. The medium (hypnotherapy sessions) is so powerful that frequently even one session of skillfully directed hypnotic suggestion can turn things around and get the client on the right tract, for the truth is that the subconscious is really a very brilliant student. The subconscious mind learns very fast.

Question No. 52 ...
WHAT IS MEANT BY IDEOMOTOR RESPOSES?

Ideomotor response is a term created by the famous psychologist, William James. It means that every thought held in the mind has an unconscious (or subconscious) muscular response occurring in the body, as a result of the thought. These responses are often so slight as to scarcely be visible, yet they are there. Ideomotor action explains how a sick mind can produce a sick body, and how a healthy mind can produce a well body, as there are muscles located in all the inner organs of the body. Thought can definitely motivate ideomotor muscular responses, and hypnosis can direct thought. Hence we gain an understanding of how the mental process of hypnosis can aid in correcting many physical diseases in the body. We teach hypnotherapists how to use ideomotor response under hypnosis, to help clients release fears and emotional anxieties as well as to activate or help to create positive emotions and or habits.

Question No. 53 ...
IS PROPER TIMING IN GIVING SUGGESTIONS IMPORTANT IN HYPNOTIZING?

Indeed yes. In connection with verbal suggestion, proper delivery of the suggestions is important to their acceptance. In this regard, tone, inflection, and phrasing of suggested words all have their place, but the major purpose and goal of the hypnotherapist is to focus the subject's attention on what is expressed. There are times when a slow pace and timing will prove most successful and there are times when a slow pace of insistence will not be as effective as a more rapid pace. There are also times when it is well to challenge the subject to try to resist the influence. The very inability the subject finds in not being able to do so enforces the effect of the suggestion. And there are times when the very opposite of challenging is to be desired, like an earnest persuasion providing the best suggestion. A hypnotist develops a certain instinct for the proper delivery of suggestions through time and professional

practice. To develop this instinct takes time, practice, and patience.
It is in the development of this instinct to use proper timing in suggestion that the real expertise of the hypnotist can be found.

Question No. 54 ...
DOES REPETITION OF A SUGGESTION INCREASE ITS INFLUENCE?

Repetition can be looked upon as the driving force of suggestion. It is important to the effective presenting of suggestions. It is cumulative in effect, and prevents the hypnotist from getting ahead too fast and out of proper timing in giving his suggestions to the subject, as well as having a certain monotony about it that is, in itself, hypnotic in affecting the mind. But don't forget that there are also physical repetitions that can increase influence and hypnotic depth. An example of a physical repetition might be "every-time that I shake your hand, you will go deeper asleep". The influence of suggestions, are increased with the depth of hypnosis. Deepening techniques can be verbal and or physical. An example of a verbal repetition might be, "every-time, I say the word sleep, you will go deeper into hypnosis". You may want to think of repetition of suggestion as being a "compounding of suggestion" whereas the suggestion intensity increases with repetition.

Question No. 55 ...
DOES THE COMBINING OF SUGGESTION HELP IN HYPNOTIZING?

The positive response to one suggestion can directly lead to the positive response of subsequent suggestions. For example, a subject is told his arm is stiff and he cannot move it. The response is positive. Then it is suggested that when he is given a suggestion for it to relax and drop to his lap, that when it falls into his lap he will go more profoundly into hypnosis then he was before. In this, it will be noted how each suggestion used in combination reinforces and next suggested occurrence. The effect is <u>compounding</u> in influence. This is an important principle to apply in producing and controlling hypnosis. A good suggestion right after you hypnotize a person might be, "Each and every exhale you take relaxes you deeper and deeper asleep and you feel your body relaxing more and more with each exhale". The compounding effect of deepening now is automatically tied into the clients breathing. You are learning years of knowledge.

Question No. 56 ...
CAN A PERSON BE TRAINED IN SUBCONSCIOUS CONDITIONED RESPONSIVENESS?

Every individual has a certain potential to the influence of suggestions. This varies in different persons and may be increased or decreased by training through graduating subconscious conditioned responses to suggestions. If the suggestion succeeds, the suggestibility ratio is increased. If the suggestion fails, the suggestibility ratio is lessened. For this reason, it is well to train the subject to respond first to more simple hypnotic phenomena before advancing to more complex phenomena. For example, to obtain a muscular cataleptic response to a suggestion prior to attempting a hallucination response. The success of the first increasing the success of the second. This is the basis of subconscious conditioned response training. In your hypnotherapy session, you might ask your client to focus on their breathing and to nod their head yes when they notice their breathing change and when they take a deeper breath in. This is a very simple and easy to follow direction, which can be given, even before you start your hypnotherapy session. Think of the game "follow the leader". The game is about one person or a group of people following and doing everything that the leader does. In hypnosis and you as the expert hypnotist, your client simply has to follow your directions and do everything that you ask them to do.

Question No. 57 ...
DOES VOLUNTARY ACTIONS INCREASE HYPNOTIC SUGGESTIBILITY?

A voluntary response to a suggestion has an influence in increasing the response to an involuntary one. The practical application of this principle lies in instructing the subject to do certain things to which he must comply before presenting actual hypnotizing suggestions. For example, telling him to be seated in a certain chair, to place his hands on his lap in a certain way, to rest his feet upon the floor spaced apart, etc. Obedience to such direct verbal commands tends to cause the subject to act upon the hypnotist's suggestions uncritically, which has a carry-over effect to subsequent hypnotic inducing suggestions given.

Question No. 58 ...
DOES DEEP BREATHING INCREASE SUGGESTIBILITY?

This is a refinement of the foregoing question of a voluntary action increasing suggestibility. In this process, the subject is told to breath in and out following a certain rhythm, as the operator directs it to be. The effect of this is to transfer an automatic action (breathing) into a voluntary action. Further, deep breathing increases the oxygen supply to the brain producing a sleepy effect rendering the subject more responsive to suggestions. Now an eastern hypnotic look at deep breathing might be the thought of breathing in energy, what is called in India, Prana. Some people believe "Prana" is brought into the subject, which combined with the vital energy of the hypnotist increases the effect of the mind-to-mind influence that hypnosis produces. Again this relates to Eastern Tradition and early Mesmerism. Deep breathing helps a person physically relax more, and physical relaxation is an important part in the process of hypnotherapy and hypnotizing a person.

Question No. 59 ...
ARE NONVERBAL SUGGESTIONS OF USE IN HYPNOTIZING?

Of course they are. Any means at our disposal in communicating is useful. In relation to hypnosis, all suggestive influences exerted by the operator, other than verbal suggestion, are used to work with and increase the power of suggestion. Such processes as passes, gestured, body movement, etc. all intensify the influence of suggestions. The using of such nonverbal suggestions is very important to the hypnotist. Even as a hypnotherapist I (Tom Silver) will say to a client who is in hypnosis in my office, "When I touch you on your forehead with my finger, you will instantly relax 10 times deeper asleep". The touch of my finger on the subject's forehead now acts as a nonverbal suggestion or physical trigger.

Question No. 60 ...
DOES PERSONALIZING SUGGESTIONS ADD TO THERE INFLUENCE?

We would say definitely "Yes" to that question. The more the suggestion can be personalized to the recipient of the suggestion, the more it will influence the suggestion. In such regard, it is even well to associate the name of the individual with the suggestion when it is possible. We always personalize the sessions that we conduct in our hypnotherapy sessions, and we tape record most of them for our clients to use at home for reinforcement.

Question No. 61 ...
WHAT IS MEANT BY VISUALIZATION AND VISUAL IMAGERY?

Visualization and Visual Imagery, is the picture-forming power of the mind. In relation to hypnosis, the hypnotherapist has the client see in his mind a visual picture of what he wants to accomplish. The client visualizes his goal in his mind while he or she is hypnotized.

The hypnotist now gives direct suggestions to the client of reaching this goal or he the therapist may give the client some positive affirmations to repeat silently to him or herself of reaching this goal. We use this principle of visual imagery continuously in our work. Visualization of a positive change is one of the most important processes we know for the production of successful hypnotherapy. Having a person visualize in their mind a goal and than seeing themselves achieving this goal all under hypnosis, has helped thousands of people achieve their goals in life. Athletes before competition utilize the powers of visualization. To use visualization, you do not even have to be hypnotized. The power of creative visualization is available for all of us to use. You should always use it in your private hypnotherapy practice because it works. Later on in our training manual we will teach you some visual imagery techniques that you will find very valuable.

Question No. 62 ...
IS HYPNOTISM SAFE AND SANE?

The hue and cry occasionally set up by ill informed people that hypnotism is harmful to the mind is ridiculous. Hypnosis is a perfectly natural function of the mind. Millions of cases of hypnotism have been conducted all over the world and not a single harmful result has been reported.

However, everything has both a positive and a negative aspect. The mind can take on harmful suggestions just as well as it can helpful ones.

As an example, look at how Hitler hypnotized the whole nation of Germany without putting them into a trance. But by and large, hypnotists are highly principled people who are out to help humanity, not harm it.

In stage demonstrations of hypnotism, the entire audience is there to witness that no harmful suggestions are presented. We believe that all stage hypnosis demonstrations and stage shows be conducted by skilled professionals who are trained and certified hypnotherapists.

Hypnotism can be looked upon as a rapid way of changing the mind. It is an effective way to produce both physical and mental changes in the body and mind of the hypnotized individual. Mind affects body and body affects mind. Correctly used, hypnosis provides a wonderful tool for mental training. If there is ever any harm, it is never from the hypnosis. Any harm must rest entirely on the scruples of the hypnotist. However, it can equally be said that the physician and psychologist are in the same boat, in relation to standards.

Question No. 63 ...
CAN HYPNOSIS BE USED TO INFLUENCE AND EVEN COMIT A CRIME?

A study of hypnotic suggestion may offer some useful ideas to the penal code that are worthy of thought. Someone or something influences everybody to a greater or lesser degree consciously, or subconsciously, or by the environment to which they are exposed too. Environment greatly enhances suggestive influence. If a man is continuously exposed to a criminal side of life and commences to feel that such is the best way to get along, he is likely to become a criminal. On the other hand, if he lives in an environment that goes along with the accepted protocol of society, he is most likely to so conform. He becomes a good citizen.

Beyond question, there are some persons that seem to have rebellious, antisocial instincts in them that lead to criminal behavior. However, even in such persons, there seems to be a countering trait of goodness that can often be developed. For example, as has often happened if a criminal is placed in the company of, shall we say, sensible and honest people who seem to be getting along okay in life, he will often revert to ways of good behavior rather than bad behavior for basically, good in humanity predominates over bad. If such a man is removed from the environment of criminality and placed in an environment of usefulness to his fellow man, often a remarkable shift in attitude will occur. On the other hand, if he is sent to jail on his first offense and placed among others far more criminally minded than himself, he is very likely to sink yet deeper into attitudes of crime. In this is seen the obvious operation of hypnotic suggestion which we have learned so well, which operates so powerfully within the mind of the individual.

By removing him from the criminal influence so often found in the penitentiary and placing him in a different environment, his mentality will, hopefully, head towards reform for the better.

Physical punishment will never reform a criminal and on the contrary, it fills his mind with hatred and malice towards mankind, and at the first chance he gets, he seeks to avenge himself. On the other hand, if the appeal is made to the subliminal self via the hypnotic suggestions and example, the spark of good that is within him may be kindled.

As was mentioned, in actual experience, good seems to predominate over bad in most people. For example, a good man, even when deeply hypnotized, will not obey a suggestion against his ingrained moral nature. The instinct of self-preservation steps in and says, No. In the same manner, a moral woman cannot be induced to perform an immoral act and if such is insisted upon by the operator will awaken from the hypnosis, frequently with a shock.

A rule of thumb in relation to hypnotic suggestions is that the subject will carry out all suggestions given by the operator providing they do not conflict with his or her moral nature, personal characteristics, or produce serious consequences to themselves. In a nutshell, it can be said that the subconscious mind of a person is basically protective of the individual.

Question No. 64 ...
WHAT'S AUTOMATIC WRITING AND DRAWING?

Often the production of such phenomena is ascribed to influence from outside entities or spirits manifesting through the subject. Whether this is so or not is hard to say.

It is generally conceded that the subconscious phase of mind has control over the body of the person, so it is reasonable to suppose that the control of the movements of the hands to write messages can come through independent of the conscious knowledge of the person.

There have even been reported cases in which automatic subconscious drawings of pictures have been recorded. Some of these drawings are really wonderful examples of artwork, normally far beyond the conscious efforts of the subject. However, again, who really knows what remarkable talents lay within the subconscious minds of some persons?

It is not uncommon even to hear great artists who consciously paint say that the inspiration for their painting came from out of their subconscious.

Question No. 65 ...
CAN A PERSON STOP SMOKING USING HYPNOSIS?

The use of hypnosis has helped many people to stop smoking. Trying to stop smoking using your Will Power is very difficult. Stopping smoking by using your subconscious motivation to stop smoking often does the job quickly. One thing we must tell you about this though, we never hypnotize a person to stop smoking unless stopping smoking is their personal wish, and never because someone outside tells them to. Smoking is a habit activated by a tobacco addiction. To master such a habit requires personal desire in that direction which motivation is amplified by the hypnotist. Cigarettes contain nicotine and sugar and it is a two chemical addiction not just one. Most people do not know that each cigarette contains about a half a teaspoon of sugar. Hypnosis can help you to let go of the chemical addictions and also to let the habit and addition go. The person who wants to stop smoking must be consciously motivated and willing to stop smoking and needs to follow the hypnotherapists program. Later on in this book I (Tom Silver) will give you some hypnotherapy suggestions that you can use on your clients to help them stop smoking and inhaling poison.

Question No. 66 ...
CAN A PERSON LOSE WEIGHT USING HYPNOSIS?

Yes hypnosis can help in directing the hypnotic motivation towards goal of regulating proper eating habits and body metabolism and to handle a smaller intake of food while increasing a person's energy.

In addition, we suggest adding a visualization mechanism such as placing a picture of an attractive person with the type of body you would like to have. Stand before it daily and allow it to form within your mind the way your body is shaping up.
This process definitely helps. You can also have the client imagine how they would look if they had already lost the weight and have them keep

that image of themselves with the weight already gone. Hypnosis can help a person separate emotions from food, increase motivation to exercise, increase body metabolism, and eat smaller portions of food and to enjoy eating healthy foods such as vegetables, and fruits. There are some very good weight loss motivation suggestions that are presented later on in our manual.

Question No. 67 ...
CAN HYPNOSIS HELP A PERSON SLEEP?

While hypnosis is not the same as natural sleep, it can definitely be a great aid in helping a person sleep. What disturbs sleep most is an over-active mind when one is trying to sleep, and an over active mind comes from an over-active body, that is to say a restlessness that comes from stress of some kind or other. The body affects the mind and mind affects the body. It is a vicious circle. Hypnosis breaks the circle. Hypnosis provides a pathway to relaxing both mind and body, and when both work in harmony, healthful normal sleep is always the result. We can definitely repeat again that hypnosis can provide the perfect cure for insomnia. In such regard, we even went to the effort of making what we call a hypnosis/sleep tape that will hypnotize a client while they are trying to go to sleep, and it will convert the hypnosis sleep to a natural deep sleep. We have given this to many persons who have requested our assistance in sleeping better. We are happy to say it has worked so well, that many report they went to sleep and slept so soundly they never even heard consciously the end of the tape.

Question No. 68 ...
WHAT IS MEANT BY HYPNOTIC RELAXATION?

This question is related to the foregoing. The entire process of hypnosis is directed towards the ends of relaxing the mind through relaxing the body.
What is meant by hypnotic relaxation is a deliberately directed process that interrupts the circle of mind disturbing body and body disturbing mind syndrome. What is very interesting to us is that just the entering of the hypnotic state alone brings about wonderful relaxation. That is what hypnotic relaxation means. It directs mind towards being at peace with itself. A hypnotic relaxation is very healthful in restoring energy and vitality.

HYPNOTIST SAVES CLIENT'S LIFE!

PICTURED BELOW IS MR. JEFF LOUDEN WITH HIS LOVING WIFE AND HYPNOTHERAPIST TOM SILVER. TOM SAVED JEFF'S LIFE BY HELPING JEFF STOP SMOKING CIGARETTES THROUGH HYPNOSIS THREE YEARS PRIOR TO A BRAIN TUMOR SURGICAL OPERATION THAT JEFF'S DOCTORS SAID HE WOULD NOT HAVE SURVIVED HAD HE STILL BEEN SMOKING!!!

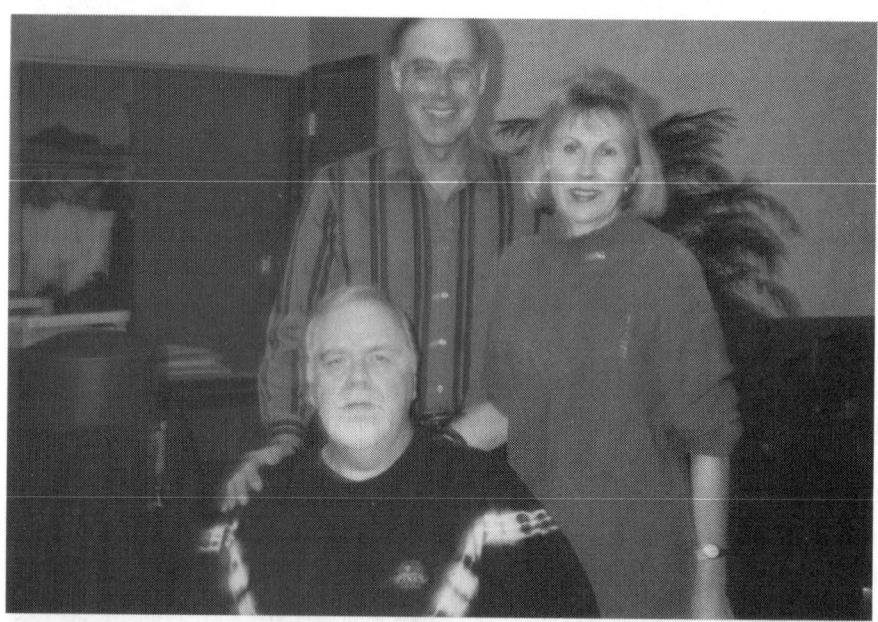

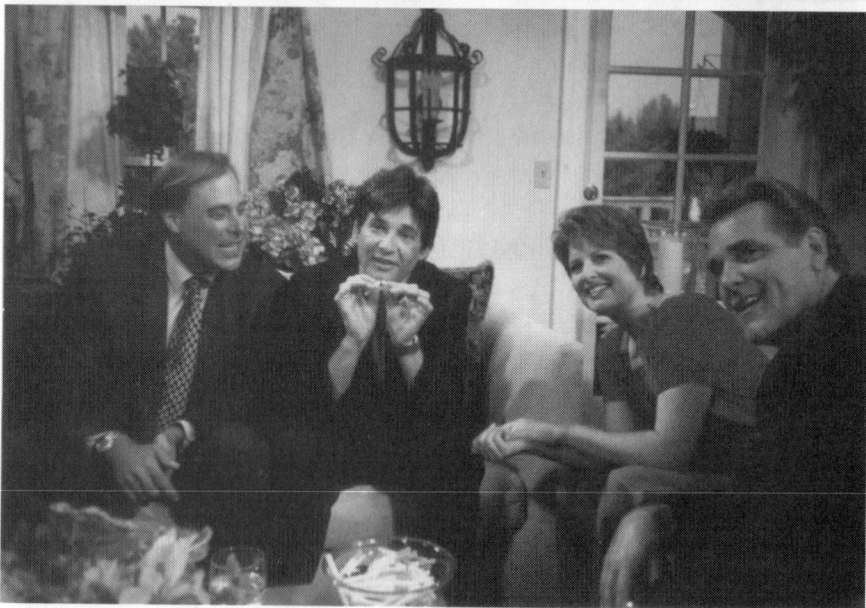

HYPNOTIST TOM SILVER HELPS ACTOR ALAN ROSENBERG TO STOP SMOKING CIGARETTES ON NATIONAL TELEVISION SHOW "THE HOME AND FAMILY SHOW"

Question No. 69 ...
WHAT IS HYPNOANESTHESIA?

Hypnoanesthesia is using hypnosis to produce an anesthetic towards pain in the body. Hypnosis has that power to disassociate pain. For that purpose it has even been used in performing major operations, childbirth, and in so many cases, and its use in dentistry is popular. Our only warning is to remember that pain is a danger signal to the body sirens that something is out-of-order and requires attention.

For minor pains it is remarkably useful. Hypno-anesthesia was used by the Mayo Brothers (medical doctors and founders of The Mayo Clinics) in the early 1900s in conjunction with chemical anesthesia and it helped tremendously in reducing death during surgery, which occurred in one out of four hundred patients, due to chemical adverse reactions to the current anesthesia that was used back then. In over 17,000 procedures conducted under the Mayo Brothers Hypno/Chemical anesthesia, not one patient died of chemical poisoning. This was because, the use of hypnosis for pain control was able to allow chemical anesthesia to be reduced to about 15% percent or less of it's normal dosage.

Question No. 70 ...
CAN HYPNOSIS HELP ATHLETES IN SPORTS?

Hypnosis can definitely increase athletic ability in sports. It removes apprehensions of failure to win and increases motivation to win. Hypnosis has been used by many famous sports figures. Hypnosis can increase focus and concentration and put an athlete "in the zone". Hypnosis in sports has become a popular use for the art. Lot's of golfers utilize hypnotism. We have helped many an athlete reach their sports goals with the use of hypnosis, visual imagery and conscious affirmation. Being involved with sports entertainment as the NBA halftime show hypnotist, I (Tom Silver) have also privately hypnotized a number of professional basketball athletes to help them be more accurate, consistent and successful in playing their sport well.

Question No. 71 ...
CAN HYPNOSIS HELP DEVELOP TALENT?

Hypnosis can very much help develop talent in persons who have talent. It's used by artists, musicians, singers, dancers and actors, and has proved wonderfully successful. Hypnosis does not create talent, but if talent is there it can amplify the talent. We highly recommend that talented people learn The Art of Self-Hypnosis. It will prove of great value to all talented people who wish to increase their talent. Hypnosis can help you to reach your true performance peak level and ability. Hypnosis can help a person let go of fears and explore their own creativity and imagination.

Question No. 72 ...
WHAT IS MEANT BY AGE REGRESSION HYPNOSIS?

Age Regression hypnosis deals with bringing forth experiences and memories, which have occurred in the subject's current lifetime. Mostly this form of hypnotic regression deals with surfacing childhood experiences and traumas which have occurred in the past and which have a bearing on the behavior of the person in their current space and time. If you have had a traumatic event in your life at any time, that event may be affecting the way you feel and act.

A regression therapy back to a negative event to let go of the emotional scars of that event may be very therapeutic. Some hypnotherapists also practice the therapy that is called Past Life Regression. We have personally conducted over 1000 past life regression therapies. This is the process of hypnotizing a person and taking them back to a past life memory so that they can learn and change from that memory. Age regression therapy is used extensively and successfully in hypnosis.

Question No. 73 ...
CAN HYPNOSIS HELP OVERCOME DRUG ADDICTION?

If the person shows enough good sense to want to master a drug habit, hypnosis can definitely help as hypnosis through the proper handling of suggestions, can increase the subject's motivation to kick the habit and to even get over the chemical addition that the drug might create. When a subject has an open mind to want to stop, while hypnotized we present a barrage of good solid reasons and suggestions of why they should stop. These are positive hypnotherapy suggestions and visual images. When such suggestions and visual images are accepted by the subconscious mind, drug addiction can often be curbed and even eliminated. There also might be a number of factors involved that have created the drug addiction. The addiction might be the symptom and the cause something else. With therapy, sometimes when the cause of a habit is revealed, the symptoms will disappear. Addiction to drugs or alcohol might just be a temporary bandage that the client is putting over the wound, which might be the emotional scar from the past.

Question No. 74 ...
DOES ALCOHOL MAKE A PERSON MORE RECEPTIVE TO HYPNOSIS?

Actually there is no need for it. We prefer to avoid its use. However, remember a little alcohol is a far cry from drunkenness. Drunkenness is a very unpredictable state, and sometimes hypnosis is difficult.

The focus and concentration of an intoxicated person is very weak. A person who is not on alcohol or drugs make the best candidates for hypnotherapy because they can focus better and as you now know hypnosis is magnified concentration and focus of attention.

Question No. 75 ...
CAN HYPNOSIS STOP A HEADACHE?

We would say that hypnosis could relieve the pain and discomfort of a headache, especially if the headache is created by stress, tension, worry, anxiety or any other negative emotion. Over 60% of all physical problems or what we call "body syndromes" which are physical pains, caused by mental anxiety. Using hypnotism has neutralized many a headache. Even some migraine headaches have been drastically reduced by also using hypnosis.

Question No. 76...
CAN HYPNOSIS BE USED IN THE FIELD OF EDUCATION?

Truly amazing results are possible. Most academic learning is a matter of recalling the learned information that has been given in the classroom. Everything you have ever learned is right there for recall in that wonderful mental computer in your head called subconscious mind. Hypnosis can bring in spontaneously recall of what one has learned. Used for educational purposes it can turn one into a scholar.

We have used hypnosis with students and professional people to increase their focus and concentration on what they study, and to increase their long-term memory. All long-term memory is subconscious. Hypnosis can help you to increase your focus and concentration when you study, it can also increase your long-term memory receptiveness.

Hypnosis has been very effective in helping students be more calm and relaxed during test taking so that the correct answers can easily come up. When my (Tom) daughter Nicole was in elementary school, I hypnotized her first grade teacher to pass a bilingual exam. A stimulating teacher, who captures the attention and emotions of her students, is practicing waking hypnosis without even knowing it.

Question No. 77 ...
IS THERE ANY VALUE IN SLEEP LEARNING!

This is an arbitrary question. Some swear by it while others doubt its value. However, the fact remains that the military did use the process during war years to teach sleeping soldier a foreign language. The method used is largely mechanical and is really quite simple. The material to be learned is on a cassette inserted in a tape player, arranged to click on at a certain time during the night while the person is sleeping. A flat little speaker is placed under the pillow of the sleeping person, and during the night while the person is sleeping, the taped instructions are softly repeated over and over again. The idea being that during sleep the learning can be picked up subconsciously. The process seemed to have worked fine in some cases where sleep was not disturbed, but many persons using the process complained that the voice from under the pillow caused them to awaken.

In our opinion, the process of sleep-learning is not to be rejected as being of possible value, but there is still further research needed in that direction. If done properly, a person can convert from a natural sleep, to a suggestive hypnotic sleep by using simple techniques. Some say that during natural sleep our subconscious is transmitting information in the form of dreams, and therefore may not be able to receive information such as might be derived from sleep-learning.

Question No. 78 ...
DO SUBLIMINAL SUGGESTION TAPES HAVE VALUE?

Some say yes, and some say no. Personally we honestly do not know what to say. A subliminal tape is one where the suggestion formula for various purposes of well-being are buried inside of the sound track beneath some surface sound, such as music or such as ocean waves, etc. Consciously you cannot hear the message being spoken, but some say it does get through subconsciously. Again, like Sleep Learning this is an arbitrary question. Our personal opinion is that subliminal suggestions are not as effective as suggestions that can be heard by the subconscious mind. We also think that the suggestions under hypnosis have to pass through the conscious mind and down into the subconscious mind. We believe in an outer and inner brain and not in the left and right brain theory that has been around for years. The inner brain can both be logical and it can be creative.

We believe that suggestions or affirmations, which cannot be registered, auditable or heard by the mind, cannot be recorded by the mind. Most subliminal suggestions are executed because of the person reading the affirmations on the program is giving themselves those same suggestions when they are listening to the relaxation music or natural environment sounds. It could be based on imagination of it working like a placebo effect.

Question No. 79 ...
DO HYPNOSIS AUDIO PROGRAMS REALLY WORK?

Hypnotic audio programs of worthwhile suggestion formulas have definite value. Both of us have hypnosis audio programs that we have created and we sometimes give to our clients. Some people do not have a clinically trained hypnotherapist in their area and a good self-hypnosis behavior modification program might work great for them. Usually these are designed to commence by a relaxation series of suggestions, which are followed by the recording of the desired suggestion formula, for purposes such as overcoming stress, developing confidence, increasing memory, losing weight, stopping smoking etc. Many such tapes or CDs can be found on the public market, and their consistent use has proves successful. It actually took me (Tom) five years to create self-help hypnosis programs that I felt were as good or even better than most hypnotherapy sessions.

Question No. 80 ...
CAN THE SEVERELY MENTALLY DISTURBED PERSON OR AN INSANE PERSON BE HYPNOTIZED?

In a sense some what we call insane people have hypnotized themselves so deeply they have lost control of the process, and the process has taken control of them. Hypnosis can produced similar effects to those seen in various forms of insanities, but the difference lies in that they are always under direct control of the mind. In insanity the mind has gone wild. Hypnotizing a mentally disturbed person, or an insane person is entirely possible, but results are rather unpredictable as such persons are pretty much wrapped up in their own private world, and really don't wish outside intrusion. Personally, we have always left working with the severely mentally disturbed people, in the hands of psychiatrists, medical doctors, and those specially trained in that field. Working with people with severe mental illness is very much a specialized field in itself, which requires years of training.

Question No. 81 ...
CAN DRUGS BE USED TO INCREASE HYPNOTIC RECEPTIVITY?

This is a field for research. Beyond question there are many kind of tranquilizing drugs. Personally we have never found it necessary to employ drugs of any kind when hypnotizing, but this does not mean that some forms of relaxation drugs cannot be an aid in hypnotizing. Personally we leave the experimenting with drugs in relation to hypnosis in the hands of the physicians.

A remarkable fact we have found is that the effects of drugs can be simulated by the hypnotic without the use of the actual drug at all. Years ago when LSD first came to public attention and was on the open market some experiments in this regard were performed. As is well known, LSD is a mind-expanding drug that appears to open up inner mental realms. The effects are produced by a chemical reaction on the brain. Without the use of any chemical at all, many of the effects of LSD on the brain can be produced directly using hypnosis alone, and some even claim that the high obtained from hypnosis is much better than that of drugs. We prefer hypnotizing clients who are not medications or drugs.

Question No. 82 ...
CAN A PERSON HEAR BETTER THROUGH HYPNOSIS?

Hypnosis can cause a stimulation of all the senses, so yes it can aid hearing as it concentrates attention upon that purpose. Equally, as mention, it can increase perception through any of the other senses of sight, feeling, taste and smelling. There has been documented research conducted in the past on hypnosis being used to increase hearing.

Question No. 83 ...
CAN HYPNOSIS ADVANCE THE ESP POWERS OF THE MIND?

ESP (Extra Sensory Perception) has been called a Six Sense. This six sense takes us into the experimental realms of psychic phenomena, telepathy, clairvoyance, telekinesis, etc. Investigation of these fascinating realms of potential mental powers lie directly within the field of experimental research. Hypnosis is frequently employed as a tool in such research.

If we were to give a personal opinion on the manner in answering this question, we would definitely reply in the affirmative that hypnosis might advance the ESP (Extra Sensory Perception) powers of the mind. The facts are not out yet either way and more proof is needed.

Back in the old days of hypnosis when it was called magnetism and mesmerism, the hypnotists use to hypnotize "sensitives" and demonstrate these extra sensory perceptions by having these subjects predict future events. Some hypnosis historians say that the whole spiritual movements, which started in the mid 1800s in England and America, were an offshoot of hypnosis and directly linked to hypnotism and the hypnotic trance. Mary Baker Eddy the founder of the religion called "Christian Scientist" was healed by a mesmerist and then created a whole religion based on the mind healing the body.

Question No. 84 ...
IS IT POSSIBLE TO HYPNOTIZE A PERSON WHO IS SLEEPING?

Absolutely. Some mothers often do this deliberately by talking to their sleeping child and softly whispering to the young one that they will do well in school, be a good boy or girl, etc. The transition from a normal natural sleep to a hypnotic sleep can be done, but it has to be performed very carefully or your subject might awaken from the natural sleep and not convert from natural sleep to the hypnosis sleep. Remember, when you are in the natural sleep, your subconscious mind is transmitting thoughts in the form of dreams.

When you convert the natural sleep, to the hypnosis sleep, your subconscious mind starts receiving and accepting suggestions.

Question No. 85 ...
CAN A PERSON LEARN FASTER WHILE HYPNOTIZED?

Learning follows the laws of attention. The more attention and emotion that is given to the material being studied the more effectively that material is learned. While in hypnosis the attention can be keenly directed, and so we can answer yes, a person can learn faster while hypnotized. Under hypnosis their focus and concentration on learning is nine times greater.

Question No. 86 ...
WHAT PSYCHOLOGICAL DISORDERS CAN HYPNOSIS HELPFULLY AID?

Here is a list of some of these disorders the correction of which hypnosis can be of great help and value:

Abandonment Issues	Addictions	Age Regression
Aggression	Agoraphobia	Anxiety
Assertiveness	Career Success	Change Habits
Concentration	Control Issues	Cravings
Creativity	Death of Loss	Dreams
Fears and Phobias	Frustration	Gambling Habit
Guilt	Headaches	Memory
Moodiness	Motivation	Obsessions
Perfectionism	Pre Surgical	Problem Solving
Procrastination	Public Speaking	Rejection
Relationship Enhancement	Resistance	Responsibility
Sadness	Self Confidence	Self Esteem
Self-Defeating Behaviors	Sleep Disorders	Stop Smoking
Stress Elimination	Study Habits	Writers Block
Helplessness	Hopelessness	Relaxation
Test Anxiety	Hypertension	Trauma

Question No. 87 ...
WHAT PHYSICAL DISORDERS CAN HYPNOSIS HELPFULLY AID?

Hypnosis has likewise been used to successful aid, through hypnotic suggestions, many kinds of physical ailments, such as:

Anesthesia	Bed Wetting	Asthma
Digestive disorders	Hair Twisting	Obesity
Loss of Appetite	Epilepsy	Pain
Impotency	Muscle Spasms	Frigidity
Labor pains	Herpes	Itching
Snoring	Warts	Nail Biting
Perspiring	Paralysis	Arthritis
Nausea	Tics	Ulcers
Headaches	Lower Blood Pressure	Health
Hypertension	Paralysis	and more!

As a human being is a mind/body phenomenon in which mind affects the body and body affects the mind, the usefulness of hypnosis is obvious, and hypnotherapy can successfully treat all manner of difficulties for the individual in detail and effectiveness. Hypnotherapy is not a cure for everything, but it helps people in many areas of life.

"INTERLINGUAL HYPNOTIC TRANCE INDUCTION"
METHOD AND FORMULA TO HYPNOTIZE A PERSON THROUGH AN INTERPRETER

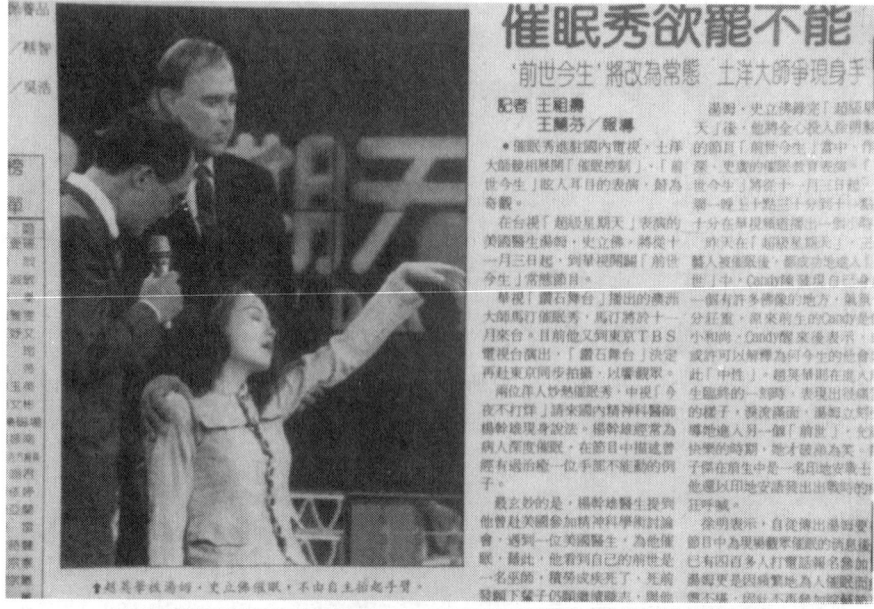

HYPNOTIST TOM SILVER AND INTERPRETER TIMOTHY HUANG
HYPNOTIZING "MISS CHINA" INTO A PAST LIFE MEMORY
TAIPEI TAIWAN NATIONAL TELEVISION SHOW "SUPER SUNDAY" OCTOBER 1994
"COCO" TAIWAN NATIONAL CELEBRITY STAR HYPNOTIZED

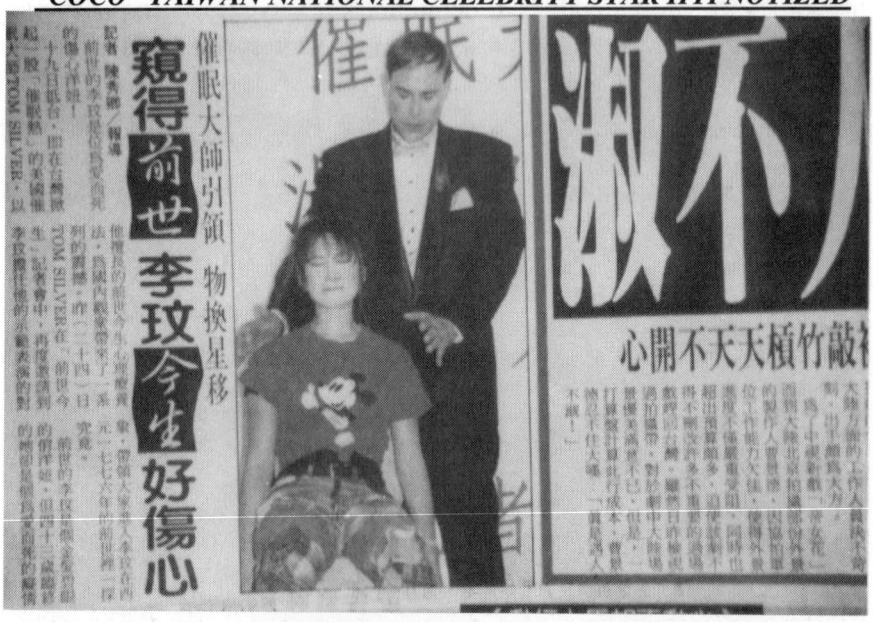

TAIWAN INTERNATIONAL SINGING STAR "COCO" HYPNOTIZED BY TOM SILVER
"COCO RELIVES PAST LIFE MEMORY ON SUPER SUNDAY TELEVISION SHOW"
TAIPEI TAIWAN * REPUBLIC OF CHINA * OCTOBER 1994

HYPNOTIST SETS "WORLD RECORD"

TAIPEI ATLETIC STADIEM
TAIPEI TAIWAN R.O.C.
AMERICAN HYPNOTIST TOM SILVER
SETS TRANSLINGUAL HYPNOSIS
WORLD RECORD!
HYPNOTIZING 3800 PEOPLE AT ONCE
THROUGH AN INTERPRETER IN
MANDARIN CHINESE
WORLD'S RECORD SHOW
JANUARY 31ST 1995
TAIPEI TAIWAN

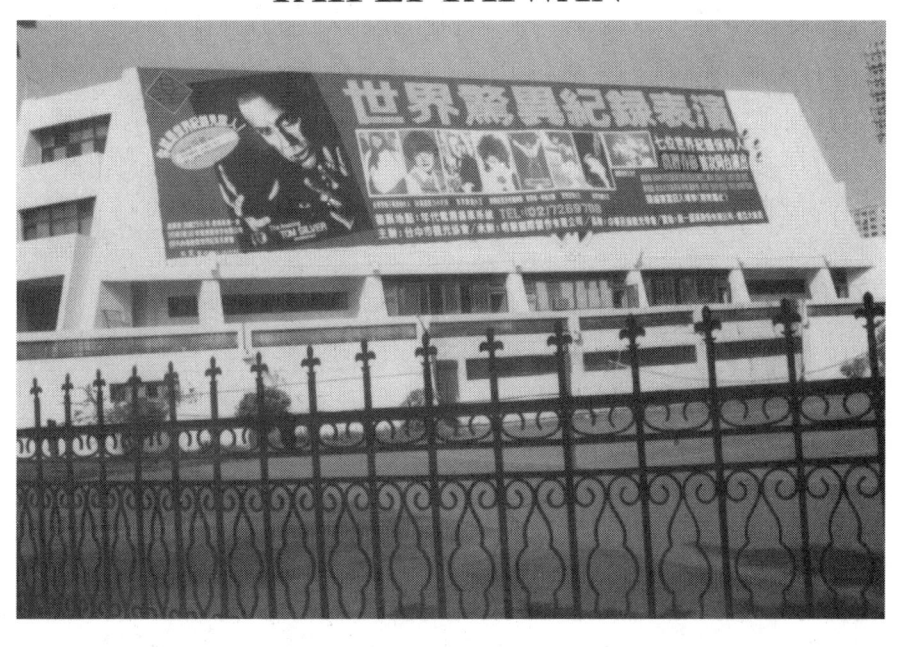

HYPNOSIS WORLD RECORD

SET BY AMERICAN HYPNOTIST TOM SILVER
HYPNOTIZING 3800+ PEOPLE ALL AT THE SAME TIME
THROUGH AN INTERPRETER IN MANDARIN CHINESE
INTERPRETER TIMOTHY HUANG
TAIPEI ATHLETIC STADIUM
JANUARY 31st - FEBRUARY 12, 1995

"INTERLINGUAL MASS HYPNOSIS INDUCTION"
CERTIFICATE OF PROOF SIGNED ON WORLD RECORD DAY
BY WORLD RECORD HOLDERS AND WITNESSES
Hypnosis World Record Witness

We, the performers of the Amazing World Show in Taipei, Taiwan, Republic of China, witnessed and verify the fact that Tom Silver, a hypnotist from Los Angeles, California, U.S.A. hypnotized the entire audience 3 shows a day from January 31, 1995 through February 12, 1995. Tom Silver hypnotized the whole audience through an interpreter in mandarin Chinese. The interpretor was Dr. Timothy D. Huang of Taipei, Taiwan. Stadium capacity is 3,800 plus per show. Interlingual Hypnotic Trance Induction Method was created by Tom Silver hypnotist.

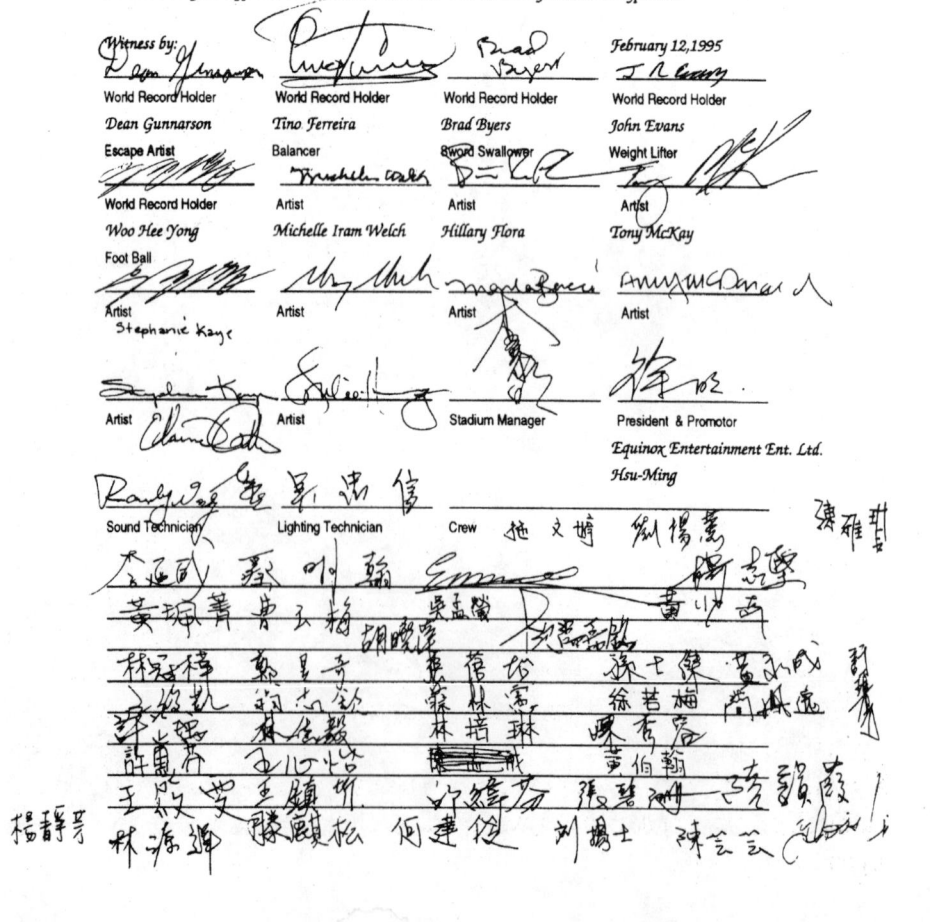

Witness by: February 12, 1995

World Record Holder	World Record Holder	World Record Holder	World Record Holder
Dean Gunnarson	Tino Ferreira	Brad Byers	John Evans
Escape Artist	Balancer	Sword Swallower	Weight Lifter

World Record Holder	Artist	Artist	Artist
Woo Hee Yong	Michelle Iram Welch	Hillary Flora	Tony McKay
Foot Ball			

Artist	Artist	Artist	Artist
Stephanie Kaye			

Artist	Artist	Stadium Manager	President & Promotor
			Equinox Entertainment Ent. Ltd.
			Hsu-Ming

Sound Technician	Lighting Technician	Crew		

CHAPTER EIGHT

LINGUISTIC QUESTIONS AND ANSWERS
INTERLINGUAL HYPNOTIC TRANCE INDUCTION
Created and Copyright in 1994 by Tom Silver
Master Hypnotherapist & Re-Educator

Question No. 88 ...
IS IT POSSIBLE TO HYPNOTIZE IN ANOTHER LANGUAGE?

This chapter deals with the art, science and practice of a method of hypnotizing people who do not speak the same language that you may speak. Most hypnotherapists or stage hypnosis performers have only practiced hypnosis or hypnotherapy on people who speak the same language as the hypnotherapist. An example of this might be an English-speaking hypnotist who hypnotizes people in the language of English. Many people who practice the art of hypnotism even think that it is impossible to hypnotize a person in a foreign language.

In 1994 in Taipei Taiwan (Republic of China) I was able to create a formula and method to hypnotize the people of Taiwan through an interpreter in Mandarin Chinese who was not a hypnotist, but just a person who spoke both Mandarin Chinese and English. During my six years of hard work in introducing the Taiwan culture to the science of hypnotism and the utilization of forensic hypnosis for investigation purposes for memory activation, I worked hard on perfecting my method of Translingual Hypnotism.

I am proud to say that the over Five Thousand Year Old Chinese Culture, the Taiwan Department of Defense, and the people of Taiwan would never have recognized the science of hypnotism or awarded me a "Gold Plate of Honor" in July of 1997, from the Taiwan Minister of Defense had I not been able to hypnotize people in a foreign language.

Hypnosis is becoming recognized and utilized Worldwide now for therapy and even in conjunction with standard medical practices. Medical doctors are even learning more about the applications of hypnosis. With the ever-growing demand for hypnotists around the world, the science and application of being able to hypnotize people through an interpreter is a system and technique that is important to all hypnotherapists.

I would like to thank Mr. Timothy Huang of Taipei Taiwan, for being my interpreter, my friend, and the key person in helping me introduce the amazing science of hypnotism to the Taiwan Culture and the people of Taiwan. Tim Huang has since become a hypnotherapist with a practice in Taipei. Tim and I have created a working Hypnosis Research Center in Taiwan to help further the scientific development of hypnotism in Taiwan, as well as to help create acceptance of this science by the medical and mental practitioners of Taiwan and all of Asia. Our research center is also developing more accurate methods of hypnotic inductions and suggestive formulas. I am proud to say that through hypnotherapy, I have helped thousands of people in Taiwan, including children, teenagers and adults become more confident in themselves, and to acquire greater health and happiness.

More people than ever before are suffering from mental illness and negative emotions. Medical Doctors say that stress, tension, worry and anger kill's more Americans than anything else, including cancer. People in the United States and in other countries commit suicide or harm other people because of the negative thoughts they think and emotions they create. More Children then ever before suffer from depression, sleep depravation, fears, angers and some of the same negative emotions and habits that adults have. When I was in Taiwan I read newspaper articles of children in Taiwan and Japan taking their own lives because the pressures in their lives were too much to bear. Hypnotherapy is a universal science that can help people all over the world and with the utilization of Interlingual hypnotism, all language boundaries and limitations are now gone. You can hypnotize people through interpreters.

I will now give you some answers to some of the most asked questions about Interlingual Hypnotism. These answers will help to give you a better understanding of what it is, and how it works. I will also give you some wonderful knowledge and insight on how to hypnotize people who speak a different language.

The information that I will give you will only be effective and will work for you, if you practice and if you are patient. I practiced for days and weeks on perfecting my methods to hypnotize people in Taiwan, through an Interpreter speaking Mandarin Chinese.
My method works!

SOME QUESTIONS AND ANSWERS ABOUT "INTERLINGUAL HYPNOTIC TRANCE INDUCTION"

Question No. 89
WHAT IS THE INTERLINUAL HYPNOTIC TRANCE INDUCTION METHOD?

"Interlingual Hypnotic Trance Induction" is the method and formula of hypnotizing a person through an Interpreter or another person who is speaking the subjects or person who is being hypnotized "Primary or Native Language".
The word Inter-Lingual relates to more than one language. Such as using the English language and using the Mandarin Chinese language combined together to hypnotize a person. Simply put it is hypnosis through an interpreter.

Question No. 90
CAN AN INTERPRETER HYPNOTIZE A PERSON?

A hypnotist is the person who hypnotizes the clients or subjects, and an interpreter is the person, who assist's the hypnotist, by using or speaking the subject's primary language. The interpreter is the hypnotist's assistant and not the actual person hypnotizing the subject. A hypnotist who is able to speak more than one language can always hypnotize a person in that language even if it is not the hypnotist's primary language and as long as the hypnotist knows the exact meaning of the words for the culture he is working with.

Question No. 91
HOW EFFECTIVE IS INTER-LINGUAL HYPNOSIS?

Interlingual hypnosis is just as effective in hypnotizing a person just as any other type of hypnosis process or induction. As long as the pacing and timing are conducted in a successful manner by the hypnotist and interpreter, the induction of hypnosis will be successful Sometimes Interlingual Hypnotic Trance Induction can be even more effective by creating what I call, "The misdirection of the Conscious Mind". This procedure is performed with a hypnosis induction in which the hypnotherapist, creates an overloading process of the subject or client's conscious mind though words, movements, suggestions, and misdirection/confusion and then instantly through a "Shock Induction" technique, converting that "Peak of Conscious Mind Activity" into a deep hypnotic or delta stage of conscious sleep.

Translingual hypnosis techniques "should" only be conducted By a trained and experienced clinical hypnotherapist

Question No. 92
WHAT SPECIAL CONSIDERATIONS SHOULD BE TAKEN INTO CONSIDERATION IN CONDUCTING THE INTERLINGUAL HYPNOSIS?

The most important consideration taken into account when conducting an "Interlingual Hypnotic Trance Induction" method or for hypnotizing people through an interpreter is the correct interpretation of the words that the hypnotist is using to hypnotize the subject. The interpreter should know exactly every meaning of each and every word that the hypnotist is trying to communicate to the subject or else the wrong meaning and messages that the hypnotist is telling the subject will be confusing and will have negative affects on the hypnotic induction, therapy and or suggestions.

The pacing and timing of the hypnotist and interpreter are also important. It must be smooth and skillfully conducted. The speaking pattern of both the hypnotist and the Interpreter are important and should match or complement each other instead of conflict and clash with each other.

Question No. 93
HOW DEEPLY HYPNOTIZED CAN A PERSON BECOME WITH INTERLINGUAL HYPNOSIS?

A person can go just as deep into hypnosis as with any other hypnosis type of induction. All the way down to delta or what is call somnambulism.

Question No. 94
WHAT HYPNOTISM DEMONSTRATIONS AND OR POSITIVE CHANGES CAN OCCUR WITH INTERLINGUAL HYPNOTIC TRANCE INDUCTION?

With the application of Interlingual Hypnotic Trance Induction, everything that can occur with the traditional forms of hypnosis and hypnotherapy can also occur with translingual hypnotism.
With Interlingual Hypnotism, you can help a person to lose weight, stop smoking, increase motivation and confidence, reduce stress, tensions and worries, increase memory retention and focus and concentration, become a better athlete and elevate a persons level of success by increasing the positive emotions in a persons subconscious mind. Interlingual Hypnotic Trance Induction hypnotherapy can be used for natural childbirth, for surgery to reduce pain, for releasing negative emotion, habits, to reduce fear and more. Translingual hypnosis demonstrations can also show pure creativity and imagination suggestions for live hypnosis show demonstrations. The subconscious mind does not distinguish between fantasy and reality. If the subconscious mind can accept a suggestion of creativity or imagination, then the subconscious mind can also accept positive suggestion to help change a person's life, or to increase the physical health of a person.

Question No. 95
HOW MANY PEOPLE CAN BE HYPNOTIZED AT ONCE WITH INLINGUAL HYPNOTIC TRANCE INDUCTION?

In February of 1995 Timothy Huang and myself (Tom) hypnotized approximately 3800 people all at the same time through an interpreter in Mandarin Chinese. Tim Huang of course was my interpreter. This was the very first Interlingual Hypnosis World's Record. Groups of people can all be hypnotized to one degree or another. Everybody's depth of hypnosis may vary, but some people in a crowd will go into very deep levels of hypnosis. Take for example a famous celebrity, or musical artists such as "The Beatles", or even a dynamic political speaker like Martin Luther Kind. They can hypnotize you into a very receptive state of emotional concentration without you even knowing that you are hypnotized. Music and Public speeches are considered a form of waking hypnosis when emotions are activated. Watching a movie can hypnotize a person and activate or create positive or negative emotions or feelings from your subconscious mind. When you watch the movie, the emotions created by the movie will automatically and without thinking, come up to your conscious mind by-passing your logic and reason, giving you feelings of feeling good, sad, happy, mad, angry, fearful and more. I can remember one movie that made millions of people afraid of sharks and the ocean. Movies are very hypnotizing.

Question No. 96
CAN CHILDREN BE HYPNOTIZED BY USING THIS METHOD OF TRANLINGUAL HYPNOTISM?

Yes indeed children can certainly be hypnotized by an interpreter by using the same hypnosis induction methods that you would use on children who speak English as their primary language.

Question No. 97
WHO MAKES THE BEST INTERPRETER?

Anybody who speaks two languages can make a good interpreter for Interlingual hypnotism, however, the better that the interpreter speaks and understands your own primary language, the better co-hypnotist he or she will be. The better their understanding of what they are interpreting, the better word translations can be used for the subject to follow and understand in order to hypnotize the subject, and to implant positive hypnosis therapeutic suggestions.

If you are working with a child and one of the parents can speak your language and the child's primary language, they would probably make the best candidate to use as the interpreter and person to help you to hypnotize that child. The more comfortable and safe and secure you make the child in this situation, the better the chance of inducing a deeper state of hypnosis for the therapy.

Now we will discuss the method formula that is needed in order to hypnotize people is another language. In order to successfully complete a deep hypnotic induction on a subject through an interpreter, it is important to:

FIND AN INTERPRETER WHO SPEAKS AND COMPREHENDS YOUR LANGUAGE WELL ENOUGH TO TRANSLATE YOUR WORDS AND SUGGESTIONS TO THE SUBJECT WITH THEIR CORRECT MEANING.

An example of this might be the word "sleep". To the average English speaking person, the word "sleep" would probably mean, when we are asleep, such as a night in our beds. Now to the hypnotist, the word "sleep" means to enter into a hypnotic sleep, not a natural sleep. Now the word sleep in another language might mean the same thing, or maybe something entirely different.

When I (Tom) first worked with an interpreter and hypnotized some subjects, I said to the subject the word "sleep" and when it was translated into the Mandarin language, the person just stood there as if they were frozen solid. I asked a person in the room, what word did the interpreter say in Mandarin Chinese, and what did that word mean, and the person said that the interpreter said a word that meant to "Freeze", as if to not move instead of sleep.

THE PROPER MEANING OF THE WORDS AND THE CORRECT INTERPRETATION OF THE WORDS THAT ARE TRANSLATED INTO ANOTHER LANGUAGE MUST BE INTERPRETED CORRECTLY.

Explain to the interpreter what hypnosis is and how hypnosis works. The more understanding of the induction process and science of hypnotism, the better the interpreter will be in helping you to hypnotize a subject. Maybe even showing your interpreter examples on video or even a live demonstration of what a person might look like when they are physically relaxed and in a hypnotic state of relaxation might be beneficial.

THE TIMING AND PACING OF THE WORDS OF THE HYPNOTIST AND INTERPRETER MUST BE SMOOTH AND SHOULD NEVER OVERLAP EACH OTHER.

When conducting a hypnosis or hypnotherapy session with a client through an interpreter in another language, it is important to make sure that there is a smooth transition from each language without overlapping, or to long of a space or rest between languages. If you and a interpreter practice together, you can create a type of rhythm of your words together and even be able to almost mirror your voices together with emotional vocal expressions which will create more of a successful hypnosis session.

ALWAYS EXPLAIN TO THE CLIENT OR SUBJECT BEFORE YOU HYPNOTIZE THEM EXACTLY HOW YOU ARE GOING TO HYPNOTIZE THEM.

Before you hypnotize your subject or client through an interpreter in a foreign language or even in the same language, you should always explain to your subject, exactly what is going to happen to them physically when you hypnotize them. The directions of how you will hypnotize them will act as a pre-hypnotic suggestion for them to follow, and that will help you to hypnotize the subject easier and quicker.

With directions to follow, the fears of the unknown of "what's going to happen to me" are gone, and so this method will lessen the subject's resistance to being hypnotized. The mind likes to follow directions.

An example of this type of pre-hypnosis induction would be as follows:

In a moment, I will ask you to close your eyes, when you do, you will enter into a hypnotic sleep. Your head will drop down and rest and relax and your whole body will become relaxed. When I touch you on your shoulder, you will open your eyes and look into my eyes. I will then look into your eyes and say the word sleep! Your eyes will close. Your head will drop down. Your body will instantly relax, and you will enter into a deep hypnotic sleep. Do you understand me?"
And get a yes or nod of the head.

Then say to the subject, "Okay, I will now hypnotize you." After that, you simply start your hypnosis formula and induction, and do exactly as you told the subject you would do, and they will enter into a wonderfully deep state of hypnosis.

Remember when conducting translingual hypnotism you are speaking only a few words at a time, and then pausing for your interpreter to translate and speak the words in the subjects own language. .

In a moment (pause-now the interpreter says the same thing in the subject's primary language, and then you continue with the sentence). I will ask you to close your eyes, (pause-interpreter speaks and then you continue, and so forth).

LITERAL SUGGESTIONS WHICH ARE SIMPLIFIED SUGGESTIONS TO THE HYPNOTIZED SUBJECT IN TRANSLINGUAL HYPNOTISM WORK THE BEST

You never want to get too complicated or confusing in your hypnosis induction or hypnotherapy sessions with translingual hypnosis because you will only confuse your interpreter and subject, and you might cloud up the positive simple literal suggestions that will be much more easily accepted. The subconscious mind understands simple directions better than confusing directions. The conscious mind uses logic and reason and is the intellectual part of the mind. The more direct and easier you present positive suggestions to the subconscious mind of the translingual hypnotized subject, the quicker and more effectively they will be accepted. This simple rule will give you greater success with your clients.

PRACTICE, PRACTICE, PRACTICE, AND YOU WILL BE ABLE TO HYPNOTIZE A PERSON THROUGH AN INTERPRETER IN A FOREIGN LANGUAGE

The more that you can practice your techniques with an interpreter, the better of a team of players you will be, as your interpreter is actually your co-hypnotherapist and partner when it comes to being successful in hypnotizing your subjects or clients who do not speak your language. This method of hypnotic induction breaks all barriers.

The more you practice together, the better harmonization between your voices, words and sentences will be obtained, and the more your two voices will sound and even become like one voice.

As long as the purpose of the process is understood, hypnosis can occur. However for a verbalized suggestion to be carried out, the person involved must understand it. There is little accomplished by speaking Chinese to an Englishman who doesn't understand that language than there is in speaking English to a Chinese speaking person who doesn't understand English. However this difficulty of communication between hypnosis operator and subject can be easily overcome by working with an interpreter. I (Tom) have presented my hypnotism shows that way hypnotizing subjects through the medium of a competent interpreter. Translingual hypnotism can increase your private practice because by using it, there are no language barriers anymore.

Question No. 98 ...
IS IT POSSIBLE TO HYPNOTIZE OVER THE TELEVISON OR TELEPHONE?

Wonderfully so. In the early years of television an experiment in hypnotizing the viewers by way of the tube was tried by BBC in England. Viewers were instructed to take a seat in front of their television set and try the experiment. A famous hypnotist was then introduced, and he went into a hypnotic induction directly into the tube. The experiment was so successful it was alarming. Hundreds of people throughout the British Isles reported being hypnotized. Immediately, regulations were put into effect that no further direct induction was to be permitted performed on TV. Hypnotic demonstrations could still be shown with subjects in hypnosis, but the actual induction from now on was always performed off camera. ABC, NBC, and CBS likewise put in similar regulations in America.

On a Fox Television Special called "Powers of The Paranormal", I (Tom) hypnotized three people two thousand miles away from me live on television. I had them become stiff and rigid as a steel bar and had a woman walk on their stomachs up to a water fountain, outdoors in the rain. Remote hypnosis can be performed. I also conduct telephone hypnotherapy sessions all the time.

Question No. 99 ...
CAN WATCHING A MOVIE HYPNOTIZE YOU?

Movies can create good positive feelings and movies can also activate subconscious fears, anxieties, and other negative emotions. Children who watched the Friday the 13th movies had fears of going to sleep after watching that movie, because the fear of being killed in their sleep was accepted into the emotions in the subconscious mind. The movie Jaws created fears of sharks and water in thousands of people around the world.

Question No. 100 ...
CAN READING A BOOK HYPNOTIZE YOU?

Reading a good book and feeling the emotions created by the book and story is hypnotic and can hypnotize you. A good book is always a book that activates your emotions and puts you into hypnosis.

Question No. 101
WHAT SAFETY CONSIDERATIONS SHOULD BE TAKEN WHEN CONDUCTING GROUP HYPNOSIS?

Some hypnotists might say that there is no harm at all to anyone who is hypnotized in a large group. We believe that you should always be careful and use good judgment when conducting group hypnosis. The safety of the subjects you are hypnotizing, should be your number one priority.

It is hard to have complete control over the situation when you are conducting hypnosis demonstrations and suggestions on a group of people all at the same time. If you hypnotize a person to show a physical demonstration, you want to make sure that the people you are hypnotizing, prior to being hypnotized has no physical problems or if you are hypnotizing females in a group, please make sure that none of the female volunteers are pregnant.

You do not want to harm or physically hurt anyone. You want to use good judgment and always give positive good healthy suggestions to benefit the subjects and not to harm them. You also want to make sure that the area where you are hypnotizing your subjects and volunteer's are safe so that no body falls or hurts themselves. Personal Liability insurance for stage hypnotism performers is also recommended.

Question No. 102 ...
CAN A PERSON PERFORM SUPER HUMAN FEATS WHILE HYPNOTIZED?

People have been known to show extra ordinary strength and performance abilities under hypnosis. Controlled breathing and the reduction of air intake under hypnosis can also be performed. Even total pain control has also been demonstrated with people under hypnosis.

Question No. 103 ...
WHAT ARE DREAMS AND WHAT DO THEY MEAN?

We usually go through three different stages of dreaming at night. Precognitive Dreams, Wishful Thinking Dreams, and Venting Dreams. Precognitive dreaming is creative idea dreaming. Wishful thinking dreaming is dreams of goals or aspirations that you have in life.

The last dream cycle is called, venting dreams, which usually occur a few hours or so before you wake up. Venting dreams are the dreams that you have to let go of previous days emotions or activity. Events from your past such as traumatic events or major emotional situations that might have affected you might be trying to be released or vented out in the forms of dreams. If you keep having the same dream over and over again, that dream might be a subconscious anxiety that you for some reason cannot release out of your mind. Even under anesthesia in a hospital with a patient being operated on by a doctor, that patient's conscious mind might be asleep, but his subconscious mind is still very much awake and hearing and even responding to the words or actions of the people around him in the operating room.

Question No. 104 ...
WHAT IS REINCARNATION?

Reincarnation is not directly connected with the study of hypnosis other than that of a popular form of hypnotherapy that has developed over the years, and is known as "Past Life Regression Therapy." In this process, the subject is hypnotized and told to go back in time to a time when he/she lived prior to their current lifetime. Often fascinating stories are revealed, which frequently benefit the person in this lifetime.

Reincarnation is really the evolution of the soul, and implies that we live lifetime after lifetime in renewed body after renewed body. Some say the "stories" produced from out of the subconscious are pure fantasies, much like dreams, while others take them as factual experiences lived through in a previous life. And the third kind of opinion on this topic is that "we can't confirm or deny this yet."

Whatever, the fact remains that this form of hypnotherapy has helped many people.

Question No. 105 ...
IS REINCARNATION TRUE?

Current Western theology does not accept it. Eastern theology has no question about it at all, and reverently states, "It is the way and every moment something within us dies and is renewed, and life goes on". "It is the way of the Universe." We are safe in saying that more than half the world believes in reincarnation as factual truth. Strictly speaking, the Christian religion believes in reincarnation too.

And it is the very foundation of that religion with the second coming of Jesus Christ. "And all believers will join Him in heaven." This is a form of reincarnation only once. However the oriental believes in multiple lives of the soul. All of these religions, no matter whether a single reincarnation or multiple reincarnations, derived themselves from a common concept of the ancient Egyptian belief of the Soul is immortal.

Question No. 106 ...
WHAT CAN BE LEARNED FROM PAST LIFE EXPERIENCES AND MEMORIES?

If it is so, we learn that death is the greatest lie in the world, and that we are immortal. That what we call "death" is but a transition from one existence to another, like the passing from one room to another room. And each lifetime after each lifetime is a school of experiences in which the evolution of the soul (our real SELF) learns and grows in a perpetual expansion of consciousness.

Question No. 107 ...
IS A REINCARNATION MEMORY OR EXPERIENCE UNDER HYPNOSIS ALWAYS REAL?

It all depends on whether one believes in the existence of past lives or not. To the subject who believes so, or who experienced such, the past life can be so "real" that he/she is a true believer. Countless extremely interesting past life stories can be the best candidates for novel or movies. So, in this sense, to the subject, it is real, or even "very real" to him or her. However, to others, these experiences may be just fantasies.

A past life memory regression might be a real experience or it can be something else. Not everybody believes that they have lived before and there still is no actual proof that we have lived lives before our current one, but there seems to be more and more people who are becoming open to the idea of past life memories. More therapists are utilizing past life memory regression as a therapeutic tool in helping a person overcome a negative emotion or habit.

Question No. 108 ...
WHAT OTHER THINGS BESIDES A PAST LIFE COULD THE REINCARNATION EXPERIENCE REPRESENT?

From our point of view, "A Past Life Regression" is just one of many methods used in hypnotherapy. Whether it is real or not is not our concern. If a subject believes on such and can be benefited by, there is no reason why we could not use this type of therapy.

Also, in our experiences of more than several thousands of "Past Life Regression", we have always asked the question right before a subject leave a "past life" memory, "What have you learned from this life?" The answer to this question is very useful. The answers usually are very heart touching, such as "Love thy family", "To be Kind", "Give to others", etc. Therefore, we think the most valuable thing about the past life experience, is what the subject can learn from a past life and use that wisdom in his or her current life.

Past life memories can be a number of different things. It might be pure fantasy. It might be a real past life memory that has surfaced up from the subconscious mind. A past life memory might also be a story or a metaphor of a past life that is not a real life but represents the present fear or anxiety that a client is trying to overcome. In other words, it can be a created or imagined past life trauma.

A memory of drowning in the ocean in a past life might also be a childhood fear created by a boating accident when the person was quite young. Maybe a past life memory might also be an opened up frequency in the human brain that is receiving a single or message of a past life that might not even belong to the person experiencing the past life. To a therapist, the regression therapy might help to neutralize or resolve an inner mental conflict, wall or barrier that is holding a person back from living life to the fullest.

Question No. 109 ...
HOW CAN YOU BE SURE THAT YOU HAVE HAD A TRUE PAST LIFE EXPERIENCE UNDER HYPNOSIS?

Frankly, you can't. Trying to prove or disprove any given past life is impossible and impractical. However, as long as we keep in mind that "Past Life Regression" is one of many hypnotherapy tools and we use it appropriately, it doesn't matter if past life memories are real or not real. That answer is still in debate. There is no actual proof of you having a real past life experience, unless we guess if you can go back to that past life place and find the facts about that life to see if they match your past life memory.

Question No. 110 ...
DOES OUR SUBCONSCIOUS MIND EVER SLEEP?

Our subconscious mind never sleeps, and in fact it is always active and operating. Like previously mentioned, even under anesthesia in a hospital with patient being operated on by a doctor, that patients conscious mind might be a sleep, but his subconscious mind is still very much awake and hearing and even responding to the words and actions of the people around him in the operating room.

Question No. 111 ...
CAN WE CONTROL OUR CONSCIOUS MIND?

Our conscious mental computer is our logic and reason part of our brain, and is also our will power and is the weakest part of our brain power, while our subconscious mind is our emotional, conditioned, habit and pattern part of our mental computer. It is the strongest and most powerful part of our brainpower and mind.

It must operate for you properly and positively, and in sync with your conscious mind in order for you to reach all your goals in life. If your conscious mind or your inner talking voice gives yourself negative words or suggestions, you will never achieve true mental power. You cannot be happy if you consciously and logically punish yourself everyday by thinking negative thoughts.

You must exercise your conscious mind to think positive thoughts, emotions and words, that you want your subconscious mind to respond to. You want your subconscious mind to respond to only positive emotions, by giving yourself positive suggestions everyday. "I'm happy, I live life to the fullest, I love myself, I am confident in every thing I do, I have lot's of energy", etc. Both of your bio mental computers need to be functioning properly and under your operation because you are the operator of your mind, thoughts, and action. You can tell your mind when to think and what to think because you are really the master of your mind. You have to start being in control of both of your bio computers, and make them work for you. Make both of your minds (conscious and subconscious), work for "You" now!

Question No. 112 ...
HOW IS OUR SUBCONSCIOUS MIND LIKE A COMPUTER?

Subconscious mind can do wonderful things, but it is not self-operating. Likewise a computer can do wonderful things, but it is not self-operating. Both require an outside operator to properly program it. This programming can be from the conscious mind itself, or from an outside operator, such as a hypnotist, via self or hetero-hypnosis.

Question No. 113 ...
WHAT IS A SUGGESTION FORMULA?

In relation to the thought of mind/brain functioning like a computer, a suggestion-formula could be regarded as the programming of one's mental computer. A suggestion-formula presents to the mind a positive affirmation that what is wanted to occur has already occurred.

When use in conjunction with hypnosis it becomes an effective way to modify behavior. Through the use of suggestion-formulas mind can be motivated to use mind to control mind. Suggestive Therapeutics was the old name for "Hypnotherapy".

Question No. 114 ...
HOW DOES OUR MENTAL COMPUTER OPERATE IN RELATION TO HYPNOTHERAPY?

What is amazing about hypnotherapy is that you do not have to know how it works to make it work. Such is very much the same in working a computer. Millions of people (even children in grade schools today) know how to operate a computer, but very few know the inner electronics, which make it work. All most know is simply that it works. Hypnotherapy is much like that. Hypnotherapy helps to reprogram our mental computer. Our mental computer represents our subconscious mind, and hypnotherapy is the key to open up or unlock our subconscious mind.

Question No. 115 ...
CAN SUBCONSCIOUS MIND THEN BE LOOKED UPON AS A SORT OF BIOCOMPUTER?

We look upon the matter in this way. The subconscious is the computer. The suggestions and formulas are the programs for the bio computer. The hypnotist is the operator of the reprogramming. We look at both of our minds as bio mental computers. They are a conscious bio mental computer and our subconscious bio mental computer.

Question No. 116 ...
HOW DO SUGGESTIONS INFLUENCE THE MIND?

Suggestions can influence the mind through any of the senses, however most commonly, in inducing and controlling the hypnotic state; the influence is through the sense of hearing. That is through the use of words. Words, and the meaning of certain words, have been conditioned into our mind through constant usage. Psychologically speaking, words can be regarded as triggers to action. As an example, you think of the word love, and you automatically get a responsive feeling of a warm and friendly nature. On the other hand, think of the word hate and just the reverse is aroused. Words are like that. Truly they are triggers to action. Words can activate emotions and emotions stimulate actions, which can be good or bad.

Question No. 117 ...
WHAT IS THE POWER OF SUGGESTION?

We will go into this subject more extensively in the coming pages but for now we should look at suggestion this way. The subconscious plays the role of supervisor over our body's physical processes.

This subconscious computer controls all of our vital organs. Automatic Operations such as digestion, assimilation, the circulation of the blood, heartbeat regulation, the action of the lungs, the kidneys are all governed by our subconscious or what you can call our Automatic Mind, because it automatically controls our entire nervous and internal systems.

The subconscious never sleeps. During sleep it seems to be more alert and active than it is during our waking hours. In the state of hypnosis suggestions become hypersensitive and hyperactive.

The two aspects of the mind, conscious and subconscious, are in perpetual interaction. If we consciously think a thought and cause it to be accepted by the subconscious, the idea will spontaneously go into action in producing the effect. If it is a healthful thought, we are so much better. If it is a diseased thought, we are so much the worse. For unlike our conscious mind, the subconscious has no selective power. Whatever is presented to it is accepted and automatically acted upon. It is in the process of the transformation of a thought into an element of our life that we make use of the power of suggestion. Since the phenomenon is a normal part of the mind's action, we can easily find evidence of its workings in our daily experiences. Think about all of the suggestions that you give yourself everyday.

Question No. 118 ...
CAN YOU TELL ME MORE ABOUT THE POWER OF SUGGESTION?

If we can get the subconscious to accept an idea, realization follows automatically. For any idea to enter the subconscious it must be charged with emotion. This is where so many of the thinking fads fall down. For it is not the thinking of ideas that is of paramount importance, but rather it is the emotional drive that is given to the idea being thought about.

For such reasons ideas that are directly associated to our personal experience are the ones most likely to carry the greatest suggestive influence. Ideas relating to health, pain, success, or a goal dear to our hearts all carry an emotional impact. The greater the operation of the power of suggestion, the more successful is the hypnotherapy.

The ready acceptance or rejection of an idea by the subconscious depends largely on the associations connected with it. Thus, an idea is most readily accepted when it ties in with similar emotionally charged ideas already seated within the mind. Suggestions all ideas that a person can relate to in their own life, will be more easily accepted. It is rejected when it is contrary to ideas previously established. This brings us to another operating law of the Power of Suggestion:

A suggestion is accepted when it is not countered by other suggestions already established in the mind. Such being the case, how is it possible to alter ideas already established in the subconscious?

On this point, consider the subconscious as a tide, which ebbs and flows. In sleep it seems to submerge consciousness altogether, while at moments of full wakefulness the tide is at its lowest. Between these two extremes is any number of intermediary levels. When we are drowsy, dreamy, lulled into a gentle reverie by music, etc., the subconscious tide is high.

While the more wakeful we become, the more it ebbs. This submergence of consciousness is referred to as the outcropping of the subconscious. This outcropping of the subconscious occurs in daily life most markedly in periods just before we fall to sleep and just after we wake up.

But it occurs to the greatest extent of all in the hypnotic state of mind, which has the advantage of being able to cause it to occur at any time when hypnosis is induced.

During these periods of the outcropping of the subconscious are the times in which to effectively implant suggestions, in relation to hypnotherapeutic benefits to the subject, such as in removing unwanted habits and establishing desired ones. During such periods, contrary associations do not seem to take place and established patterns in the mind lose their strength to resist change via the influx of new and desired suggestions.

The power of hypnotically inspired suggestions is such that in-rooted, unwanted ideas may be weeded out from the soil of mind and fresh ones planted, so that on the return to normal consciousness, a new plant of thought (behavior) will be growing in place of the old. For a suggestion to carry power it must be accepted by the subconscious, and no amount of willing on our part will bring about the desired results; for willing only makes the conscious aspects of mind more active and submerges deeper the subconscious. A person trying to use his will to implant ideas in his subconscious is attempting the impossible. A sick man tries consciously to think he is not sick, and he still remains sick. Indeed, often instead of feeling better he feels worse, for the ideas only serve to bring him to a fuller realization that he is sick. Consequently he finds himself contemplating the exact opposite of what he desires. He battles with his will to repress the aroused thoughts of illness but it seems the more he tries to repress them, the more the unwanted ideas possess him. Which brings us to the basic law in the operation of the power of suggestion like I have mentioned earlier in this book. It is worth mentioning this valuable information to you once again.

WHENEVER THE WILL IS IN CONFLICT WITH AN IDEA
THE IDEA INVARIABLY WINS THE STRUGGLE

Thus it will be recognized, willpower is incapable of mastering subconscious power for as fast as will brings up its big guns, thought captures them and turns them against itself.

This is known as the Law of Reverse Effort, viz.:

> When the imagination and the will are in conflict, the imagination invariably gains the day. The conflict between the will and the imagination is in direct ratio to the square of the will.

Thus, the will turns out to be not the commanding monarch of life, as many people would have it, but a blind Samson capable of either turning the mill or pulling down the pillars.

Using hypnosis, mastery between ideas and our will is obtained. Wrong thought can be replaced by right thoughts, not by resisting the unwanted thoughts but by overcoming (overpowering) the unwanted by the wanted. This in no way devalues willpower; it merely relegates it to its proper place. Will is under the direction of conscious mind and it must be used in accordance to its capacities, i.e., it can locate ideas that are unwanted, it can locate thoughts that are needed, it can direct the deliberate process that will result in the removal of the undesired and replace same with the desired, but always remember that the actual performance of the process takes place as a subconscious operation and not a conscious one. And hypnosis is the key to deliberately directing the subconscious.

Hypnosis provides our gardening tools for the successful cultivation of the fertile field of the subconscious to raise a full crop of living life, as we desire it to be.

CHAPTER NINE

HOW I CAN DEVELOP A PEACEFUL MIND
By: Ormond McGill

Question No. 119 ...
HOW CAN I DEVELOPE A PEACEFUL MIND?

Just changing your attitude about a few basic things can go a long ways to giving you a peaceful mind. Take this in ...

> THE MIND BECOMES PEACEFUL BY CULTIVATING ATTITUDES OF FRIENDLINESS TOWARDS THE HAPPY (SUCCESSFUL), COMPASSION TOWARDS THE MISERABLE, JOY TOWARDS THE VIRTUOUS, AND INDIFFERENCE TOWARDS EVIL.

We will explain a little how this applies to you in bringing about a peaceful mind, viz.:

On the surface, cultivating an attitude of friendliness towards a happy person seems easy, but it is not. Actually it is far easier to feel friendliness towards an unhappy person than towards a happy one. Why?
Because a happy person is a successful person, and the uncontrolled mind invariably feels jealous of the successfully happy person, as though, somehow, his success and his happiness should be yours, not his. However, if you would truly obtain a peaceful mind, you must change this attitude and commence feeling friendliness towards the happy. Now go on ...
The mind becomes peaceful by cultivating attitudes of compassion towards the miserable. To understand this, you must understand the difference between sympathy and compassion. Compassion is a totally different quality from sympathy. Compassion means you would like to help the other come out of his misery, but in so doing you do not allow his misery to become your misery. In other words, when a person is miserable around you, you would like to do whatever is possible to help him come out of his misery, but while you are not happy about his

misery, at the same time you are not miserable about it either.

<u>Just between the two exists compassion</u>. Out of compassion you can help the person, but your own SELF remains peaceful. Such is the dynamics of the operation of mind.

The mind becomes peaceful by being joyful towards the virtuous. Mind is very suspicious of virtue. When you find somebody who is virtuous, the ordinary attitude is to be suspicious of the virtue. Then much criticism goes on. For your own peace of mind, when you find somebody who expresses they are virtuous: promote it instead of discouraging it.

The mind becomes peaceful by cultivating attitudes of indifference towards evil. Evil is the negative side of good, and the mind tends to gravitate towards the negative for the negative is easier to accept than is the positive. Just remember that when you become negative to that which is good you are not harming that which is good, you are harming yourself. If you would have a peaceful mind be joyful towards the virtuous and indifferent towards the evil, which is an entire reversal of the attitudes of the average mind.

Using hypnosis these attitudes can be implanted (conditioned) as your new attitude for life. It will open a peaceful mind for you, and with a peaceful mind your life becomes filled with sunshine.

Question No. 120 ...
CAN HYPNOSIS BRING SUCCESS TO A PERSON'S LIFE?

Hypnosis can bring optimism into a person's life. Optimism is the first ingredient of success. Also, Creative Mind is a process of bringing abundance into the life of every person and hypnosis can motivate your Subconscious Creative Mind to create success. Turning imagination into reality.

Question No. 121 ...
IS HYPNOSIS SIMILAR TO BRAIN WASHING?

Brain Washing, so it has been called, was developed during the war years when psychological/physiological methods were used in spies to break them down to reveal military secrets. It is a <u>forced</u> process upon the individual often including the use of drags. Hypnosis is just the opposite. It is never forced upon the individual. The individual always uses it in complete acceptance.

Brain washing someone implies something forceful and against someone's will. Hypnosis works by a person's conscious desire to be hypnotized and not by force.

Question No. 122 ...
IS THERE A CONNECTION BETWEEN HYPNOTISM AND TELEPATHY?

Some people believe there is a definite connection between hypnotism and telepathy. I look upon it as the possibility of the influence of mind-upon-mind.

As you have learned, mind is a process for producing thoughts, and thoughts are forms of energy arranged in certain patterns. These patterns are known, as thought forms. The more effectively you learn how to use your mind, the more powerful the thought forms you can produce and powerful thought forms carry influence across space. This is telepathy. However, we are still waiting for the scientists to show us the concrete conclusion.

The brain acts like an electrical transformer in stepping up the current, while the nervous system provides the wires, which conveys the current throughout the body. To put it concisely, mind produces thoughts, which the body amplifies. The stronger the amplification the more powerful is the thoughts, which can influence others directly.

The operation is like the process of induction, in which two coils of wire are spaced apart. One coil is electrically charged with an impulse and it is transmitted through space to the other Coil. Each resonates to the same frequency (call it tune), as it were.

Some have called this transmission of thought from one person to another thought projection. Our current understanding of how our brain function is something like this. Our brain functions by electro-chemical reactions between neurons. Therefore, if there is a strong magnetic or electrical field influence on our brain, this will throw our normal signal passages out of whack, say if a visual signal is received by the olfactory (smell) nerve, it won't be able to understand the visual signal, and may interpret it as ghost signal. This is the case when people see the ghost. As whether our brains can transmit (broadcast) very low frequency brainwave to the space, we don't know because we don't have a way to measure it yet. We certainly can measure brainwave thru contacting electrodes, but not as a radio receiving radio wave yet.

CHAPTER TEN

QUESTIONS ABOUT SELF HYPNOSIS

Question No. 123 ...
CAN A PERSON LEARN HOW TO HYPNOTIZE THEMSELVES?

Absolutely. In fact, learning how to hypnotize yourself is one of the most important skills the hypnotherapist can develop. In mastering Self Hypnosis you can learn how to disassociate one part of your mind, which is the conscious presenting the desired suggestions, while the other part of the mind your subconscious, becomes subjective and receptive to responding to the suggestions self-presented. You will be given detailed instruction of how to hypnotize yourself in a latter section of this manual.

To use an analogy, the subconscious aspect of your mind possesses the power like the atomic bomb in it is the energy to destroy us or to build a better life. Self-hypnosis is the means of controlling and directing that energy in a positive way.

The technique of self-hypnosis that we are going to give you has within it all the laws of suggestion and hypnosis you have previously asked about. All are artfully combined allowing you to harness the atom-like power within your subconscious.

Question No. 124 ...
WHAT IS THE DIFFERENCE BETWEEN HETERO-HYPNOSIS AND SELF-HYPNOSIS?

Hetero-hypnosis involves two persons working together. The operator taking the objective role while the subject plays the subjective role. It is the most frequently employed way of being hypnotized, as all the subject has to do is become passive and allow the suggestions from the operator to take effect. Self-hypnosis involves you becoming both the operator and subject at one and the same time inside yourself.

One part of your mind remains objective (more or less) throughout the process, while another part of your mind becomes subjective. Both hetero-hypnosis and self-hypnosis are important to the art/science of hypnotism.

Question No. 125 ...
WHAT IS THE DIFFERENCE BETWEEN AUTOSUGGESTION AND SELF-HYPNOSIS?

Both are related states of mind. However autosuggestions is employed mainly during awake states of awareness, while self-hypnosis aims for deeper levels of hypnosis.

The term, AUTOSUGGESTION was coined by the French hypnotherapist, the late Emile Coue'. This innovative operator showed the way to use suggestions in personal benefit during all periods of one's life. He had his clients repeat out loud or to themselves each morning upon awakening and each night before falling asleep this special formula:

EVERY DAY AND IN EVERY WAY
I AM GETTING BETTER AND BETTER

That generalized auto suggestion-formula pretty well covers everything. The suggestion. IN EVERY WAY was the key to its success, and many people throughout the world who used that formula were helped in everyway. Think of Autosuggestion as a conscious waking affirmation and suggestion.

Question No. 126 ...
IS THERE A GOOD METHOD OF HYPNOTIZING WITHOUT MENTIONING SLEEP?

Yes there is. We will devote an entire chapter to this technique as not only is it an excellent method of hypnotizing, but also provides an opportunity for us to give you a consideration of some basic principles that we have found important to successful hypnotic induction. You should have this knowledge. Even the progressive relaxation induction can put a person into deep hypnosis without using the word sleep and simply using the words relax, relaxed and relaxation.

If you are creative, you can think of lots of inductions methods and suggestions that you can use instead of using the work sleep.

CHAPTER ELEVEN

THE FIVE-MAIN FUNCTION OF MIND

Question No. 127 ...
FROM WHAT CENTERS DOES MIND FUNCTION?

There are five main functions of mind, which you can use to either your advantage or disadvantage. Learn these for yourself so you can instruct others likewise.

The five main functions of mind are right knowledge wrong knowledge, imagination, sleep, and memory

The value of mind depends upon how it is used. Mind is there in everyone, and it is neither your enemy nor your friend. You can make it a friend or you can make it an enemy, it is up to you. "YOU" who stands behind the mind. If you can master your mind and use it as the superlative instrument it is designed to be, it can become the means through which you can accomplish great achievements. That is what you must teach your subjects.

As you have learned, mind is an instrument for thinking, but many have lost control of it. It is running wild, as it were. For example, you want to sleep, but your mind remains restless. You say Stop to your mind, but your mind continues right on. It seems not to listen to you, and you can't seem to do anything about it.

Why?

Because you have allowed your mind to direct you rather, than you directing it, your mind may not be working properly. Think of the predicament you would be in if your hands and feet behaved like that. And mind is far more powerful than your hands and feet can ever be. You must learn to use your mind just like you use your hands and feet. You have perfect control over them, and they work for you, rather than against you. You must get your mind under similar control.

The five main functions of mental activity, right knowledge, wrong knowledge, imagination, sleep, and memory all act upon and interrelate to each other. We will consider each of these functions in turn.

The first main function of mind, right knowledge, is an innate capacity to intuitively know what is right (what is true) when it is used correctly. It is a searchlight of truth, and wherever it is focused becomes immediately clear to you. It is a most remarkable mental faculty. When you know how to use it, right knowledge will be instinctively revealed. Conversely, without knowing how to use this faculty you will often be wrong, or at best have a 50% chance of being right.

The second main function of mind is wrong knowledge. It is a faculty to be aware of and avoid, as it can accept what is untrue as being true. When the mind's faculty of wrong knowledge is functioning, then whatever you choose will be the wrong choice; whatever you decide will be the wrong decision. Further, when you are focusing in the wrong, the mind tends to find wrong everything. This is the basis of pessimism. Also, of course, there are minds, which are in between, and such minds are sometimes right and sometimes wrong, such is the status of the average man.

As you work with your clients, you will note many who are suffering from using this faculty of wrong knowledge rather than right knowledge. You will find that directing such clients towards using their faculty of right knowledge instead will prove an excellent psychotherapy.

The third main function of mind is imagination. Imagination is the creative function of the mind. It is very powerful. All that is beautiful originates in the imagination including art, music, dance, inventiveness, breakthroughs in science, etc. But, likewise, everything that is ugly comes equally through the imagination. If imagination is used in the wrong way, it can be very harmful to you and/or your clients.

Imagination is a form of visualizing pictures in the mind, which mental-pictures, are caused to become transformed from the unreal to the real. Some say that when mind energizes these imagined images form a kind of matrix in space, which starts a process of direct creation. At all events, imagination must be recognized as a great mental power, and one must be careful to use it correctly.

The fourth main function of mind is sleep. Much research has gone into the study of sleep and it appears to occur in various stages. In the lighter stage (Rem) dreams occur. In the deeper stages brain activity slows down and opportunity is afforded for bodily rejuvenation.

Sleep is beautiful and life giving, and if you know how to use sleep fully, it can become a source of inspiration.

In this kind of sleep your consciousness remains awake while you sleep. The body falls asleep, but the <u>witnessing consciousness</u> remains. Many a solution to an innovative creation has been born in the mind during this kind of sleep.

<u>Memory</u> is the fifth main function of the mind. Memory can be used either correctly or incorrectly. If memory is misused, it creates confusion. Actually, memory is not completely reliable. You can add many things to it. Imagination may enter into it. You may delete many things from it, and all manner of assorted things may be done to it. When you say, this is what I remember, you may be assured that much of what you conjure up from out of the past is not real at all. It operates in this manner:

Memory is distorted, as instead of allowing it to be based upon true experiences, it is possible to drop many things from it. Mostly one drops that which is disagreeable and hangs on to that which is agreeable. This is a major cause for inaccurate memory.

To achieve accurate memory, you must be totally honest with yourself. Only then can memory be right. The secret for achieving right memory is to accept whatever has happened, be it good or bad, and don't change it. <u>Know it as it is</u>! If you correctly remember your past, then there comes in no urge to repeat it in the present, and the memories of the past but help you live the present better. This is why processes such as hypnoanalysis and previous-life regression psychotherapy are of value, for they compel the mind to bring in right memories. In other words, when memories are faced squarely they can be dropped. Buried memories can be a source of much disturbance; when they are surfaced via hypnosis.

Question No. 128 ...
HOW ABOUT MORE ON THE FUNCTION OF MIND?

In relation to hypnotherapy, the importance of the five main functions of mind merit further study.

1   <u>Right Knowledge</u>

Right knowledge is a direct perception of what is true. It is one of mind's most important functions. It means that mind is capable of a direct perception of what IS, without any in between agents. Not even the senses are used, as the senses can report inaccurately. All senses (sight, hearing, feeling, taste and smell) are mediators for conveying information to the mind, but you must be questioning of the accuracy of what they convey.

Direct perception is the mind a function for directly perceiving truth. In other words, mind has the ability to automatically knee what is right. In this mental phenomenon, you (as the knower) and the information (as the known) meet directly. In this intimacy of perception, truth is directly conveyed to the mind. Right knowledge arises out of your Inner Self.

2   Wrong Knowledge

We contribute greatly to mind's faculty of wrong knowledge because we carry within us many prejudices. Prejudices think for us before we even start thinking. They come in and interfere with one's instinctive knowing of what is right. To counteract this and aid in acquiring right knowledge, you must put aside your prejudices. And this has to be done continuously, as ever-repressed prejudices arise anew unless they are kept under watch. Only in so doing will you be freed from wrong knowledge.

3   Imagination

In relation to imagination, be cautious of words, as imagination can operate just through words. Through speech and the written word can be created things which seem to be, but are not there as a reality. Words can produce a mental image so powerful as to deceive even yourself. Words can so stimulate imagination that you come to believe what is not so as being so.

Hypnosis proves this.

If you hypnotize a person and suggest the appearance of a hallucination, that image appears, within the subjects mind, being real. And mind can be hypnotized in so many ways while living in the world.

Hypnosis is an excellent way to train the mind when what is presented is what is wanted; but, conversely, the hypnosis must be cleared away when what is presented is not what is wanted. Likewise, you must learn to separate fact from fancy.

Every hypnotist knows the power of words. But we use them so continuously that we often forget their power. In truth, words are triggers to action. That is, we have become conditioned to respond to words, frequently without even considering why we are responding. It has been truthfully said that that the right word, spoken at the right time, can change the world.

Hitler almost did it.

Imagination has to be understood, because it is very susceptible to being influenced by the words of others. Remember that others teach words, and through words many prejudices are born. Through words false beliefs, untruths, everything can be stimulated via the imagination. One must be very cautious of words, for it is not uncommon for them to lead you to wrong knowledge rather than to right knowledge.

4 Sleep

In deep sleep you are largely freed of awareness; or, it can be said that you are largely unconscious. That is the way of the ordinary mind. But, for the exceptional mind deep sleep provides a very special state in which you sleep with awareness. <u>Sleeping with awareness is one of the great goals of mental achievement.</u>

To become aware while you sleep, you have to learn to be more aware while you are awake. And then try to be aware while you are dreaming. When you manage to do that, you are on your way. Only if you succeed with the waking state and then with the dreaming state of mind will you be able to succeed in the deep sleep state. Experiment with learning this control of the mind.

First, try to be aware while walking on the street. Don't just go on walking automatically. Be alert to every movement your legs make in walking: the muscles rippling under the surface skin of the legs, the feel of your feet upon the ground. Let your walking become a conscious experience. Next, while you are eating, become aware of the taste of the food in your mouth, the feeling of the chewing, and the way you swallow. Do the same with drinking.

Next, take your conscious awareness to your breathing, and become aware of the breath going into and out of your lungs.

Next, become aware of whatever you are doing, whatever you are hearing, whatever you are seeing. Whatever you are experiencing, become alert to the experiencing.

The practice is to make you more aware while you are awake.

Then, in the night, while you are falling asleep, try to remain aware. Various thoughts of the day will be passing through your mind. Watch these. Remain alert and try to fall asleep with awareness. It is not easy because of old mental habits you have in relation to falling asleep, but if you persist the time will come when you will be asleep and aware simultaneously.

When you can do this, the experience is a transition into higher realms of consciousness. It is a very precious moment to become aware of when the waking state goes and the sleeping state comes to the mind. In that neutral moment, just between waking and sleeping, old habits of the mind drop away, and you soar upward in consciousness. In that moment, one becomes aware of their true nature.

There are two of these in between moments that happen continuously; one in the night when you go from the waking state of mind to the sleeping state of mind, and another in the morning when you go from sleeping to waking. In these moments, if you can become <u>aware</u>, your whole life will change, and you will have laid the foundation for discovering your SELF.

Having mastered the foregoing, then add this technique to your practice of sleeping awareness:

Just before falling asleep visualize something you love in your mind. For example, visualize the image of your sweetheart. See your beloved vividly in your mind, and just as you are falling asleep go on thinking that in your dreams, also your sweetheart will be there. Visualize the image completely; see your sweetheart in every aspect of being. Make it a vivid experience in your mind, and with that fall asleep.

After performing this technique for a few nights, you will find that you will be able to bring the image of your sweetheart into your dreams every time you sleep.

This is a great success because you have deliberately created at least a part of your dream. You have started on your way toward the mastery of your mind, while it is in the sleep state. And the moment you see the image of your sweetheart in your dream, you will simultaneously remember that it is a dream – even while you are asleep.

There is no need to do anything else because the image and the awareness that this is a dream become associated, and when that happens the whole quality of the dream will change. You have become alert in sleep, and you have mastered the secret of dream creation. And through deliberate dream creation you can totally change the structure of your mind. And when you succeed in dreams (dreaming is a partial sleeping state of mind), then you can succeed in complete sleep, because through dream creation you will learn to be aware, and awareness can be carried on into sleep.

It is a compounding process, which once started, will sweep you on toward mastery of mind.

In relation to hypnotherapy, that is why suggestions of sleep are important to use, as profound hypnosis is a state of mind related to sleeping with awareness, which automatically brings in control of ones mind. This is one of the great secrets for successful hypnotherapy in helping your clients.

5 Memory

Memory is the recalling of experiences from out of the past. Learn to use it without distortion. This rule is easy to understand and appreciate because memory is continuously operating. Whatever happens to you becomes instantly stored in your memory. Just recognize that memory can distort the truth of happenings in various ways. That distortion can be either good or bad, as the case may be. But it is distortion, and you should not allow distortion, for distortion is not truth.

Becoming aware of this distortion is the way to remove the distortion; and, as you gain mastery over your memories, you will gain a skill of being able to drop your memories whenever you please.

Dropping memories does not mean that you will cease to remember. Dropping memories simply means that you will be able to drop their constant interference and/or intrusion into your life. When you need the memories you will be able to bring them back into focus; but, when you do not need the memories you will be able to just let them be there silently, rather than having them coming continuously into your mind unbidden.

Disturbing memories, buried in the subconscious, can be a cause for discomfort in your present-day behavior. That is the value of regression hypnotherapy which surfaces buried memories, so you can face them squarely. When they are faced squarely, without distortion, amazingly their power over you disappears.

The disturbance they cause often vanishes on the instant. If memory is right it can free you from past influences even influences from past lives. Then one desire will grow within you: to transcend all the nonsense that belonged to the past. But far too many think the past was wonderful and that the future is going to be terrific, and only the present is mundane, If you live like that, you can never really live fully at all. The truth is that only the present is real. There is actually only one way to live, and that is to:

APPRECIATE YOUR LIFE THAT YOU ARE LIVING IN THE HERE AND NOW!

NOTE: When you can hypnotize your subject and/or client so they can use these faculties correctly, you advance from being a hypnotist to being a great hypnotist.

CHAPTER TWELVE

THE MASTERY OF DESIRES
By Ormond McGill

Question No. 129 ...
HOW DO I BECOME MASTER OF MY DESIRES AND STILL HAVE DESIRES?

Frustrated desires are a cause for much mental disturbance. The hypnotist can greatly help his subjects by assisting them to master their desires rather than being mastered by them. To do this the best way is to obtain a peaceful state of mind that is freed from desires. Constant desiring makes the mind restless and unhappy. Desirelessness on the other hand, makes the mind happy and contented.

The first step is to follow this rule:

<u>Drop, desires from mind and end the constant search to find happiness by indulging jn sensuous pleasures in the world.</u>

To do this takes a recognition that one's real source of happiness is to be found inside oneself rather than outside oneself.

The second step is to follow this rule:

<u>Having recognized where your real source of happiness is coming from, discover therein your SELF. It is then that you will find the real happiness that is your true nature.</u>

There is nothing moralistic about these rules. They offer no criticism of behavior in seeking pleasure. There purpose is to point the mind in the right direction to find ones source of real happiness.

Your real source of happiness emanates from your Inner Self. This recognition comes through achieving desirelessness, as it is then that you come to recognize your true nature.

<u>When you recognize your true nature you discover real happiness because real happiness is your true nature.</u>

Desires place demands upon the individual that call for satisfying. And so one satisfies the desires, often with self-indulgent or sensuous pleasures. Then one seems satisfied, but not for long. Very soon the desires arise again and demand even greater quantities of satisfaction. And so the process goes on and on. It is a vicious circle.

The reason desires constantly plague one is because desires are old habits set in the mind. A mental set is much like a program set in a computer and once it is started it plays on its own. Desires are like that; they play on their own. In other words, they are involuntary acts (habits of behavior), and in order to drop them they have to be <u>reconditioned</u> into voluntary acts, and then you can deal with them.

The trouble with habits is that they command you rather than you commanding them. Desires are habits of behavior that bring you satisfaction, in one-way or another. There trouble is not the satisfaction they bring you, but is in the fact that they distort your perception of where your real source of happiness is.

To correct your direction towards the happiness of your true nature, follow these five points for mastering desires:

Point One:

Consciously think in terms of your mind becoming master of your desires rather than adhering unconsciously to old habits and desires.

Point Two:

Appreciate that nothing is against you for enjoying life to the fullest in the world in anyway you wish. Just appreciate that your real source of happiness is far deeper than is the superficial happiness found in satisfying worldly desires.

Point Three:

Appreciate that you will be far happier when your mind is free of desires than it is when it is cluttered up with ideas to try to figure out how to satisfy desires.

Point Four:

Appreciate that your real source of happiness is to be found in your inner world (inside yourself) rather than in the outer world (outside yourself).

Point Five:

Discover your SELF, which dwells within your inner world. When you do this, you discover your true nature, which is so complete in itself that you have nothing further to desire. You have all already.
Thus desirelessness comes.

It is easy to understand these steps, which lead you to desirelessness, but it takes conscious effort to take them. Old habits resist changing. But change them you must, if you would discover your true nature. And the use of hypnosis is one of the most effective ways to change old habits.

So,,,

Let's study your nature, as then you will know what you must do to change your direction of searching for happiness outside yourself rather than inside yourself.

The effort for mastering desires is not a struggle against your right nature, it is a struggle against your wrong nature, as it were. And the effort to master desires must be made as an effort without effort. That is why hypnosis is so effective as a psychotherapy. As you simply relax and drop off into a reverie state the hypnotherapy suggestions change your mind.

Understand ...

You are not fighting yourself; you are fighting desires, which your undisciplined mind has conjured up as being your nature. If this is not understood, then your whole effort is valueless. Once your start fighting yourself, you are fighting a losing battle.

Who is going to win and who will lose? You are both sides. There is no great division between your so-called lower self and your higher self. The truth is there is nothing lower or higher about your-self.

You are both; there is no need to divide yourself.

Understand ...

The fight is not against your nature; the fight is for your nature. The fact is that you have accumulated many non-purposeful habits of behavior during the course of life, and because of these your true nature cannot move spontaneous. These habits have to be destroyed, but they are only habits. They may seem like your nature because you are addicted to them, but the truth is they are not you.

This distinction has to be clearly understood otherwise you can misinterpret these instructions for achieving desirelessness. The basic purpose for mastering desires is so that whatever has come into you from without that does not truly bring you real happiness can be put under control, so that that which is within you that can truly bring you happiness can flow.

Also, the concept of desirelessness can possibly lead you in the wrong direction unless you carefully understand the finesse of the meaning. You must remember that these rules are not laws they are simply directions. This means that they are not to be followed like an obsession; they are simply to be understood so their meaning can take on significance. Then, that significance has to be carried into your life, both physically and mentally, if you would achieve mastery over your desires; which is really mastery over yourself.

Desirelessness is a direction. If you pursue it as an obsession then you start killing all desires. On the surface, it seems a logical way to go about mastering desires. True, then you will be without desires, but you will also be lifeless. You will be committing inner suicide because desires are not only desires – they are the flow of life energy.

Desirelessness is to be achieved with more life, not less life. Unless you can appreciate the significance of the methods rather than the performance of the methods, they could well lead one into deeper confusion than one already is. Wrongly used they can suppress your life. Rightly used they can give you boundless life.

When you are filled with overflowing energy, your overflowing energy can lead you into many desires. However, since desires are basically but outlets for energy, two ways are available to handle them:

One is to drop your desires while allowing the energy to remain, and the other is to drop the level of your energy to cause the desires to disperse. This instruction is for the former and against the latter.

In doing this, you achieve a state of mind in which you master your desires, and yet you are still filled with energy. Just follow this rule:

Don't destroy energy destroy desires

Understand ...

Use conscious effort to drop desires from your mind and cease your endless search to find happiness from pleasures in the world by recognizing that real happiness comes to you from inside yourself rather than from outside yourself. Recognize that happiness outside can only be as a mirror reflecting your inner happiness, to the degree to which you have recognized your happiness to be. Or you might say, you have narrowed your happiness potential in not fully recognizing the tremendous potential for happiness, which you possess inside yourself. To become aware of that potential fully is the value of obtaining desirelessness.

To obtain true happiness, conscious effort is needed, so whenever you feel that a moment of pleasure is at hand and you become a witness to the situation.

To help you do this, close your eyes and look within, and see from where the pleasure is really coming. Then you will see the truth about the pleasure, and your perception will be accurate. This moment is precious to your training in mastering your mind.

This moment is precious as it can cause a quantum leap in your awareness (consciousness), and then you will know the truth about your real source of happiness, which is your true nature. In this you discover your SELF, and then you will automatically stop searching for outside pleasures. Then all the frustration you felt in searching for desires that were not fulfilled, will wither away on their own, and then you will give the desires no further attention.

You have the basis for wonderful hypnotherapy here in helping your clients overcome their desires (old habits): desire for smoking, desire for over eating; desires for non-helpful things of every kind. Learn the method first for yourself and apply it to your own life.

CHAPTER THIRTEEN

ADVANCING TO Optima CONSCIOUSNESS
By Ormond McGill

Question No. 130 ...
HOW DO I MAKE THE QUANTUM LEAP FROM SELF CONSCIOUSNESS TO Optima CONSCIOUSNESS?

To advance man in the direction of optima consciousness is to make him master of his mind. Through mind, consciousness is known. When man becomes master of his mind, he will know his true nature, which is in harmony with all that IS. It is KNOWING.

The hypnotherapist can bring about this state of mind in his clients by advancing consciousness, and he can do it best when he attains to this advanced degree of consciousness for himself. For this purpose, we will consider some details about optima consciousness.

Optima consciousness is like a bright light, which reveals the truth of everything upon which it is turned. The moment you begin to recognize your SELF – your true nature – you begin to advance your consciousness from self-conscious to optima consciousness. This recognition can begin as an intellectual realization, but it must become completed as an <u>experiencing</u> from deep inside your-self. When this happens, your consciousness advances in a great quantum leap, and you realize the immortal being you truly and are directly linked with the TOTALITY of all that is.

The experiencing of optima consciousness, when it first bursts upon one, seems to manifest in different ways. Some report a sort of bombshell effect, in which everything about them seems to be illuminated with a bright light and/or sparkling colors. Others say it seems like a delightful swimming sensation, as though they had dropped into a warm pool of utter contentment. Others say it seem that somehow they seem to know whatever everything is all about, and that things are right in the universal scheme of things, in harmony with each other. This form of consciousness (awareness) is wonderful to experience.

To obtain optima consciousness one must advance from learning to KNOWING. Making use of the following four processes of mind will advance the stature of mind to realization of optima consciousness.

ONE
Using mind for reasoning, optimism, reflection, and clarity of thought allows optima consciousness to come into the individual.

TWO
Allowing mind to cease being a clutter of thoughts and become silent, while waiting an outside input of knowing, allows optima consciousness to come into the individual. And this <u>knowing</u> can be very personal as an intuitive recognition of one's true nature.

THREE
In attaining to optima consciousness, a person comes to recognize their immortality; they cease to so closely identify themselves with the body they inhabit in the current lifetime, and even with their bodies in previous lifetimes. The realization dawns that they are a consciousness, which exists entirely independent of the body, and that consciousness is not bounded by the 3-dimensional space of the physical world.

FOUR
Some attain optima consciousness through faith, effort, recollection, concentration, and discrimination.

Understand these ...

Mind is a process through which optima consciousness is formed into thoughts, which may be expressed, when mind is advanced to that degree. For such <u>direct perception</u> to enter mind, mind has to be cleared of the many things that cause it to perform with imperfection.

For this purpose, these superior ways of using mind are suggested, to aid you to <u>condition</u> mind for optima consciousness attunement. As a hypnotherapist, you know that mind in body functions mainly on two levels which conscious and subconscious. Both of these levels have to be clarified and made receptive to optima consciousness input.

Start with conscious mind ...

Reasoning, reflection, optimism, and clarity of thought are all conscious mind activities. Set your sights high to improve these mental processes. When reasoning, reason with your mind in a positive manner rather than in a negative way.

Positive reasoning unclutters the mind from disturbances, and then you can really commence to think. Be an optimist because an optimist accepts life with a positive attitude rather than a negative one. The fact is that an attitude can create heaven or hell out of whatever occurs in life. Optimism directs attitude, and attitude directs thoughts.

If you allow thoughts just to continue without being controlled, you can become possessed by them rather than being the master of them. Only when you move in the direction of positive reasoning can you really become capable of thinking. Thinking is a capacity; thoughts are not.

<u>Thinking, you have to learn for yourself</u>.

Thinking is a quality of your inner being. A really thinking man uses his consciousness each time there is a problem he wishes to think about. He encounters the problem, and then there arises within him a thought, which is not part of memory.

If you ask a question, which is <u>new</u> to a man of memory (such as someone who has learned much from the thoughts of others), he will be at a loss to answer it. Only when you ask a question to which he has been told the answer will he be able to answer it. This is the difference between a university graduate and a sage. The former repeats what he has learned, while the sage uses his consciousness to bring in the answer. This latter is the meaning of wisdom, and is directly related to optima consciousness.

Next is the matter of reflection. Positive reasoning leads to reflection, and reflection brings you closer to optima consciousness. Reflection provides you with a glimpse of truth; it is only a glimpse, it will come and go, but for a moment the mind is flooded with insight. This glimpse of truth is important, as through it you come to recognize your possibilities. It shows that you are heading in the right direction. Reflection on the experience produces a state of pure thought. You are on your way to attaining optima consciousness.

Next is the matter of the mind becoming silent. This will happen to you automatically when you clear your mind of a ceaseless barrage of thoughts, which are not under your control.

A mind that is silent is a mind that is receptive to optima consciousness. <u>The experience is like being aware of awareness</u>.

You will find a great difference in the way you think, as it will seem as though you no longer have to try to think.

Thinking occurs on its own. That is the beginning of KNOWING, and, in this stage, much of that knowing will be personal and involved in recognition of your true nature.

As you come to recognize your true nature, you will find yourself thinking more and more about your immortality, and how little your body actually has to do with the real nature of yourself in this current lifetime in which you exist; and, also, in relation to the universe, and feel the smallness and insignificant of oneself, which is the prime thrust for one to live his/her life to the fullest.

The concept that you have lived life after life is that of reincarnation. Some people believe in it and some do not. Belief or non-belief is irrelevant. The key point is that memories of past are allowed to flow up from your subconscious you will know, and KNOWING is truth.

This recalling of past is important to your cleansing of your mind, for memories of many things that in the past have been disagreeable become buried in the subconscious, and often unbidden spring forth to disturb the enjoyment of one's present.

The technique of recalling past memories is to use hypnosis to direct the subconscious to probe its memory banks. The mind is just allowed to drift and form whatever pictures that come in to unfold. Such are just <u>witnessed</u> as adventures flowing out of the subconscious. The value of this psychotherapy lies in the removing of repressions.

Repressions cause tensions within the mind, and make a noisy mind. When the repressions are released the mind become more and more silent In this technique, both conscious and subconscious phase of mind becomes silent, and a silent mind is open to optima consciousness.

The skill of the hypnotherapist comes into play in the way the adventures are probed out of the client's subconscious guided by the hypnotherapist. When memories are released that are right on target, remarkable cures and healing can be affected.

The use of faith, effort, recollection, concentration, and discrimination are additional means for attaining optima consciousness. Consider these each in turn:

FAITH

Usually faith is something others hand you and insist that you accept. That kind of faith has no value in relation to expanding your consciousness, as it constricts rather than expands you. The kind of faith that is created for yourself, actually it is faith in yourself.

It is your own creation, and you grow into it. Optima Consciousness brings in that kind of faith in accepting all that "You" are and all that "YOU" exist in, as being "YOU".

EFFORT

Effort, in relation to optima consciousness (advancing consciousness) means energy. It is bio-energy. It is your total energy phenomena of BEING. Without energy consciousness is not and your very SELF is based in energy. The entire universe is an energy phenomenon, and you are part of "IT".

RECOLLECTION

In relation to optima consciousness, recollection means self-rememberence. Many people remember many things, but they go on continuously forgetting themselves. Self-remembrance is important to the advancement of your consciousness, so here is a technique you can use for that purpose:

Whatever you do, remember deep down inside yourself that I am doing the doing. As an example, you are walking. While walking, remember deep down It is I who am walking. From your center of being witness the walking. Do not just repeat it in your mind; such means nothing, such mental verbalizing is not remembrance. What is needed is to become aware that I am walking. I am eating. I am talking. I am listening.

While doing whatever you do, the "I" inside yourself should always be remembered. This is not self-consciousness. It is consciousness of SELF.

The process is not as easy to master as it sounds, because it is easy to remember the object (what is being done) and forget your SELF (which is doing the doing). The opposite is, also, not too easy: in which you remember yourself and forget the object. But even that will not do. In this process, you must associate the two together, which is the object and the doer. It is then that you begin to have self-remembrance.

Self-remembrance should become so much a part of yourself that it becomes your way of looking at life, and relating yourself to life. For the start, even if you succeed in attaining this dual perception of your SELF doing only for a single moment, you will have had a flash of Optima Consciousness. This is a start towards complete awareness.

CONCENTRATION

Optima consciousness is advanced awareness, and once this quality of awareness comes, you become concentrated in it. That to which we most turn our attention (concentrate upon) is the way in which we develop; and, the development grows continuously within ourselves. It becomes a 24-hour experiencing, and once started it never stops and it becomes a concentrated experiencing of the universe in which you exist, and your relationship to it.

DISCRIMINATION

In relation to optima consciousness, you develop a very special kind of recognition in discriminating your true nature. It is a KNOWING awareness of your SELF.

The hypnotherapist can use Power Hypnosis to implant these principles for advancing consciousness into the subconscious mind of his or her clients. The subconscious is completely programmed for optima conscious experiencing. It merely has to be motivated in that direction. The subconscious then goes into action to make such the way of life for the client and even for yourself.

CHAPTER FOURTEEN

HYPNOTISM, WILL POWER, AND YOU

Now that you know some of the most asked questions about hypnotism, let's consider how learning "How To Hypnotize" can contribute to success in daily life. Let's consider its personal value to yourself. There is no better way of learning anything than by personal application.

In recognizing that hypnotism is induced through communication between people on both physiological and psychological levels by induced suggestions or commands from one person to another, while full attention is given to the process in which acceptance of the suggestions is emphasized, it becomes obvious that similar results in varying degrees can be produced in everyday communication. Indeed, it has been our finding that it is not necessary to induce trance (sleep-like and/or somnambulistic state) in a subject in order to produce hypnotic phenomena With proper procedures it will be found that persons can be hypnotized in the waking state while fully conscious of what they are doing yet still be unable to resist the established influence. This is illustrated by the popular " Hand Locking Test", which Coue' sometimes used in his clinic when working with patients, in which the subject's hands are fastened together so firmly by suggestion that he cannot release them from each other until the hypnotist gives the command that they will come apart when the suggestion is given for them to separate. Full directions for performing this "Hand Locking Test" will be given in a subsequent chapter.

To produce effective experiments in waking hypnosis, the operator must know how to positively direct the suggestions. The basic secret is this. The hypnotherapist knows how to influence the subjective (subconscious) mind of the person while the latter does not know how to resist it and as a consequence obeys the commands even when such are contrary to his conscious judgment.

Hypnotizing is not a question of a weak mind verses a strong mind. It is not a question of willpower. Becoming an expert hypnotist comes from learning how to effectively influence subconscious mind activity while bypassing conscious mind non-acceptance. Willpower comes solely as the directive aim of the hypnotist. Directive aim of the mind to accomplish anything in life is the key to success. In such regard, learning the art of hypnotizing is a key factor to success in accomplishing whatever you will yourself to accomplish. In relation to hypnosis, such can almost be likened to a direct telepathic influence of mind upon mind, while the verbalized suggestions affirm the inner mental purpose of the hypnotist is to effectively influence the subject. In a nutshell, effective hypnotizing of others comes via the hypnotist knowing with positive assurance that what the hypnotist suggests will be performed or carried out by the subject.

Learning how to hypnotize automatically increases one's willpower, and willpower properly directed will cause things to come one's way with half the difficulty compared to one who does not use this remarkable mental gift.

For example, some people do things by the sheer force of will. Two merchants started in the same line of business on opposite sides of the street at the same time. Each had an equal chance to do business. Within a few years, one of them had prospered tremendously and had to build a larger store to accommodate his business. The other was still in the same little store doing about the same amount of business as when he first started. Why? The prosperous merchant had used his will to succeed, while the less successful merchant was too lazy to use his will. The successful merchant used the power within himself to attract new customers and continued to keep them. He was always alert and his mind is constantly working and influencing people to buy from him. Learning the art of hypnotism trains you in that skill.

To succeed, you will have to shake off that lazy feeling of "I wish that I could" and transform it to "I know that I can". The will can be trained by mental exercise, the same as the body can be trained by physical exercise. The development of your willpower is part of the training you will gain from this "How-To" Training Manual. Following the lessons will develop a wonderful power within you. Indeed, it may even seem like you are awakening from a long sleep. You will find yourself a changed individual at the end of this training. Every person has the same power of potential within him or her. All that is needed is to learn how to cultivate and use it.

Some people naturally have a magnetic personality and use that power to influence others unconsciously. It is a talent. However, it is something everyone can learn to do by training the mind in that hypnotic direction. Just follow the instructions as they are given to you in this book and you will acquire the power. It is a power beyond your wildest dreams. It will brace you up. You will walk erect. Your eyes will clear and you will look everyone head on. All shyness will vanish like a drop of water on a hot tin roof. In place of fear you will have confidence. With a mind that is positive instead of negative, you will radiate a force that is practically irresistible to the people with whom you come in contact with. This is the power you will develop, as you become a hypnotist.

Of course, do not expect to influence everybody because there are some people whose magnetism is antagonistic to you, but you will be able to influence a full seventy-five percent of those you try to hypnotize. You can hardly call that percentage bad. Learning how to hypnotize is like everything else in life. Persevere. If at first you don't succeed – try, try again – and it is guaranteed you will. Hypnotizing your first subject is the first hurdle you must pass. Once you have had your first success, you will advance by leaps and bounds.

Have confidence in yourself. Learn your lessons well. Practice what you learn. Persevere and as surely as the sun comes up each morning you will succeed. You will become a hypnotist.

As you learn the art and science of hypnotherapy and hypnotizing others it will make you a master of yourself because you will know how your mind works and how to operate it.

CHAPTER FIFTEEN

MOVING ON TO HYPNOTHERAPY AND VARIOUS EVERYDAY APPLICATIONS OF HYPNOTIC SUGGESTIONS

SUGGESTIVE THERAPEUTICS AND HYPNOTHERAPY

As mind affects the body, just as body affects the mind, in a circling of influence, it is entirely possible to aid in the treatment of physical ailments as well as psychological ones with hypnotherapy, as you will learn in this chapter. However, the hypnotherapist must not invade the domain of the physician. He works with clients, never patients, and never diagnoses.

During the Victorian Age on through the 1920's, what you will now study was called "suggestive therapeutics". Today, hypnosis used for therapeutic purposes is called "hypnotherapy" and is recognized by the American Medical Association (AMA) as a valuable ally in the treatment of disease (dis-ease).

Hypnosis used as hypnotherapy is unquestionably its most important usefulness. The mind of the hypnotized person being in a subjective state is ready to accept any and all suggestions as true, provided they are not in conflict with his moral nature. The hypnotist must remember this rule:

The strongest suggestion implanted in the subject's subconscious will be the most effective suggestion.

Unless otherwise directed, the subject is in rapport with the hypnotherapist only, and he readily accepts suggestions from that source as they are given him.

Hypnotherapy sessions may employ posthypnotic suggestions beneficial to the subject, which are usually complied with following awakening or sometime later, as directed. Many people have been helped to overcome their physical and mental distress without the aid of medicine using the process of hypnotherapy. The major requirement being that the client must be willing to allow the hypnotherapist to help them overcome their ailment or life situation. The client must cooperate with his or her Hypnotherapist one hundred percent.

We will later on describe in detail a number of ailments, fears, negative emotions and habits, which appear to respond to positively to hypnotic suggestion. You must learn how to give suggestions positively with conviction and precision in order to be a great Hypnotherapist. Since you are now going to gain some confidence in yourself, here's an exercise you can use to give you that confidence:

Go into a private room by yourself and talk out loud to an empty chair, table or whatever you wish to talk to. It makes no difference. Its only purpose is to provide you with a personal exercise to present suggestions most effectively. Suggestions that are most effective are suggestions that influence and suggestions that most influence are invariable POSITIVE SUGGESTIONS!

To help a person overcome an ailment, it is often not necessary to induce hypnotic sleep, as a suggestion properly presented in the waking state will greatly benefit. In hypnotherapy, a good deal depends on your pre-hypnotic suggestions and the consultation given to the patient when he or she first comes into your office for their hypnotherapy session. If you can inspire in him faith and confidence in your ability to help him, you have advanced already towards the cure. You must be sincere in helping people overcome obstacles in life.

Never state impossibilities in relation to "miracles" occurring, but affirm you can definitely be a great help, as testified by the many people you have helped in the past.

In relation to hypnotherapy, never tell the client that profound hypnosis will be necessary to help him. Tell him honestly that there are many different stages of hypnosis and it makes little difference whether he enters a light stage or a deep stage. Your treatment will benefit him just the same.

If you wish, you can tell the client of some of the cases you have treated, similar to his own that have been greatly benefited. Your aim is to establish confidence that you can aid and help your client. If your client should ask how long it will take to help him, tell him one cannot tell; some clients respond fully in only one session while others take a small number of sessions. It all depends on the nature of the problem or habit, and the responsiveness of the client to your suggestions and to hypnosis.

In hypnotherapy, you have no opportunity to be selective of those who seek your service. As you are able, induce as deep a state of hypnosis as is possible but be willing to work with whatever depth of hypnosis the client enters into.

Everything in life is based on some type of suggestion, whether the suggestions be verbal or non-verbal, conscious, or subconscious. Let's take for example:

SUGGESTIONS IN SALESMANSHIP

Suggestions are the essence of salesmanship. Examples are constantly in evidence. Most everyone has at sometime or other bought something they did not know they wanted yet they bought it, and it was not until later that they decided they did not want what they had been persuaded by suggestion to buy. The buying came about through the power of suggestion on the part of the person or advertisement, which induced the sale.

SUGGESTION CHANGES OPINION

Frequently, people change their opinions regarding certain matters when new ideas are suggested to them. The remark, "Well, now that you speak of it, I believe it is so," is often heard. Such is directly the result of exercising the power of suggestion.

To some degree, everybody uses the power of suggestion, some consciously and some unconsciously. Some use it conclusively and some inconclusively. The more one knows how to deliberately use this power, the more effective is the power. Training in hypnotism brings mastery of this power to change the opinions of others.

In some persons, the use of the power of suggestion seems almost an inborn talent. They automatically use it to good effect. This is why such persons are called "natural born salesmen". Their use of the power of suggestion is naturally effectively and it is there for the use of everyone. Used consciously in a definite direction to produce a desired result, suggestion is a limitless asset to what can be accomplished.

SUGGESTION FOR HEALTH

Suggestion can be used to help sick people get well. The value of cheerful and optimistic expression in the sick room to improve the health of an ill person is well known. The successful doctor uses the power continuously to heal his patients the fastest. It is often referred to as his "bedside manner". Persons in all walks of life use the power. Politicians, ministers, physicians, attorneys, salesmen, actors, etc., all use the power of suggestion. The study of hypnotism trains you most effectively to use this power in all walks of life actively.

SUGGESTIONS IN THE HOME

Parents should know how to use the power of suggestion in bringing up and molding the character of their children. Children are very responsive to suggestion. It is foolish to inflict punishment on a child every time they do not behave or if they have acquired a bad habit. Find out who or what is responsible for suggesting such a wrong direction.

For example, if a youngster comes home and starts using profanity, do not punish him.

Simply take him to one side, look deep into his eyes and ask him where he heard such language. Usually it is not of his-own origination; it comes via an outside source. While holding his attention, suggest that he discontinue such language. Show him the difference between right and wrong. Convince him you have his welfare as a parent in your heart, and that he ceases accepting such suggestions from outside companions.

Well-trained children are the result of proper suggestions on the part of their parents and teachers. In giving suggestions of behavior patterns to a child, be direct and emphatic in your suggestions, and do not change your mind, as your own vacillation of ideas will confuse the child.

Learning how to give effective suggestions to the child is a must for successful parents. Some parents even take advantage of talking to the child while sleeping which directly implants suggestions of well being into the subconscious, as the natural sleep can be transformed into hypnotic sleep by careful handling. A study of hypnosis by thoughtful parents is excellent.

SUGGESTIONS IN THE SCHOOL

Suggestion in the field of education can be of great value. Teachers would do well to study the laws of suggestion and apply them to the classroom. A positive suggestion is like a command and it produces results automatically. It is easy to note that some teachers are far better than others. Why? Largely it is because the successful teacher knows how to appeal to the responsive minds of their students. Their teaching is in accord with irresistible suggestions of successful learning. They are magnetic and students like them. Ask a student's opinion of a teacher and you will get an "aye" or "nay". If he doesn't like him, he will not do as the teacher instructs and will learn poorly. On the other hand, if the student likes the teacher, he will learn well. Teachers do well to master a study of the power of suggestion.

INCREASING THE POWER OF SUGGESTIONS

There are basically two forms of hypnotic (suggestive) influence as has been previously mentioned. One is the mesmeric approach of implanting the suggestion in the subconscious through the use of human energy power. This is the mesmeric approach, which was made famous as Mesmer's "Animal Magnetism". The other is the verbalized approach of using the psychological method of the power of words. Words have been conditioned in our mind to produce automatic responses. That is to say: Words are triggers to action. The most effective form of using the power of suggestion comes through a combining of the two methods, viz.:

Form the thought within the mind first before it is spoken and think of it in terms of being directly transferred into the mind of the recipient. Then follow directly into a verbalized affirmation of the thought. Such handling greatly increases the power of suggestion and gives what you express hypnotic impact.

CHAPTER SIXTEEN

PREPARING TO BECOME A HYPNOTIST

Having learned of the Power of Suggestion, you are now ready to prepare yourself in the direction of exerting this power in a directed hypnotic way. In other words: to become a hypnotist. For a start, it is well to appreciate these fundamental facts:

ANYONE CAN MASTER HYPNOTISM

Whoever you are, whatever you are, or wherever you are, you can master the science of hypnotism. And once you learn the science, you can learn the art of its performance. Such is why hypnotism is often referred to as a science/art.

The power to hypnotize is within each person. Naturally some have more talent for it, just as some persons will have more talent than do others for singing, as an example. But the power is there inside of each and everyone to be developed. It is the purpose of this book to show you how.

Hypnotism is the foundation of all mental phenomena. The science of hypnotism is universal and has always been a part of human relationships. Each day in our current computer age the power of hypnotism is advancing. With study, the great majority of people can, in a surprisingly short time, produce results that are far beyond their expectations. This book shows you how through a very practical way of producing the phenomena instead of merely theorizing on the subject.

WHO IS HYPNOTIZABLE?

Every human being is hypnotizable to some degree or other. Fifteen to Twenty percent of the population is capable of entering deep hypnosis (somnambulism) on the first attempt. Others take more repeated hypnosis sessions. People who are mentally challenged are difficult to influence so such persons are best avoided. Quick-witted, impulsive and intelligent people make good subjects. College students and military trained personnel are excellent. Even more so are artistic and creative individuals. Working with persons between the ages of 15 and 45 is the most desirable. Children are readily hypnotized, but the state is unstable in its lasting qualities. Older persons are also good candidates for hypnosis, as long as they are willing to be hypnotized.

QUALIFICATIONS OF A HYPNOTIST

The qualifications of a hypnotist are first of all confidence, a strong will, and the desire and knowledge to use both. It is not uncommon for a person to think they have a strong will because they are stubborn. Stubbornness is of no value. A strong willed person is one who knows how to direct his thoughts to accomplish the product of his thoughts. In such regard comes SELF-CONTROL. You must learn first how to control yourself before you can expect to control others. Self-control to the hypnotist means never to lose one's temper, to speak with a clear voice, have a healthy attitude, good morals and a willingness to do one's best.

One's clothes should be neat and clean, and being personally immaculate is a necessity. Show good taste in all you do and say. Do not try to convince skeptical people you can hypnotize them against their will. You must motivate people to work with you in cooperation, not opposition. Do not expect to hypnotize every person you come in contact with. Be satisfied with a fair percentage at first. Your percentage of success will increase as you advance in experience and build up your confidence.

REQUIREMENTS FOR HYPNOSIS

The essential thing to the induction of hypnosis on the part of the subject is attention to the hypnotist's suggestions, plus a willingness to be hypnotized. Generally speaking, a person cannot be hypnotized against their conscious will, although this does not mean they cannot be hypnotized if their subconscious is willing.

Mainly, all that is necessary in a good subject is the willingness to be hypnotized, willingness to pay attention to the suggestions given by the hypnotist, and willingness to relax the physical body. In seventy-five percent of such persons you will be able to induce hypnosis in one form or another. One's desire to be hypnotized plays an important factor.

DEVELOPING YOUR HYPNOTIC EYES AND VOICE

It is well for the hypnotist/hypnotherapist to develop a steady and earnest gaze. If you use your eyes in hypnotizing, the less you blink your eyes the better. Getting a hypnotic gaze like this takes practice.

Just before going to bed at night, stand in front of a mirror and look steadily at your eyes. Keep your eyes from blinking for as long as you can stand it, which will be for about a minute on the first trial. The second time you practice you will be able to look longer without blinking. At first it makes your eyes smart, but this will pass in a few days as you practice developing a hypnotic gaze. Keep practicing, a bit at a time, until you can keep your gaze steady, without blinking, for up to five minutes.

Now acquire a steady eye. That is, don't let your eyes move from one point to another as most people tend to do, but when you look into the eyes of your subject, keep your gaze in a concentrated stream into their eyes.

Looking a person straight in the eyes builds immediate confidence between hypnotist and subject. The eyes have been called the "windows to the soul" or innermost consciousness. They show character, willpower, determination and strength of the individual.

It is well for the hypnotist to develop a voice that expresses self-control and power. A squeaky, uncertain voice will not present suggestions effectively. The hypnotist should speak in a pleasant, yet commanding way that automatically demands acceptance. Practice the development of your voice, just as you practiced the development of your hypnotic gaze.

Stand in front of a mirror while looking at yourself and state to your image:

"I am going to succeed and become a Hypnotist. My voice is becoming perfect to most effectively present suggestions that will be accepted. Day by day, in every way, my voice becomes increasingly more powerful in what I say and the way I say it."

Learn to speak in a pleasant, even tone. Keep the pitch low. Talk to yourself as if you were conversing with a friend. It is not necessary to talk loud. Use just an ordinary tone, as in conversation.

An even toned voice can accomplish wonders, whereas a jerky, squeaky voice will not make a good impression. A hypnotic voice always makes a powerful impression.

Learn to speak positively, in a manner that demands acceptance. Perhaps you have heard the drill sergeant tell a line of soldiers, "Attention!" Notice how he says it. It is positive. It is a command. It expects obedience. A suggestion given positively is equivalent to a command. It is speaking in a POSITIVE MANNER, and behind it is the thought that what is spoken will be followed and obeyed. Practice this positive way of speaking. For practice, you can go into your room and look at a piece of furniture and imagine it is a client. Give your client positive commanding suggestions. Talk to your imaginary person as if they are accepting every commanding suggestion. Say to him:

"You WILL do everything that I ask you to do instantly!"

"Your Subconscious Mind accepts every SUGGESTION I give you!"

"GO DEEP ASLEEP NOW!"

Speak these phrases in a forceful manner several times over to your imaginary person. Do it seriously. Do not be afraid of being too strong or forceful, or even too maternal, as you are only practicing for yourself. Do this for at least a week once a day. Then practice the same on people you come in contact with. Naturally you will not use the above statements, but use the same commanding way. Use your will power and speak with confidence in yourself as if you can actual project each word you say into reality. Words create triggers to emotional reaction and emotional reaction is the driving force to physical and mental action. Look at words as a form of energy and look at energy as creating action from the words that you say.

If you ask a person to do something for you, say to him or her, "I WISH you would do this for me." Lay emphasis on the word WISH and it will sound just like WILL. There is all the difference in the world in how this is spoken to gain immediate obedience. When spoken positively it sounds like a command. When said weakly it sounds like you are pleading. This faculty of giving positive suggestions is essential to hypnotizing.

Study and practice these instructions for developing your hypnotic eyes and voice. They are important to your success as a hypnotist.

OBTAINING SUBJECTS TO PRACTICE ON

As a beginning hypnotist, you will need persons to practice with. With a little diplomacy you can easily obtain willing subjects. For this purpose, invite some congenial friends to your home who are interested in psychology. You can discuss psychology with the group without especially mentioning hypnotism at first. Turn the conversation upon the value of relaxation for removing stress from the body. You can mention that some persons who think they know how to relax really don't know how to do so. You propose a test the group can try:

Have each person in the group take a comfortable seat and give attention to the experiment you suggest. Each person is to raise his or her left arm up at a right angle out in front of his chest, then extend the fingers of his right hand and place it directly under the palm of his left hand. In such a position, the extended fingers are ready to support the entire weight of the left hand and arm.

Now tell the group to completely relax their left hand and arm letting the extended fingers of the right hand being the sole support of that arm. The participants are thus in a position that requires the relaxing of the left arm while, at the same time, concentrating on holding it up with the extended fingers of the right hand. In this you have produced a situation requiring both concentration and relaxation at the same time. A condition very similar to that required for the induction of hypnosis.

Now tell the group, for each person to be sure they have relaxed their left hand and arm completely, in this testing for relaxation. At the count of "three", they are to quickly draw the right hand support from under the extended left hand.

You then slowly count, "*One, two, three.*" What happens?

If the volunteers trying the experiment have truly relaxed as you instructed, the moment support is withdrawn from under the hand that arm naturally drops limply to their lap. Such is the expected result, but as sometimes happens, the left arm of some persons will still remain suspended even when the finger support beneath is removed.

When this happens, explain that it indicates the person has not really relaxed even when they thought they had. So repeat the experiment. A second time around most everyone will have learned to fully relax.

It is a simple experiment, but it is interesting and gets the group participating in some demonstrations with you. You can then turn the discussion to William James's effect of Ideomoter action, that every idea of motion held in the mind produces an accompanying unconscious motor-muscular response in the body of a minute nature.

To demonstrate this, hand each person a pendulum (simply a small fishing weight tied to the end of a length of string). Instruct them to hold the top end of the string in their right hand, allowing the weight to dangle down as they hold it with arm outstretched. Tell them to think of it being still. It will become still. Now tell them to think of it swinging back and forth and just the thought alone without making any conscious muscular effort to move it. It will begin to sway back and forth.

Next tell them to think of the pendulum swinging around and around in a circle and it will so respond. Response to this pendulum test will give you a good idea as to whom in the group is the more responsive to suggestions.

These simple experiments will quickly capture group interest and you can now proceed to trying some experiments in waking hypnosis (as you will be instructed) such as Falling Backwards and Forward Tests, Fastening Hands Together, etc.. When you feel the group is ready for it, you can suggest trying a few experiments in hypnotism.

If you are serious about learning hypnotism, and join a hypnosis school of training, you will have plenty of eager students for you practice on in the training workshops that you will be attending. In these class programs, you will also feel what it feels like to be hypnotized as the students practice on you.

In practicing hypnosis with your friends, it is often best not to mention hypnotism at first, but generally lead up to it. And never mention that you are a beginner and just practicing.

This initial practice with friends in experimenting with hypnotism is very important, as it is desirable for you to achieve good results right from the start. To be a successful hypnotist, nothing is more important than to have confidence in your ability to hypnotize, and nothing advances your confidence in your ability to hypnotize more than having success with your early experiences in hypnotizing.

These tests are considered to be what we call responsiveness tests, or suggestibility tests. These tests are great for helping you to become confident in turning words into action, as well as they will tell you who is following your directions, and who might be resisting your directions or suggestions. People, who are more responsive to these types of tests, tend to be more responsive to hypnotic suggestions and deeper depths of hypnosis.

CHAPTER SEVENTEEN

DIFFERENT METHODS OF HYPNOTIZING

All people are not affected by the same method of being hypnotized. People differ in their responses. While one person will respond best to an authoritarian (father) approach, another will respond to a gentle (mother) approach. The art of becoming an expert hypnotist comes in learning which hypnotic method will best influence the specific subject being worked with. It is an art that comes only through experience. It is almost an intuition as to what is best to do. Here is a generalized list of the most popular methods of hypnotizing:

1. By verbalized suggestions (oral techniques)
2. By mental suggestions (mesmeric techniques)
3. By fixation of the gaze upon a bright object (Braid)
4. By fascination
5. By contact passes with the subject
6. By noncontact passes over the subject
7. By monotonous procedures
8. By loud and unexpected noises
9. By the lulling effect of soft music (lullaby techniques)
10. By the use of mechanical devices such as revolving spirals and flashing lights
11. By a combination of mesmeric and suggestion techniques
12. By autosuggestion to one's self (self-hypnosis)
13. By a physical induction method
14. By a shock induction method

There are countless variations of these methods, but these procedures are the basics.

HEAVY HAND AND LIGHT HAND SUGGESTIBILITY TEST

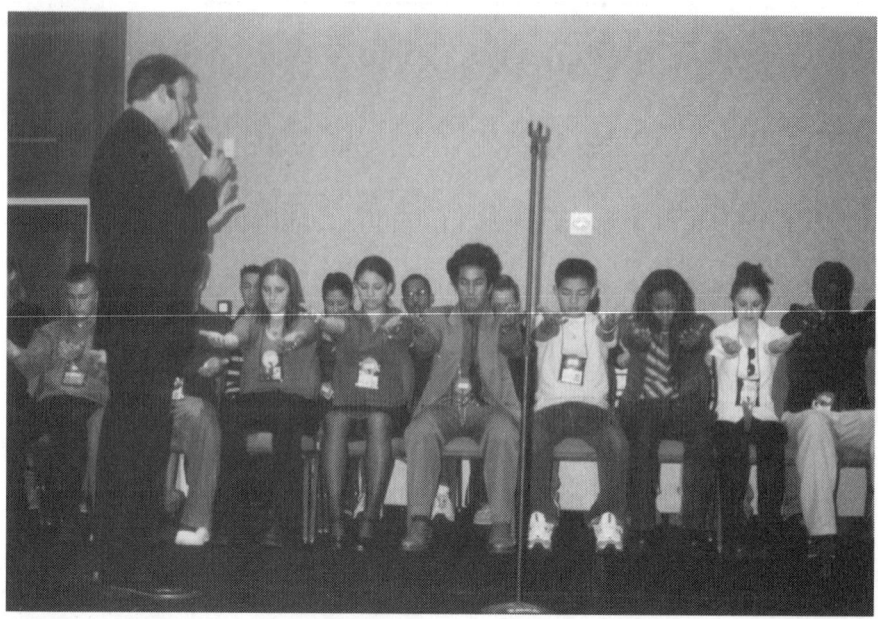

THE SUBJECTS ARE ASKED TO IMAGINE THAT THERE IS A TWENTY POUND WEIGHT IN THE PALM OF THEIR LEFT HAND AND THAT THEIR RIGHT HAND IS ATTACHED TO A LIGHT AIR BALOON

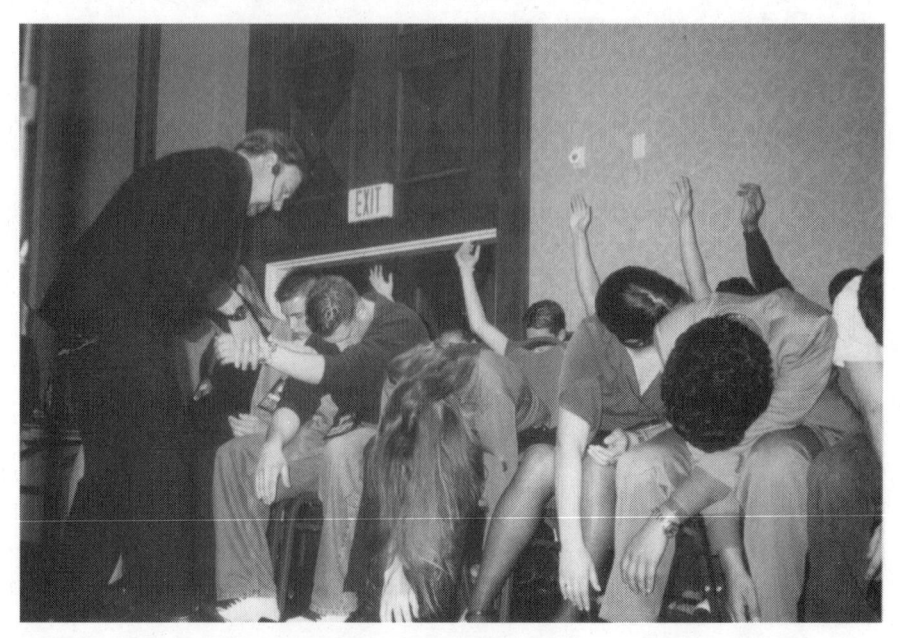

THE HYPNOTIST NOW PULLS DOWN ON THE SUBJECTS HAND AND ARM THAT IS UP IN THE AIR AND SAYS THE WORD "SLEEP"!

CHAPTER EIGHTEEN

THREE PRELIMINARY TESTS IN WAKING HYPNOSIS

Now that you have background knowledge for understanding hypnotism and the laws of its operation, instructions for developing your hypnotic eyes and voice combined with methods to present suggestions that influence, you are ready to perform some preliminary test demonstrations in hypnotism. It is the method of experimenting with experiencing. In other words, the most effective way to learn hypnotism is by hypnotizing.

If you were to study mathematics, you would start with arithmetic before you advance to calculus. It is the same with mastering hypnotism. Start with the less complex and advance to the more complex.

There are three good preliminary tests following with which you can begin your practice.

Waking hypnosis experiments are good to begin with, for while the basic subconscious phenomena are the same, we are more familiar with our waking state than we are with our sleeping state of mind.

In this HOW TO BOOK OF HYPNOTHERAPY, you are instructed in exactly how to present each experiment, inclusive of the detailed word-for-word formula of suggestions to be used to successfully accomplish each test. Nothing is left to guesswork for you; do exactly as you are instructed and you will accomplish amazing things.

To successfully accomplish these experiments, at all times use this threefold formula of visualization, affirmation and projection. That is:

1. VISUALIZATION
   Form within your mind a mental picture of exactly how the subject is going to respond in being hypnotized for the performance of the test.
   See it happening.

1. AFFIRMATION
   Verbalize, in a positive manner, the suggestions that cause the subjective mind of the subject to perform exactly as you have visualized.
   Tell it as you see it.

3. PROJECTION
See in your "mind's eye" the hypnotic response you have visualized and affirmed as being projected into the subconscious mind of the subject automatically causing the hypnotic effect to be accomplished. Project it as you tell it.

Perform these experiments with a willing subject in the order given: 1 –2 – 3. Understand! You are set! You are ready! READY, SET, GO ...

EXPERIMENT ONE
CAUSING A SUBJECT TO FALL BACKWARD

This pre-hypnosis induction test and procedure can help you to have your client prepare to be hypnotized. It helps you to take control of the situation by directing the subject or client to follow your instructions. This physical test also can show you if the person you will be hypnotizing in going to resist from being hypnotized. Have him stand up, facing towards a wall, and tell him to place his feet together[1]. Arms should be at the sides of his body. Have him hold his arms at his sides with hands open fully. Ask him to relax his entire body. That is, he should stand naturally upright sensing within himself that the muscles of his body are free from all stiffness – they are relaxed. By standing behind him and pulling him back with your hand on his shoulder, you can tell if he has done as requested. If he comes back easily, he has obeyed you; if he resists, he has not followed your instructions and done as you requested. In such a case, explain that for this experiment in waking hypnosis to successfully operate for him, it is essential that he relax his muscles as he stands erect.

Having obtained the right conditions in your subject, say:

"Now, THINK that your body is going to start swaying backward – that you are going to fall over backwards. Think of nothing else. You will soon feel as if something compelled you to fall back, but do not be afraid.

---

[1] You can perform all hypnotic experiments with either sex. In these instructions, the masculine gender is used for literary convenience some of the time.

I am standing right behind you, and as you fall I will catch you. When you feel the impulse to fall do not resist it, but just let yourself go."

Then have him hold up his head and tell him to close his eyes. Now, stand directly back of the subject. Stand at a distance of about three feet behind him, just so far that your hands reach easily to the temples of his head from behind and tip his head back slightly towards yourself so your fingertips rest on the crown of his head, base of the brain (nap of the neck). Then continue on moving your hands down the spine to the hips, on to the very end of the spine. This is called a "contact pass".

It should be made lightly, using just enough pressure so as not to distract the equilibrium of the subject. Make three of these contact passes down the spine. A contact pass can increase your focus and concentration on succeeding in this test but it is not necessary.

Then return both hands and place them at the temples on each side of the head and verbally suggest:

"When I withdraw my hands from you, you will slowly fall backwards."

Repeat these suggestions until he topples over backwards into your waiting arms. Catch him safely and immediately return him to his feet.

Be sure during all of this process to concentrate your mind on the one idea that he will fall backwards. Use your willpower. The more firmly you believe that you can draw him backwards, the quicker the results will be obtained.

As you learn how to perform this experiment, study every step in sequence so you know exactly what to say and do in 1-2-3 order. Learn this lesson well, the movement and the words, so you can perform it in complete confidence that it will unfailingly operate. Be sure to withdraw your fingers slowly from the back of his head and present your suggestions of his falling slowly and positively.

It is important to learn how to perform this test perfectly as it sets the pattern of effectively influencing subjects in the waking state that you will use in the many forms of waking hypnosis you will learn how to do.

If the subject should feel a little dazed after falling backwards, snap your fingers close to his ear and say, *"All right ... you are just fine"*.

When you have successfully performed this first test, you are ready to perform the second.

EXPERIMENT TWO
CAUSING A SUBJECT TO FALL FORWARD

In this pre-hypnosis procedure and physical suggestibility test, you cause the subject to fall forwards, is a little different than the first test. The handling is very similar to your handling of the first test, except in this instance you use the hands to pull the subject towards you. With this test, you will tell your subject the following suggestion:

"In a moment you will close your eyes when I touch you on your shoulders. When I lift up on and off your shoulder, you will fall forward. You are safe and will not fall, because I am here to catch you. I simply want you to trust me and just fall forward when I lift my hands up and off you shoulders." "Nod your head yes, to do everything I ask you to do".

Have the subject stand facing you. His eyes should be in the shadow while facing you and your eyes in the light while facing him. Tell him to relax his muscles and look you straight in the eyes.

Ask him to think of nothing but falling forward. Touch your subject's shoulder and tell the subject to close his or her eyes and to keep them closed until you ask them to open them up. Look him squarely in the eyes, concentrating your gaze at the root of his nose at the central point between his eyes. Keep a sober, earnest demeanor and have the subject do the same. Say to him:

"When I lift up on your shoulder and you will fall forward instantly... Imagine it... and let it happen".

(Now lift up off the shoulders while you slightly pull the subject towards yourself. If your subject is not resisting you to hypnotize him, they will fall forward with the back heels of the shoes or feet leaving the floor. The higher the backs of the shoes or feet lift up in the air, the more willing is the subject to have you hypnotize them.)

Speak positively to him. Command him.
Tell him (subject) exactly what you want him to do.

"When I remove my hands from your shoulder you will fall forward. You are safe and I will catch you, simply let it happen, fall forward."

As you give these suggestions, withdraw your hand forwards from his shoulders and let your movements gentle and keep on saying:

"Falling forward. Falling forward. You are safe. I will ...n you. Fall forward now!"

Repeat these suggestions over and over until he falls forward into your arms. The repetition of suggestions has a compounding effect in developing power. Draw your own body slightly downwards while withdrawing your hands. Catch him firmly when he falls.
Properly performed, your success with this experiment in waking hypnosis will be excellent. This test also looks great when performed in front of a live audience.

EXPERIMENT THREE
HEAVY HAND AND LIGHT HAND SUGGESTIBILITY TEST

This test I (Tom Silver) will usually conduct in my office prior to my hypnotherapy session. This suggestibility test helps to increase a person's hypnotic suggestibility and also their concentration. It involves an ideomotor muscle response which is "a subconscious suggestion tied into a physical movement". This ideomotor muscle response is connected to the subconscious mind and is a physical subconscious involuntary muscle movement. This suggestibility test will also act as a pre-hypnosis type of induction that if performed correctly will also be a "post hypnotic suggestion" for hypnosis. I have my client sit back in a chair with their hands resting on their lap. I have them focus their attention on their breathing, and to nod their head yes, when they notice their breathing change and they take a deeper breath in. I tell them to close their eyes and to hold their hands straight out in front of them with their fingers extended straight out in front of them and the palms of the hands facing the sky. I then say to them in a direct and focused way:

"When I count to three, I want you to imagine with your eyes closed that I am placing a very heavy object in the palm of your left hand. A steel ball that ways 25 pounds. When I count to three, you will feel your left hand and arm getting very heavy and dropping down onto

...ap. When your hand touches your lap, it will become totally and completely relaxed. Imagine it is now going to happen".

"One...Two...Three...A steel ball in the palm of your left hand....your left hand getting heavier and heavier, tugging and dropping down....heavier and heavier as though there are two steel balls now that weigh 50 pounds in the palm of your left hand...dropping down...heavier...tugging dropping heavier down until it touches your lap and relaxes on your lap and then you will feel your right hand and arm lifting up into the air, as though your right hand and arm was attached to a dozen light air balloons as it goes higher and lighter, up and up".

"Your left hand now gets three times as heavy and now four times heavier as thought there are four steel balls in the palm of your left hand that weigh 100 pounds. Let that hand drop onto your lap now and now let your right hand and arm now lift all the way up into the air until your right hand and fingers are pointing up to the sky, as though there is 4 dozen light air balloons attached to that arm and your hand and arm now lifts up all the way in the air now".

The ideomotor response as you keep on repeating the suggestions over and over again will take hold and if the person is concentrating properly without physical or mental resistance, their hands and arms will move to in the directions that you suggest them to move.

After the subject's left hand has relaxed on their lap, and their right hand has lifted all the way in the air, you can say to them while their eyes are still closed and they are concentrating on your words,

"You have now reached your peak of concentration and suggestibility to allow me to hypnotize you. I will give you a post hypnotic suggestion that, when I ask you the next time, to close your eyes and relax, and I say the word "sleep", you will enter into a deep hypnotic relaxation and you will become deeply hypnotized. You will do everything that I ask you to do and you have perfect concentration to go into a deep restful hypnotic sleep. You are doing perfectly. When I count to three, you will awaken and open your eyes and look at your wonderful concentration. One...Two...Three...now open your eyes and look at your perfect concentration".

Now say to the client or subject:

"Your right hand in the air represents your subconscious desire to let me hypnotize you. I have given you a post hypnotic suggestion to enter back into hypnosis when I hypnotize you and say the word "sleep". Do you understand me? Good, I will now hypnotize you".

THE FAMOUS HAND LOCKING TEST

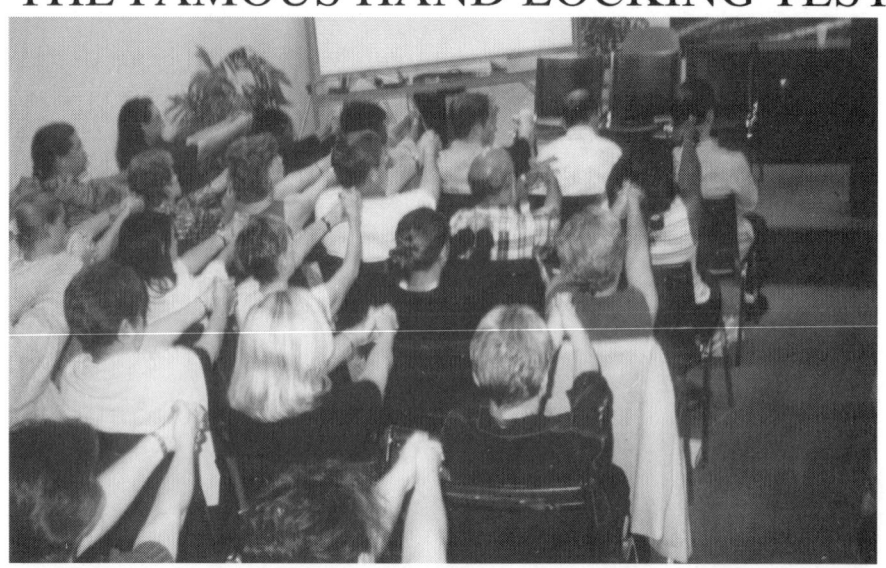

TOM SILVER PERFORMING HAND LOCKING TEST IN TAIWAN WORLD RECORD SHOW 1995

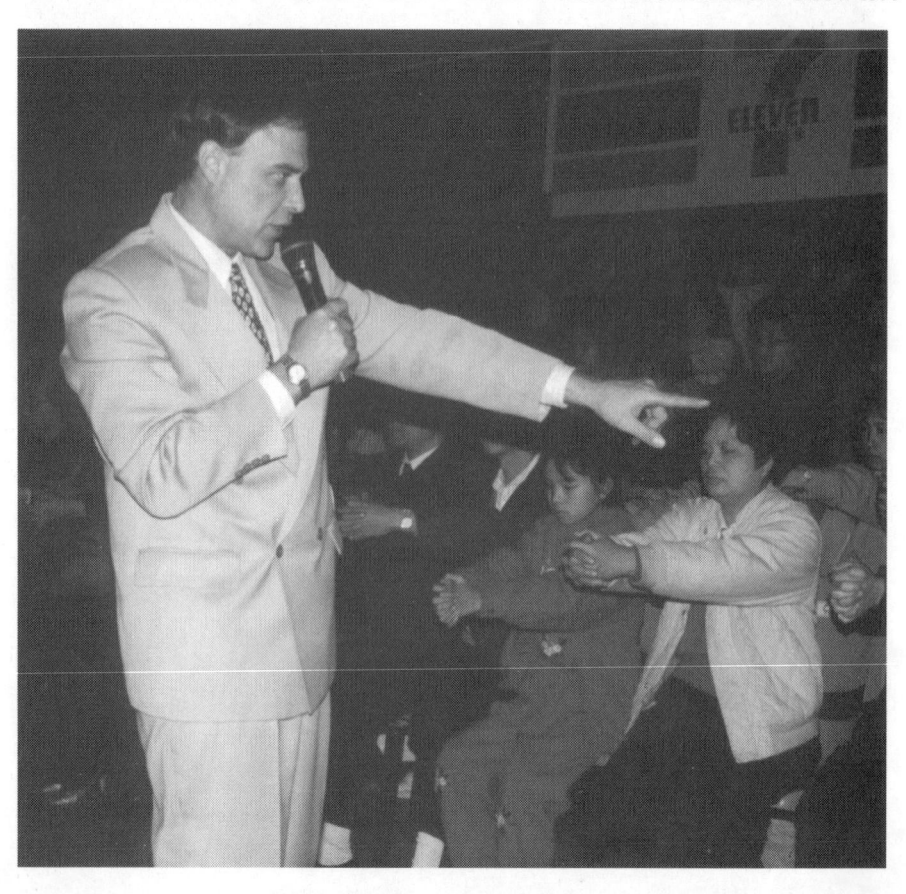

CHAPTER NINETEEN

THE FAMOUS HAND LOCKING TEST

Having successfully performed the three foregoing preliminary waking hypnosis suggestibility tests, you are ready for the fourth. The Hand Locking suggestibility test was made famous by the French psychologist, Emile Coue' who demonstrated it in all his lectures and used it as a method to test his client's responsiveness to autosuggestion in his clinic. Rumor has it that Emile never accepted a client unless they past the hand locking test that he conducted on them.

For this test, have the subject stand in front of you and concentrate upon your eyes. Ask him to put his hands together with palms clasped and fingers interlocked. Have him straighten out both arms and make them stiff. Then suggest:

"Squeeze .. your .. hands .. tightly .. together .. and .. think .. that .. you .. cannot .. pull .. them .. apart. As..thought..I..am..tightening....a vice...or..clamp..alround them..... They .. have .. become .. locked .. so .. tightly .. together .. that .. you .. cannot .. pull .. them .. apart .. no .. matter .. how .. hard .. you .. try. Pretend... they.. are.. now ..stuck... together...Try hard. .. Your .. hands .. are .. locked .. so .. tightly .. together .. you .. cannot .. pull .. them .. apart .. no .. matter .. how .. hard .. you .. try. .. Pull ... pull. Try .. try .. try. You .. cannot .. unlock .. your .. hands .. with .. all .. your .. might. Your .. hands .. are .. locked .. together. You .. cannot .. get .. your .. hands .. apart."

If your subject has been following your suggestions with earnest concentration, his hands will have become so firmly locked together that struggle, as he will he simply cannot pull his locked hands apart.

After the subject has tried in vain to release his hands, snap your fingers beside his ear and state:

"All .. right .. now, .. the .. influence .. is .. all .. gone .. now. Relax. You .. can .. take .. your .. hands .. apart .. now."

In presenting suggestions to subjects in performing waking hypnosis experiments, speak positively, slowly and distinctly, becoming more and more forceful as the test proceeds towards its climax.

Throw your energy into the performance of these tests. Having succeeded with these four experiments, you will gain confidence in your ability to hypnotically influence people. Mastering the art of how to present suggestions that influence will put new life into your whole personality. All tests of this muscular nature in waking hypnosis follow this pattern.

CHAPTER TWENTY
BY TOM SILVER

SUGGESTIONS FOR A HYPNOTHERAPY PRACTICE

SETTING UP YOUR HYPNOTHERAPY RELAXATION ROOM

When you have a private hypnotherapy practice, you want to have your office set up so that your client can rest on a recliner or some comfortable furniture. You want to possibly have a desk in your office facing your client, so that you can converse with your client easily. You will also want to have a chair in the office so that before you have your client sitting down on the recliner to be hypnotized, you can have them sitting in a chair right next to your desk. This way you can easily explain to the client what hypnosis is and what you are going to do for them, once they sit down in the recliner to be hypnotized. I also recommend that you do some of the pre-hypnosis suggestibility tests to increase the client's focus and concentration before you hypnotize them.

The heavy hand and light hand and arm induction is a very good ideo motor response test you can do while your client in sitting in the chair. You might want to have some soothing pictures on the wall and some soothing lighting in the office. The more comfortable you make your office for a client, the more responsive they will be when you hypnotize them.

OBTAINING DOCUMENTS OF COMPETED HYPNOSIS COURSES

It is important that when you start a hypnotherapy practice that you have in your office some of your certificates of educational courses in hypnotherapy that you have completed. There are many one to four day courses in specific areas of hypnotism that will present you with a certificate of completion after you take that seminar or workshop.

There are also longer educational programs that can even up to a year or more in hypnotherapy training. All of these courses will present you with a certificate of completion after you complete the program, course or workshop. These certificates are your client's proof of your continuous training and education as a clinical Hypnotherapist.
Start with one course and continue your hypnosis training.

CLINICAL HYPNOTHERAPY DIPLOMA
CLINICAL HYPNOTHERAPY TRAINING CERTIFICATION
TOM SILVER "CLINICAL HYPNOTHERAPIST" JANUARY 1ST, 1986

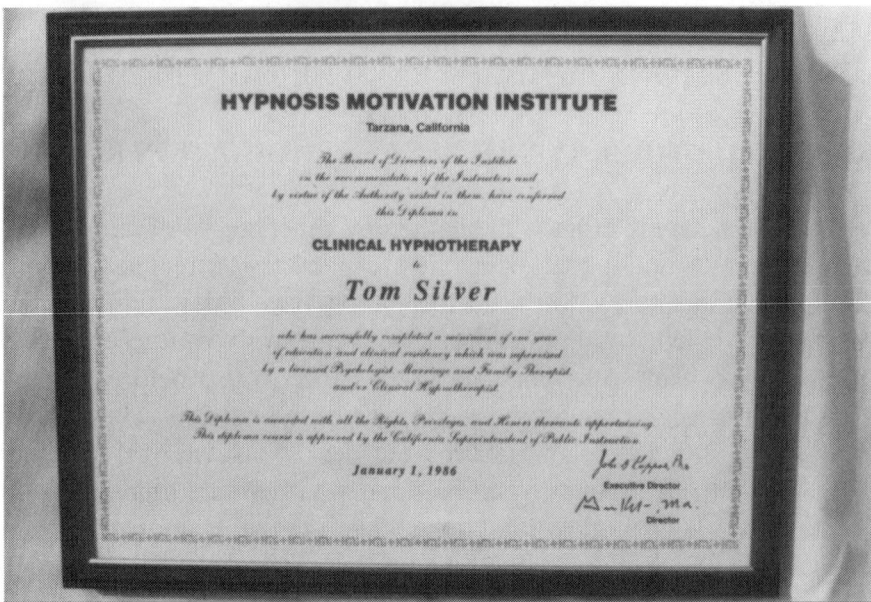

CLINICAL HYPNOTHERAPY CERTIFICATION PRESENTED TO TOM SILVER FROM THE FOUNDER OF THE HYPNOSIS MOTIVATION INSTITUTE DR. JOHN KAPPAS

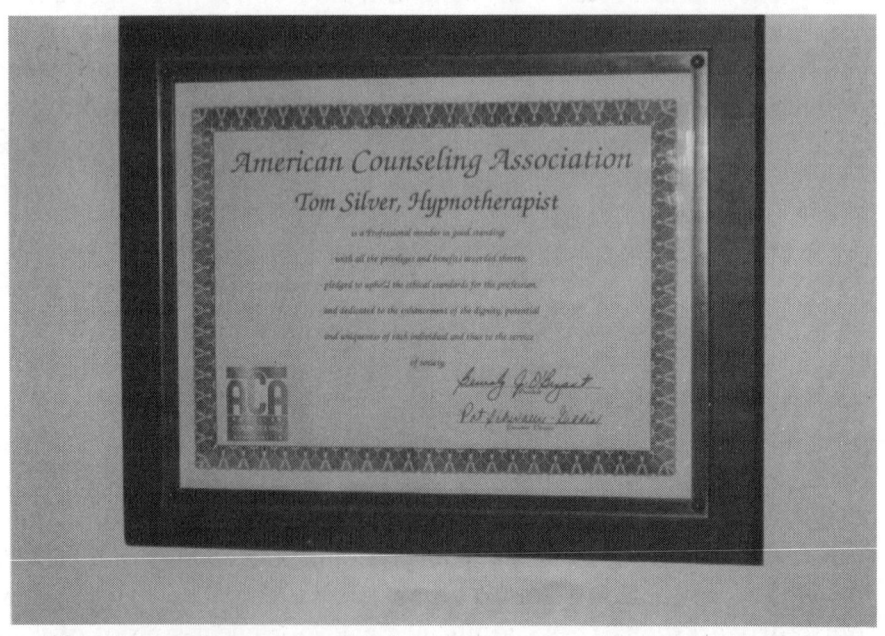

"THE AMERICAN COUNSELING ASSOCIATION"
TOM SILVER HYPNOTHERAPIST "MEMBER IN GOOD STANDING"

MEMBERSHIPS IN HYPNOSIS ORGANIZATIONS

I recommend that any person wanting to become a Hypnotherapist should join one or a few of the various hypnosis organizations and or hypnosis Guilds that exist throughout the United States and other parts of the world. Being part of a national hypnosis organization adds credibility to your practice and can also help increase your education as a Hypnotherapist, by attending the national conventions and workshops that they may offer. There are some really great hypnosis organizations that offer memberships to beginning and seasoned hypnotists.

These organizations also will present you with a membership certificate that you can place on the wall or door of your hypnotherapy office. If you go into a doctors office or even a lawyers or accountants office, just look at the wall in their office and you will see there awards and certificates which verify their credibility in what they do.

YOUR FIRST HYPNOTHERAPY PRIVATE PRACTICE SESSION

INTRODUCTION AND BACKGROUND OF YOURSELF

When your client comes into your office and sits down to talk to you about what they want to accomplish by being hypnotized, it is good to introduce yourself and to give your client some background information on yourself. How you became interested in hypnosis. If you have been practicing hypnotherapy for many years, it's good to let your client know that. You want to convey to your client, that you are an expert in helping people through the scientific application of hypnosis. The more your client gets to know you, the more trust they will have in your ability to hypnotize them and to help them.

EXPLAIN TO YOUR CLIENT WHAT HYPNOSIS IS AND WHAT HYPNOSIS IS NOT

The next beginning part of your hypnotherapy session should include what I call your life script programming. You now can explain to your client about how we are programmed from early childhood and how our subconscious mind can be filled with negative emotions and habits. "From birth to about 3 or 4 years of age, everything that goes into our mind, goes directly into our subconscious mind. We take in message units or bits of emotional information. Love, trust, security, fear, misdirection, pain, confusion and so forth, and these emotional positive and negative feelings can stay with our whole life, unless we change them.

"Hypnosis is a great way to change your negative habits, patterns and emotions because all of these are in your subconscious mind and hypnosis helps you to reprogram your subconscious mind to work for you".

Tell your client that all hypnosis is, is magnified concentration and that this magnified concentration in about nine time stronger than a conscious suggestion. Let your client know that 15 minutes of hypnosis sleep is equal to about 5 or more hours of a natural sleep. Let your client know that hypnosis and sleep are two different things. Give your client enough information on hypnosis so that they can believe in you and your knowledge of hypnosis. "Hypnosis has been used in the Western World for over Two Hundred Years, and that some of the top medical doctors in Europe were also "Hypnotists" or what they called "Mesmerists". Say that with hypnosis you help people, lose weight, stop smoking, release stress and tension, and increase focus and concentration and many other wonderful positive changes.

Tell the client that the A.M.A. officially recognized hypnosis back in 1957. That's why they come to see you, because you are the expert in hypnosis to them, so you can motivate and stimulate your client by educating them on hypnosis before you ever hypnotize them.

TALK ABOUT ENVIRONMENTAL HYPNOSIS

Ask your client or subject, if he or she has ever been hypnotized before? If they say yes, that means that they are already use to the experience. If they say no, tell them that each and every one of us has been hypnotized before.

"When you drive your car, you are hypnotized and your subconscious mind is doing the driving for you while your conscious mind is day dreaming or just drifting in thoughts. Have you ever driven your car and then wondered how did you get to your destination? You were hypnotized". "We all go into hypnosis every day".

You can tell your client about how movies and sports events also hypnotize them. This information about environmental hypnotism is in the questions and answers part of the book. You will find a lot of good useful information that you can use in the questions and answers section.

FIND OUT WHAT YOUR CLIENTS GOALS ARE

Before you start your hypnosis part of the therapy session, you need to know exactly what your client in coming in for and what he wants to accomplish by being hypnotized. If you as a hypnotherapist can give your client consciously and subconsciously (through hypnosis) what he tells you he's wants from being hypnotized, you will find tremendous success in your practice.

You need to be a good listener and take some good notes during the cognitive part of your hypnotherapy session. What I do is I ask my clients before they come into my hypnotherapy office to see me, to write on a piece of paper in their own words what they would like to accomplish through hypnosis. I say to them that, "If hypnosis was a miracle type of cure all thing in their life, what would your goals be in your own words in writing". I ask for writing because I feel that handwriting comes more directly from the emotions of the subconscious mind.

WRITE A MENTAL PRESCRIPTION FOR YOUR CLIENT

A mental prescription is my custom formula and suggestions that I create as I am talking to my clients and when I read their written hypnosis "wish list". If you think of what you do in a medically scientific type of way, you will realize that your mental prescription is your hypnosis suggestive formula that you are creating and giving to your client while they are hypnotized. You might have certain hypnosis phases and suggestions that you have memorized and that you use in specific sessions, but a this type of individualizing and spontaneous suggestive response by mirroring their desires by to them, works really well.

It may take some time until you can feel comfortable enough to be completely spontaneous with your client, but with practice it will come. Find out in their own words what they want, and simply give it back to them under hypnosis in yours and their words. As your knowledge in hypnotism increases, so will your inner wisdom in creating spontaneous mental prescriptions and therapeutic suggestions and visual imagery techniques. The next part of this hypnotism textbook will be on asking the client some key questions that will determine if the client is suggestible to suggestion and if the client is natural somnambulist.

KEY QUESTIONS TO DETERMINE NATURAL SOMNAMBULISM SUGGESTIBILITY

I have a few key questions that I ask my clients before I hypnotize them. This might tell me if they are a natural somnambulist, (a person who automatically goes into deep hypnosis), and if they are physically suggestible. This also tells me if they are a person with mixed emotions.

My first question is always:

Question Number One:

"Have you ever walked in your sleep at all during your life"?

If the answer is yes, it will tell me if this client is a natural somnambulist and will probably go into a very deep state of hypnosis the first time that I hypnotize him or her.

Question Number Two:

"If you were to imagine sucking on a sour, bitter, juicy lemon, would you notice your mouth start to water"?

If the client says yes, then you know that they are physically suggestible and that they respond best to physical suggestions. It also says that they are very visual.

Question Number Three:

"As a child, were you more affected by the looks that your parents gave you, or by the negative words that they said, or by the tone of voice of your parents"?

If the client says that they were affected by the tone of voice more than the words that would tell me that this person is very emotionally suggestible and positive emotional suggestions might be the triggers that work best the them.

MAKE A PARTNERSHIP AGREEMENT WITH CLIENT

I always make a "Partnership Agreement" with my clients. It is important for you to make a Partnership Contract (Agreement) with your client or with anyone that you are going to hypnotize before you hypnotize them. This Partnership agreement will give you more of a commitment from the client to allow themselves to follow your directions and not to think about the process, but to just let it happen easily. If the person or client does not go into a receptive depth of hypnosis, or resists from following your directions or suggestions, then the client has not lived up to their end of the agreement. You must live up to your end of the agreement by using the correct methods to hypnotize this person. This agreement method will insure you much more cooperation and desire from you client to allow you to hypnotize him or her and not to analyze the process.
Your agreement can go something like this:

"I am here to hypnotize you and to help you. I promise to take good care of you. You are safe and secure and you want me to hypnotize you. I want you to agree to do everything that I ask you to do without instantly and without thinking, and I will hypnotize you to help you to overcome this obstacle that is standing in the way of your health and happiness. Do you understand and agree to allow me to hypnotize you"?

Your client must say "Yes".
Then say to your client:

"We now have a Partnership agreement with each other". "I will hypnotize you to overcome this obstacle in your life, and you will instantly and without thinking, do everything that I ask you to do. Do you understand"? "Good. I will now hypnotize you".

Even trained clinical hypnotist sometimes have difficulty in deeply hypnotizing clients. These hypnotists may be suffering from insecurities and self-doubts. Some hypnotherapists may be even skeptical of how powerful hypnosis can be and they doubt the science, so there success rate with their clients may be low. Even the greatest hypnotist's in history had sometimes failed because they lost their confidence in themselves. It is therefore important for you to be 100% confident.

HYPNOSIS INDUCTION AND THERAPY

After you have made your partnership agreement with your client, you can start your hypnotherapy session. For your first hypnotherapy session, you might want to start with a progressive relaxation induction by having the client imagine with their eyes closed relaxing every muscle, nerve and fiber in their body. You might want to say to the client that with each and every exhale of air that you take will relax them and send them deeper asleep.

After you have successfully hypnotize your client into a deep hypnosis relaxation, you can then give your client the positive suggestions and visual imagery suggestions to help them overcome the obstacles that they came in to overcome. We will get much deeper into hypnosis inductions and deepening techniques using suggestion and visual imagery in the coming chapters of Hypnotism "The Real Questions and Answers".

LOWER JAW RELAXATION
DEEPENING TECHNIQUE TO RELAX JAW MUSCLES
BY: HYPNOTHERAPIST TOM SILVER

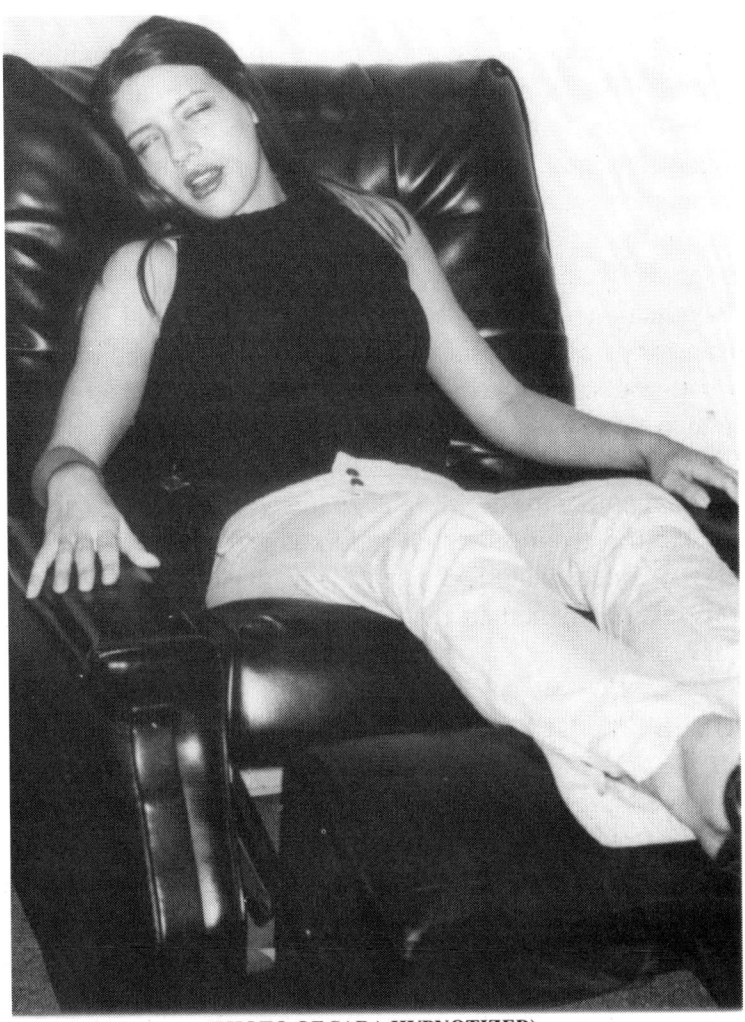

(PHOTO OF SARA HYPNOTIZED)

"I WANT YOU TO RELAX THE MUSCLES IN YOUR JAW AND JUST TO LET YOUR MOUTH DROP OPEN AND RELAX YOUR MOUTH AND LOWER JAW"
(THINK TO YOURSELF)
"I GIVE MYSELF PERMISSION TO OPEN MY MOUTH AND TO RELAX THE MUSCLES IN MY LOWER JAW AS MY MOUTH OPENS UP MORE AND MORE RELAXED"
"YOUR LOWER JAW RELAXES NOW EVEN MORE"

CHAPTER TWENTY-ONE

HYPNOSIS INDUCTIONS AND DEEPENING TECHNIQUES:

We will be discussing a number of very powerful hypnotic inductions that you can use to hypnotize a person. These are called, rapid, instant, and shock inductions. They take some time to learn how to perform them smoothly and with confidence and precision. The first hypnosis induction that every hypnotist should learn is called the "Progressive Relaxation Induction". This method is based on suggestions of relaxing a person's body and mind.

This induction was used for many years and is still taught as one of the main forms of hypnosis induction methods. We believe as a skilled hypnotist, you should have a number of hypnosis induction techniques to use at your disposal because not all people can be hypnotized by the same method.

Some hypnotherapists who have limited knowledge in inductions always use the progressive relaxation as a hypnosis induction method and also as a deepening technique for hypnosis. Some hypnotists think that this relaxation method is a thing of the past, but we both feel that it does have merit.

PROGRESSIVE RELAXATION METHOD

When working with a first time client we sometimes recommend to first start off with a "Progressive Relaxation" techniques of having the client image that their entire body is slowly becoming bathed in relaxation.

The hypnotherapist has his client imagine their toes and feet becoming relaxed, and bringing that relaxation slowly up the legs, stomach muscles and into the clients back, relaxing all the way up to the top of the clients head.

You can use visual imagery such as having your client imagine that their body was made out of a thousand lose and limp rubber bands, or that they are relaxed, like a rag doll, or just floating on a cloud of relaxation. The progressive relaxation method to hypnotize a person is a very soothing method based on breathing, relaxation, visualization techniques and imagery.

After performing a progressive relaxation induction on a client, you may want to give the client a post hypnotic suggestion that "the very next time you hypnotize them, they will become ten times more deeply relaxed and hypnotized.

SELF-HYPNOSIS PROGRESSIVE RELAXATION

This Hypnosis induction technique and method is called the "Self Hypnosis Progressive Relaxation Method" and it is a wonderful elf hypnosis relaxation technique that will help relax and revitalize you, and it is also a great way to implant your own positive suggestions into your subconscious mind.

All you have to do is to find yourself a comfortable chair or recliner to sit on. You can also sit on the floor in a comfortable position. Place your hands face down on your lap, look down at your hands and focus your attention on your breathing. Take three slow deep breaths in and out and think of the word "Relaxation". Hold each breath in for about five seconds before your exhale. As you exhale, imagine yourself relaxing a different part of your body, such as relaxing the muscles in your toes and feet. Relaxing the muscles in your stomach, or relaxing your shoulders and back, or relaxing the muscles around your eyelids etc. On your fifth exhale, close your eyes and imagine a wave of relaxation moving from the top of your head all the way down to the tips of your toes.

Now imagine with your eyes still closed, that you are in a beautiful place or relaxation, like lying on a beach, in a meadow, at the park, by a stream or mountain or some other place of beauty and peace. Just imagine yourself really there and use your child like imagination or even just pretend that you are there.

Once you are there, then it is time to give yourself positive suggestions such as, "I'm a happy person", "I love myself ", I'm a success in everything I do", "I have lot's of energy", "I am calm and relaxed", or give yourself, your own positive suggestions. To awaken, simply count to your-self from one up to five, and then say to yourself out loud a few times, "I'm wide awake with lot's of energy"!
Open your eyes and wake up with a big smile.

COUNTING BACKWARDS FROM 100 DOWN MISDIRECTION

Once you have a person is a relaxed state of hypnosis, you might want to try this deepening technique that works great with intellectual people who might consciously try to figure out every word that you are saying. As you are doing your progressive relaxation technique, have give the client the suggestion of counting slowly, silently to themselves from one hundred backgrounds trying to get down to zero.

Tell them that "with each exhale you take think to yourself, deeper asleep, and with each exhale you take, the numbers will grow further and further away from your mind and memory and simply just disappear, as though they were being wiped off the a chalk board in a classroom and before you reach number 27 the numbers have gone, and you go deeper into the hypnosis sleep".

As the client is breathing in and out and thinking of numbers, start giving his or her positive suggestions or even some more suggestions of relaxing their body and mind. This technique creates conscious confusion and can be the breakthrough in hypnotizing a resistant subject. It also helps to put a person's conscious mind on the back burner by giving it busy work to follow and therefore allowing the hypnotist to communicate to a person's subconscious mind with conscious interference or conscious resistance.

TOUCHING THE TOP OF HEAD DEEPENING TECHNIQUE

Another way to sometimes create a very deep level of hypnosis is to suggest to your client after you have hypnotized them and performed a progressive relaxation technique or another deepening technique, is to say to the client:

"In a moment, I am going to touch the top back of your head. When I touch the top back of your head, I want you to imagine with your eyes lids still closed, your eyes looking up towards the top back of your head right where I am touching. When I touch the top of your head, simply allow your eyes to look up with your eye lids still closed, imagine that it is going to happen and when I touch your head, allow it to instantly happen"

This physical deepening technique can work well at producing somnambulism and very deep hypnosis. An indication of deep hypnosis is R.E.M. and also when the eyes balls of a subject moves up as though they are looking up at the top of their head. You can sometimes notice the whites in their eyes and may not even see their eyeballs because they are looking up.

Most hypnotherapists have never heard of this type of counting backwards technique, as it is one of the many techniques that I have thought of over the past years.

ARM DROPS ON LAP DEEPENING TECHNIQUE

This is a very simple deepening technique that you can use. First you hypnotize the subject and say to them after they are in a reasonable depth of hypnosis that you are going to come up to them and lift up their left (or right) hand, and that you want them to keep their hand and arm very relaxed and not to help you lift it up in the air. You will tell the subject that when you drop their hand down unto their lap, they will go 10 times deeper asleep.

"In a moment, I will come up to you and I will lift up your left hand and arm. I don't want you to help me lift it up; I want you to completely relax it like a loose limp rubber band. When I drop your hand onto your lap, you will go 10 times deeper asleep, and every time that I lift your arm and hand up, it will become more and more relaxed and you will go deeper and deeper asleep. I will now lift up your hand and arm at the wrist and you make it completely relax. You are doing perfect. Relax it more, and now when I drop it down on your lap, you will go Ten Times deeper asleep". (Drop the hand down and when it drops onto the subject's lap say) *"Sleep. Deeper and deeper asleep."*

EYE LIDS STUCK DEEPENING TECHNIQUE

Once you have hypnotized a person, tell them that you want them to imagine that their eyelids are stuck and glued together and that the harder they try to open them, the tighter they will squeeze and shut.

"When I count to three, I want you to squeeze your eyelids shut so tight, that they will become stuck and locked together. Stuck and locked together. On the count of three, squeeze your eye lids shut tight and locked tightly together, as though there is a vice and clamp around them getting tighter and tighter stuck together".

"One...Two...Three...Now squeeze your eye lids shut tight, locked together as though they are glued shut and stuck tighter and tighter

and tighter and tighter and even if you wanted to open them, you can't and won't because they stick tighter locked together as though there is a vice and clamp holding them stuck together and let that tightness in your eyelids represent stress and tension and on the count of three, I want you to relax your eye lids and drift 20 times deeper into the hypnosis relaxation".

"One...Two...Three...Now relax your eyelids and let your lower jaw muscles relax and go 20 times deeper a sleep with each and every exhale you take".

LOWER JAW RELAXATION

Every time that I hypnotize a person in a private hypnotherapy session or on a national television show, I always have the client/subject relax the lower jaw muscles. Some hypnotist might miss the boat, if they do not relax a persons jaw muscles. The jaw is usually one of the first places on a person's body to tense up and one of the last places on the body to relax. After I conduct a progressive relaxation on a client I might suggest to the client the following:

"I will now count from five down to zero and when I reach zero, I want you to relax the muscles in your lower jaw and simply let your mouth drop open. Imagine a feel as though you have a little weight, attached to a string attached to your lower jaw and that this little weight is tugging and pulling down on your lower jaw to open and relax now. Five, feel your lower jaw and mouth opening up and relaxing.... four...as though there two little weights attached to two strings attached to your lower jaw and mouth. Your lower jaw and mouth are opening and relaxing more and more with each exhale. Three think to yourself now, "I give myself permission to relax my lower jaw and to open my mouth. My lower jaw and mouth are more relaxed and my mouth is opening more and more" "Now two, you are deeply relaxed and hypnotized. One, your lower jaw is totally and completely relaxed and open as you go into a deep hypnotic sleep".

STIFF & RIGID ARM TEST

This provides a good test that the subject is in hypnotic trance.

When you think he is sleeping soundly, lift up his right or left arm to a horizontal position and say to him:

"Your.. arm .. is .. suspended .. up .. and .. you .. cannot .. drop .. it .. try .. as .. hard .. as .. you .. will. Try .. try .. hard! You .. cannot .. move .. it .. at .. all."

If it remains up against his efforts to lower it, you have a good indication that he is hypnotized. This arm-stiffening test for hypnotic sleep can also be used to deepen the trance state. Suggest:

"You .. cannot .. move .. your .. arm .. because .. it .. is .. so .. stiff .. but you .. will .. find .. it .. begins .. to .. feel .. so .. tired .. it .. is .. commencing .. to .. slowly .. drop .. down .. to .. your .. lap .. and .. as .. it .. drops .. down .. you .. will .. go .. deeper .. and .. deeper .. asleep .. in .. hypnosis .. and .. when .. it .. finally .. reaches .. your .. lap .. you .. will .. be .. deeply .. asleep .. in .. profound .. hypnosis. You .. will .. be .. profoundly .. hypnotized."

POSTHYPNOSIS

One of the most important phenomena is posthypnotic suggestions. These are deferred suggestions given to the subject during a hypnosis session that will take effect after the subject wakes up from hypnosis.

The subject, while in trance, is given a suggestion that he is told he will perform after he is aroused from the trance. The deeper the hypnosis, the greater will be the success of posthypnotic suggestions. When he is recalled to his waking state, he has no recollection of having received any instructions, but at the time stated or when the circumstances arise, he will proceed to do what has been suggested to him while he was hypnotized.

The suggestion is carried out by the subject usually by them accepting or thinking such as being his own motivation for performing the action. All phenomena that can be hypnotically produced while the subject is in hypnosis can equally occur as a posthypnotic experience. Posthypnotic suggestions are invariably used in all forms of hypnotherapy in which the client is given suggestions that carries over into his daily life for personal benefit.

It is marvelous that this is so otherwise the use of suggestive therapeutics would be extremely limited. That is to say, if suggestions only had influence over a person while in trance, their therapy value would be limited. It is through post-hypnosis that the value of hypnotic suggestions can carry over to aid in the daily art of living.

HOW TO AWAKEN A SUBJECT FROM THE HYPNOTHERAPY SESSION

Since hypnosis is induced by a process of suggestion affirming ideas of going to sleep, it stands to reason that reversing the process by presenting suggestions for the removal of sleep and awakening from the trance is bound to remove the hypnotic condition, i.e. awaken and/or arouse the hypnotized person.

The arousal from hypnosis should always be a gentle process, just as you would want if someone were to awaken you from a deep sleep. Just keep in mind that in inducing the hypnotic condition, you presented your suggestions slowly and with care so apply this same gentle calm approach to the removal of the hypnotic sleep. Remember also, as a hypnotist it is your obligation to always arouse the subject feeling fine and well in every way.

Having caused all the suggestions of your hypnotic experiments to fade away from the mind of the subject and suggesting that he is sleeping peacefully present these suggestions:

"All right, I'm going to count from one to FIVE. When I reach the count of FIVE you will be wide-awake feeling fully refreshed. One, you feel very calm, peaceful and relaxed. Two, feel your breathing start to slowly change as you take a deeper breath in. Three. Breath in a feeling of feeling so good, so refreshed, and so relaxed, and feel your energy slowly coming back. Four, starting to awaken up with a great big smile feeling so good and peaceful and now, five, open your eyes and wake up feeling great. Eyes open and wide awake feel so good and with lots of energy, wide awake".

Under the influence of these suggestions, your subject will gradually open his eyes, move about, stretch himself and awaken feeling fine.
Occasionally, you may run into a subject who enjoys being in hypnosis so much they do not want to arouse from hypnosis right at that moment and that is okay. That is of no concern. You can say to the subject that, "when you are ready to awaken, you will simply open your eyes and wake up. Just allow an opportunity for some more moments

for the hypnosis to be enjoyed. Left entirely to himself, the subject will soon pass from the hypnotic sleep into natural sleep and will awaken on his own accord exactly as he does on arising each morning following a refreshing night's sleep. If left alone in hypnosis, a person will also convert from hypnosis to a natural sleep and will than awaken from the natural sleep feeling fully refreshed.

STANDING SHOCK INDUCTION HYPNOTIC TRANCE

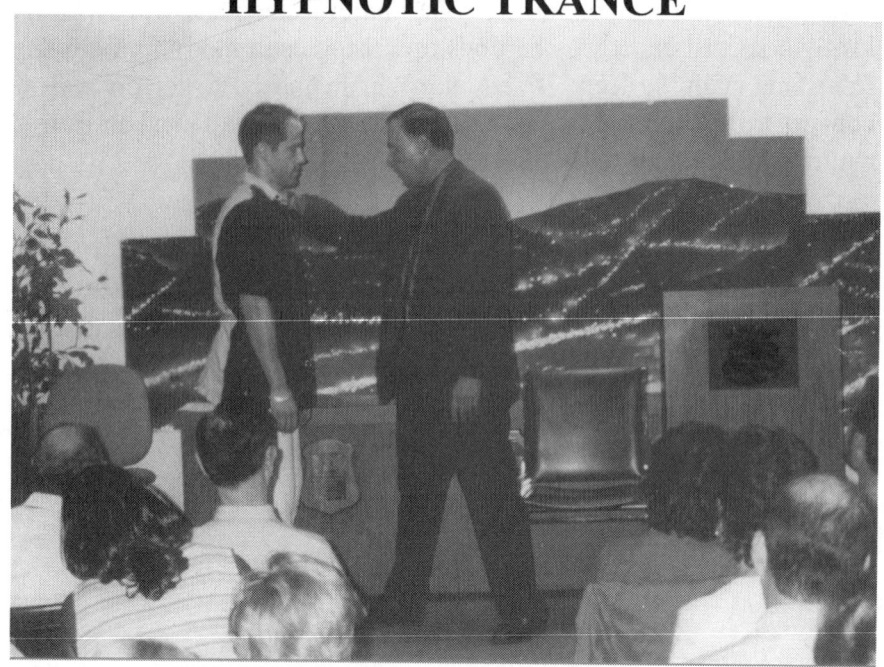

(INSTANTLY HYPNOTIZED BY TOM SILVER)

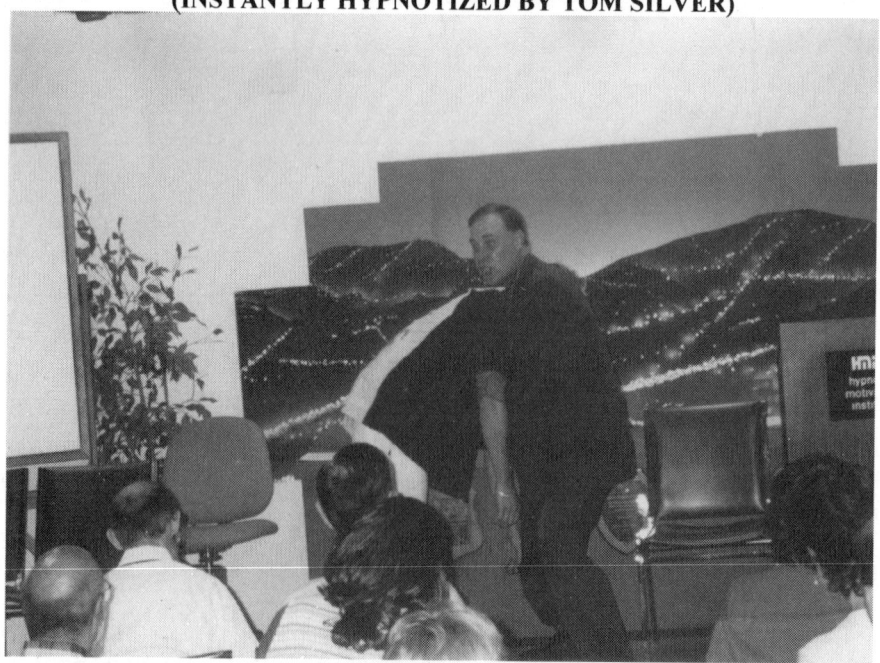

TOM "PULLS" THE SUBJECT INTO INSTANT TRANCE

CHAPTER TWENTY-TWO

INSTANTANEOUS METHODS OF HYPNOTIZING RAPID * PHYSICAL * SHOCK INDUCTIONS

To be able to hypnotize instantly shows that the hypnotist has become a master of giving suggestion-like commands. Such methods must be given with complete confidence. The entire process is forceful. It is well to learn how to induce hypnotic sleep at first by slower methods; when you have developed complete confidence in your ability to hypnotize, then you can try these methods.

HANDS PULL TOGETHER SHOCK INDUCTION

Have the client sitting down in a chair facing you and tell him/her to hold their hands straight out in front of them, their palms of their hands facing each other. Their hands and arms straight out in front of them palms and hands facing each other with their fingers straight out facing straight ahead. Tell the subject/client that you are going to instantly hypnotize them, and get their permission to be hypnotized. Make the agreement that I had spoke about.

Tell the subject/client to take 3 breaths in and out and on the third exhale close both of their eyes. Once the subject/client closes their eyes, tell them to imagine that there is a large magnet in the middle of their hands, and that this is a powerful magnet, and to imagine that their hands are coming closer and closer together. Keep repeating the suggestions that their hands are moving closer and closer together.

Then say that as soon as you pull on their hands they will instantly become hypnotized. As soon as their hands are about ready to touch each other, quickly pull on both of their hands and shout the words "sleep" as you pull on their hands towards you, the client will drop down forward in their chair. Then say "You are now deeply hypnotized, going deeper and deeper asleep with every exhale".

When I lift up your hand, and let it drop down, you will enter down 10 times deeper asleep. Now you are using a deepening technique.

LOOK INTO MY EYES INSTANT RAPID INDUCTION

Tell the subject that you are going to hypnotize them instantly.
Have the subject seated in a chair and place palms of hands on their lap.

Have the subject close his or her eyes and say to them the following:

"In a moment I will touch you on your shoulder, and when I touch you on your shoulder, you to open your eyes and to look into my eyes". "When you look into my eyes and I say the word "sleep", your eyes will close, your head will instantly drop down, your body will instantly relax and you will enter into a deep hypnotic sleep".

"As soon as I touch you on your shoulder you will open your eyes, look into my eyes, I will say the word sleep and your eyes will close, your head will drop down and you will become instantly deeply hypnotized".

Now touch the subject on their shoulder and tell them to look into your eyes. As soon as they open their eyes, you look directly into their eyes with your face only a few inches away from theirs and say the word "SLEEP" and at that same time, you push down on either their left or right shoulder in a firm manner and say, *"eyes closed, head and body relaxed and deeply hypnotized".* The subject's eyes will close and their body will instantly drop down into a deep relaxed sleep.

HAND PULLS OUT OF CLIENTS HAND SHOCK INDUCTION

Have client hold one hand out palm facing downwards and your hand out under theirs with your palm facing upwards. Tell the client that you are going to instantly hypnotize them. Have them push down on your hand with theirs as hard as they can and say that you will push upwards on their hand with your hand.

Tell them next to look directly into your eyes and then say.

"Feel your eyes getting heavy, droopy, drowsy, sleepy, closing, closing, closing", and then suddenly slip out hand out from under theirs and as you do that, snap your fingers of the other hand and at the same time, say "sleep" and push down gently on the top of the clients head with your hand. This rapid overload process works really well at

inducing deeper stages of hypnosis very quickly.

THE REVOLVING HANDS INDUCTION

Have the subject/client sit in a chair and tell them that on the count of three, you want them to start revolving their hands around each other going towards them and say that when you say the "reverse" they will reverse the movement of their hands going around each other away from them and every time you say reverse, they switch the direction of revolving their hands and when you ask them to enter into hypnosis, their hands will instantly drop down and they will go deep asleep.

Then say

"123 start revolving your hands around and around and around"
Look at your hands going around and around, faster and faster, now (snap finger) reverse the movement. Going faster and rounder and faster and faster. (Snap Finger and say) Reverse the movement, (Snap Finger); Reverse the movement and now faster and faster, (Snap) reverse the movement, (Snap) Reverse the movement, now "Sleep".

The key to this being that after they reverse the movement, you say to the client, faster and faster, reverse, faster and faster, reverse, reverse, reverse, faster and faster, reverse, reverse, reverse, faster, reverse, reverse, then touch their forehead with one hand and push lightly down on the back of the head and command the word "Sleep" you are deeply hypnotized". This is an overloading rapid hypnotic induction that creates confusion and great results.

HAND CLASP PHYSICAL "PUSH DOWN" RAPID INDUCTION

Perform the handclasp demonstration by having the subject look at his hands as he clasps them tightly together. Suggest to him to squeeze his hands tightly together. Squeeze them so tightly together that his hands are becoming stuck and locked together. So tightly stuck together that even if he wanted to open them he can't because they are stuck like a vice or clamp and keep suggesting, getting tighter. As you are repeating these words quickly, go up to the subject and push his locked hands down quickly unto his lap saying at the same time. "Sleep" and when the subject hands fall onto his lap say "Deep Asleep" and push the lower back of his head gently down. Rapid hypnosis.

HAND PULLS INTO FACE INDUCTION

Have the subject seated in a chair and tell them to lift up their left hand and place it about one foot away from their face with the palm of that hand facing their face.

Have them look at it and say the following:

"Now close your eyes and imagine or visualize that there is a powerful magnet in the palm of your left hand and a powerful magnet on your forehead and face and that your hand and arm is pulling closer and closer to your face as though it is magnetically drawing closer and to your face and forehead and when your hand touches your face, it will rest and relax on your face and be stuck to your face and you will then reach your peak of concentration to allow me to hypnotize you".

"You notice your relaxation in your other hand and arm resting on your lap as your left hand and arm pulls and tugs closer and closer to your face as though there are five strong powerful magnets on each of your fingers of your left hand, lifting, rising, pulling and tugging closer and closer to your face".

"When your hand touches your face, let it relax on your face or forehead and imagine that it is stuck and glued to your face. If your hand has already touched your face or forehead, let it rest and relax on your face and if it is not touching your face now, let it come closer and closer, pulling, lifting, tugging closer and closer and now just let your hand touch and rest on your face".

When the subject's hand touches their face, you say:

"You have reached your peak of concentration to allow me to hypnotize you and when I touch your shoulder, your hand will instantly drop down on to your lap, your neck muscles will relax and your head will instantly drop down and relax, and you will enter into deep hypnotic sleep, becoming instantly deeply hypnotized".

Now touch and push down on the subject's shoulder and say the word "sleep" in a forceful manner. If the subject is receptive to your induction, their hand will instantly drop onto their lap, their head will drop down, as there neck muscles relax, and they will be instantly hypnotized.

REVOLVING PENDULUM PHYSICAL INDUCTION

Have your subject hold a pendulum up in front of them while they are sitting in a chair and tell them to concentrate as they are looking at the pendulum to start moving back and forth, in and out, back and forth and in and out. Tell them to think of nothing else, except the pendulum moving back and forth. Tell them to close their eyes and to really concentrate on the pendulum going back and forth and inn and out.
Say the following:

"The Pendulum is moving now, more and more. Getting bigger and wider, moving more and more, and now it's moving in a circle going rounder and rounder, and bigger and bigger, and rounder, and rounder as though the pendulum is now moving in a circle getting bigger and bigger and rounder and faster and bigger and rounder and faster and faster".

As you notice the pendulum moving more and more, it means that the subject is really now concentrating and ready to go into a deep hypnosis sleep.
Tell the subject

"In a moment I am going to have you open your eyes and look at the pendulum moving which means that you are ready to get deeply hypnotized".

"When I say the word "Sleep" and tell you to close your eyes, your eyes will close, your head will drop down and you to enter into a deep hypnotic sleep. Now open your eyes and look at the pendulum"!

As soon as the subject opens their eyes and looks at the pendulum, say as you touch the top back of the subject's head *"Sleep"*, close your eyes, *"Sleep"*, deeply hypnotized as you push down on the client's head or shoulder and they drop down instantly asleep.

THREE HANDSHAKE INDUCTIONS

A famous hypnotherapist named Dave Elman use to teach this method to medical doctors and dentists. It goes something like this.

Tell the subject, who is seated facing you in a chair, with knees close to yours, but not touching yours:

"What I am going to do is to hypnotize you by shaking your hand three times. The first time I shake your hand, I want you to allow and imagine your eye lids are getting heavy and that you are getting relaxed, but don't close your eyes". The second time I shake your hand, you will feel your eyelids becoming very heavy and you will have a strong desire to want to close your eyes, but don't". The third time I shake your hand, your eyes will instantly close, your head will instantly become lose, limp and relaxed and you will enter into a very deep hypnotic sleep becoming deeply hypnotize. Do you understand? Good. We will now begin".

"Look into my eyes and now shake my hand. Feel your eyelids getting heavier, imagine it and let it happen. Okay your doing perfect. Now shake my hand again and look into my eyes. You are becoming very relaxed and sleepy and you want to close your eyes but you can't until I shake your hand again. Getting very sleepy and tired. Imagine it and let it happen".

Now stop shaking the subject's hand and say to the subject as you look deeply and directly into their eyes.

"I will now instantly hypnotize you. Shake my hand".

Grab the subject's hand and pull on it hard, kind of jerk it but don't hurt them and command)

"Close your eyes"!
"Sleep, deeply hypnotized".

"Deeper and deeper asleep with every exhale as your body becomes loose and limp like a rag doll. Every time I shake your hand, look you in the eyes, snap my finger or say deep a sleep, you will enter into this deep peaceful hypnotic relaxed sleep".

THE ONE HANDSHAKE INSTANT INDUCTION METHOD

I have modified this induction into a simpler method that I call The One Handshake Instant Induction Method.
I say to the subject:

"I will instantly hypnotize you by shaking your hand and look into your eyes. When I shake your hand and look into your eyes, your eyes will close, your head will drop down, your body will pull forward and relax, and you will instantly become hypnotized. Nod your head "yes" to allow me to instantly hypnotize you by doing everything that I ask you to do without thinking.

If the subject nods his or her head "Yes", you are now ready to instantly hypnotize them in just one simply handshake and you simply say to the subject now:

"Look into my and shake my hand now".

When the subject looks you in the eyes, shake his or of course her hand and as you shake their hand, pull their hand towards yourself and say in a commanding and controlling voice, *"Close your eyes, Sleep!"*

EYES OPEN AND CLOSED RAPID INDUCTION

Tell the client that you are going to hypnotize them by having them close their eyes and when you count to three they will open their eyes. When you snap your fingers, they will again close their eyes. Every time you count to three, they will again open their eyes, and then close them when you snap your fingers again.

Every time you snap your fingers, the subject will close their eyes. Next you start to confuse your subject by counting one, two and then pausing for a moment (Subject may open eyes) and then quickly say three and snap your finger.

What you want to do is to confuse your subject by counting and pausing and snapping. When you think that you have created enough overload, touch the subject shoulder with one hand and put your other hand on the subjects front top of head and say sleep.

The subject will relax his head forward and drop it down into your hand. Next you might rub the lower back of the neck muscles to relax the neck and head. Tell the subject to relax every muscles, nerve and fiber in their body and allow their body to go lose and limp.

INHALE AND EXHALE RAPID INDUCTION

Tell the subject that sit in a chair with their hands resting on their lap and to look straight ahead of them. Tell the subject that you will lift up your hand and arm up and down in front of them and that each time your hand and arm goes up, to take a deep breath in, and each time your hand and arm goes down to exhale the air out, and that when you tell them to close their eyes, their eyes will close, their head will drop down instantly and they will enter into a deep hypnotic sleep. Now begin and each time you move you hand and arm up or down, say the words, inhale, now exhale, inhale, exhale, inhale, exhale.

Do this maybe five to seven times and then say in a commanding directing voice, *"Close your eyes! "SLEEP"!* And while you say sleep, push gently the top of their head down with one of your hands and put the other hand on the subjects shoulder or low on the lower back of the subject's neck and say *"Relax every muscle, nerve and fiber in your body and allow your body to go lose and limp like a rag doll"*.

THE EYE CLOSURE METHOD

This method is dominated by the suggestion, *"Close your eyes, you are asleep."* You must give the command in a quick voice. Capture the attention of the subject fully and do not remove your eyes from him until he is in trance. If the suggestions are given in a quick voice in a positive manner, accompanied by a steady gaze of the eyes to those of the subject, this rapid method of inducing hypnosis works wonderfully.

THE SUDDEN SLEEP METHOD

Use a subject you have hypnotized previously and have him take a seat in a chair. Ask him to look you in the eyes. Look at him steadily for about fifteen seconds without saying a word, and then suddenly shout, "SLEEP!" positively. You can make a pass as you say it with both hands directly before his eyes. His eyes will close and he will drop instantly into hypnosis.

THE CHAIR "BUMP" METHOD

Tell the subject you are going to cause him to fall back into his chair and go to sleep. This is the suggestion. Have subject stand in front of his chair. Make sure the chair is directly behind him so he can fall back into it safely. Ask the subject to close his eyes and to concentrate on your suggestions:

"Your chair is right behind you. Think of falling back into it. Already you feel an impulse pulling you over backwards to sit in that chair. You are going to fall back. Your knees are bending and you are falling back to sit in that chair. Sit down in the chair. Back, back you go. Sit down! Sit down! Sit down!"

The subject will begin to sway, falling backwards. Emphasize that he bend his knees so he can fall right over backwards into his chair. He will drop into his chair with a decided "bump". The moment he experiences this "bump" in dropping into his chair, shout:

"SLEEP! GO .. TO .. SLEEP .. THIS .. INSTANT!"

The bump causes a jar. Immediately grip the subject's head and rotate it around several times. This deepens the instant hypnosis.
Then push his head down into his lap and state:

"You are in deep hypnosis now. Sound asleep."

These hypnosis induction techniques are very good at producing profound hypnosis in just a few minutes or less. After you have mastered these inductions, you will have a library of knowledge and techniques that you can successfully use on your clients to produce deeper stages of hypnosis, and we believe that the more profound the depth of hypnosis, the more receptive is the subconscious mind for accepting positive suggestions and emotions.

HANDS PULL TOGETHER INDUCTION

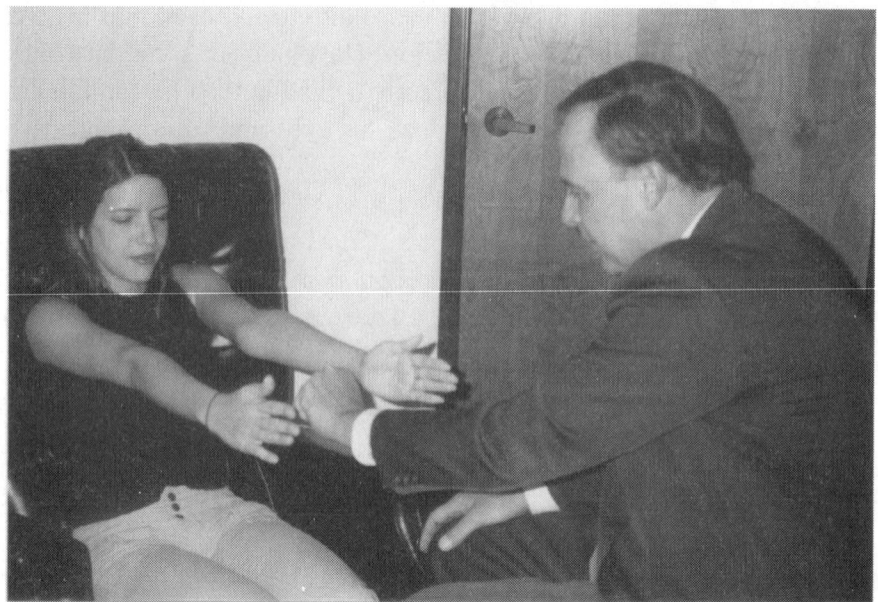

SUBJECT IMAGINES THAT THERE IS A POWERFUL MAGNET IN THE MIDDLE OF BOTH OF HER HANDS CAUSING HER HANDS TO PULL IN

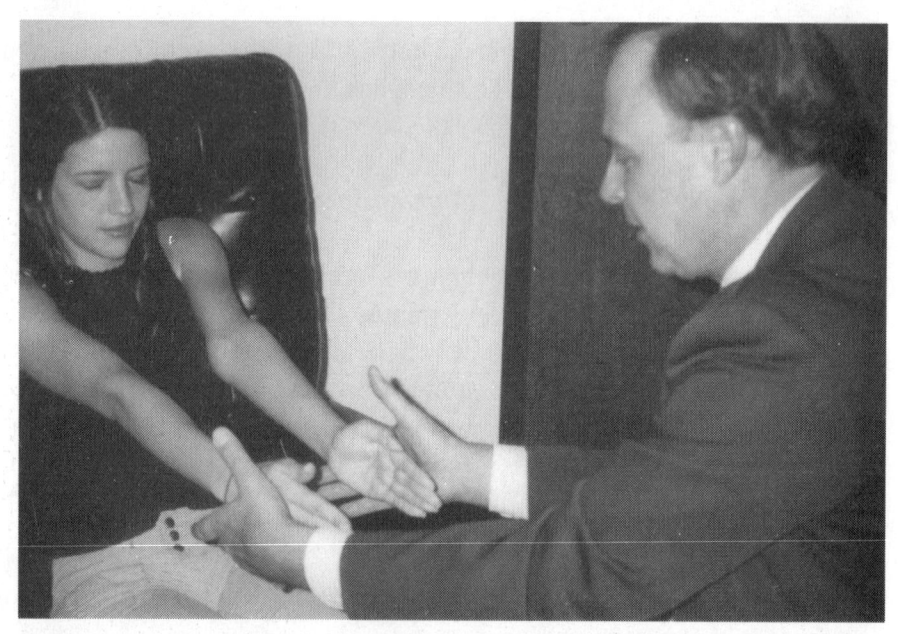

HYPNOTIST PLACES HIS HANDS ON THE OUTSIDE OF THE SUBJECTS HANDS AND GIVES SUGGESTIONS OF THE SUBJECTS HANDS TUGGING AND PULLING CLOSER AND CLOSER TOGETHER

HANDS PULL TOGETHER INDUCTION

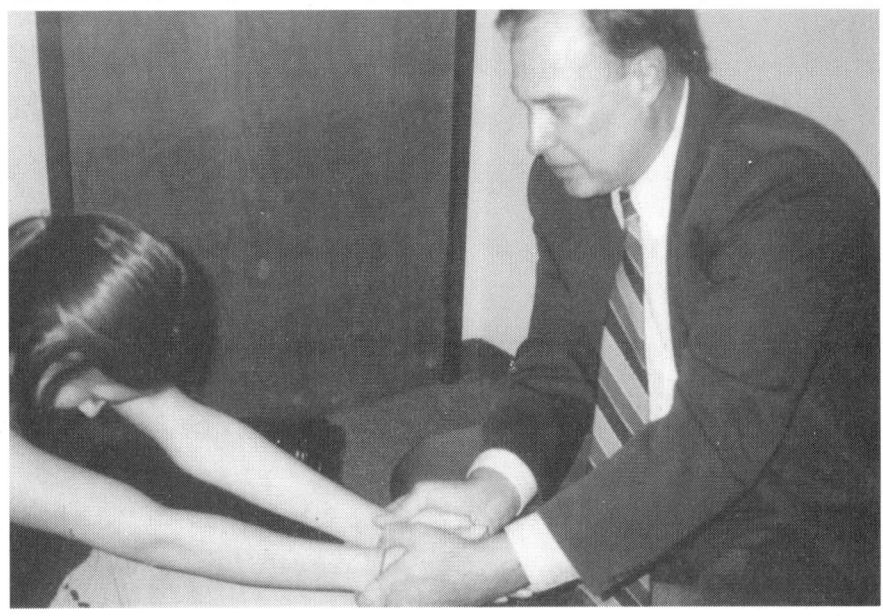

PHOTO THREE
AS THE SUBJECTS HANDS ARE READY TO TOUCH EACH OTHER THE HYPNOTIST PULLS ON THE HANDS OF THE SUBJECT WHILE PULLING THE HANDS TOGETHER AND DOWN ANS SAYS "SLEEP"

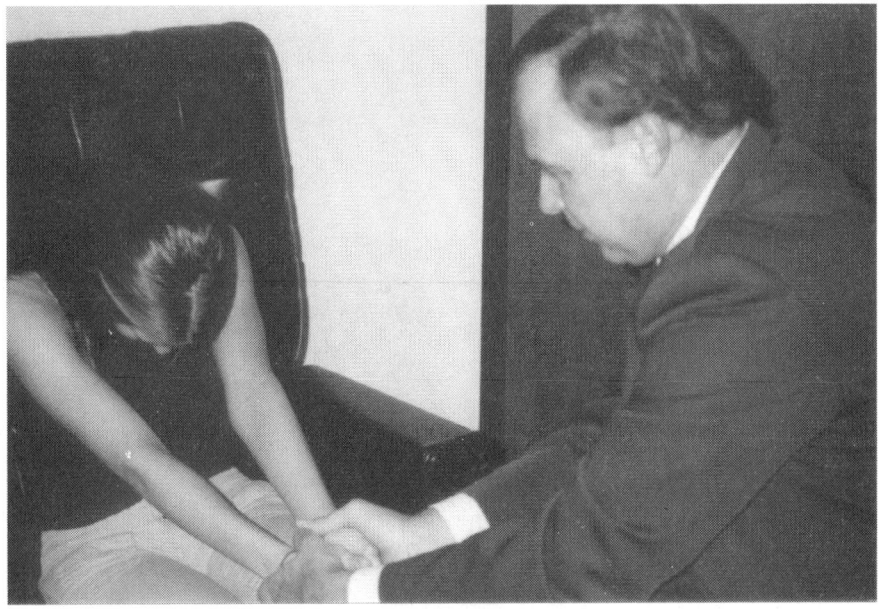

PHOTO FOUR
THE SUBJECTS HAND'S DROP ONTO HER LAP AS THE HYPNOTIST GIVES THE SUGGESTION AND COMMAND OF GOING DEEP ASLEEP

THE REVOLVING HANDS INDUCTION

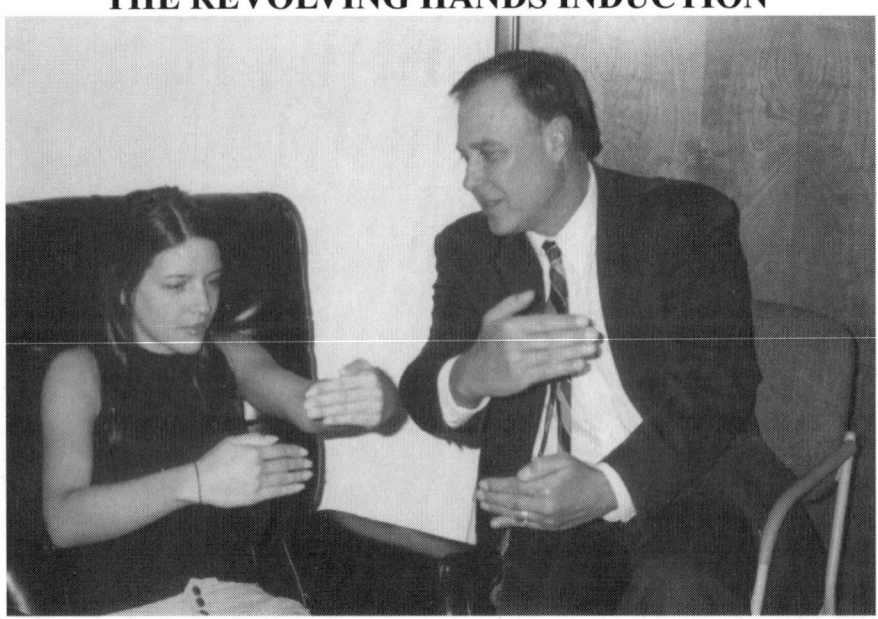

PHOTO ONE
HYPNOTIST ASKS SUBJECT TO LOOK AT HER HANDS AND TO REVOLVE HER HANDS AROUND IN A CIRCLE TOWARDS HERSELF WHILE SHE IS GAZING HER FULL ATTENTION ON HER HANDS MOVING IN A CIRCLE

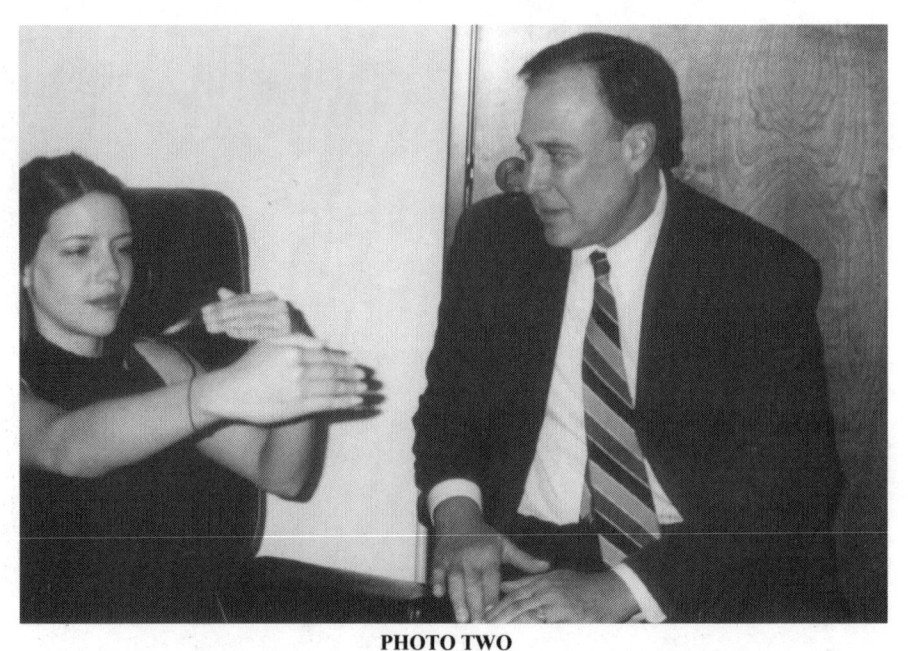

PHOTO TWO
HYPNOTIST ASKED THE SUBJECT TO REVERSE THE MOVEMENT OF HER HANDS EVERY TIME HE SAYS THE WORD "REVERSE" AND TO MOVE HER HANDS FASTER EVERTIME THE HYPNOTIST SAYS THE WORD "FASTER"

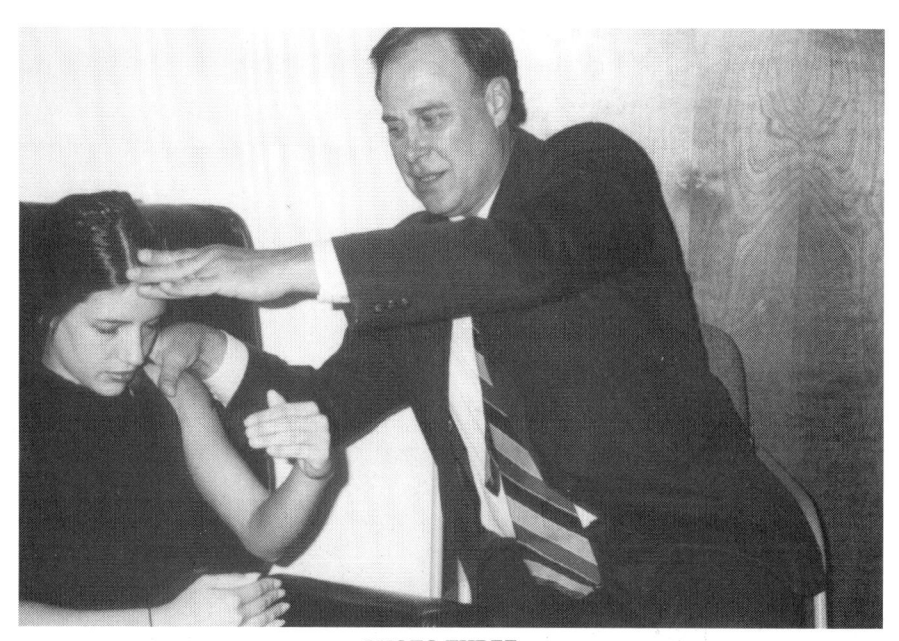

PHOTO THREE
THE HYPNOTIST SAYS TO SUBJECT "AS SOON AS I TOUCH YOU ON YOUR SHOULDER, YOUR HANDS AND HEAD WILL DROP DOWN AND YOU WILL INSTANTLY ENTER INTO THE HYPNOTIC SLEEP AS YOUR BODY RELAXES"

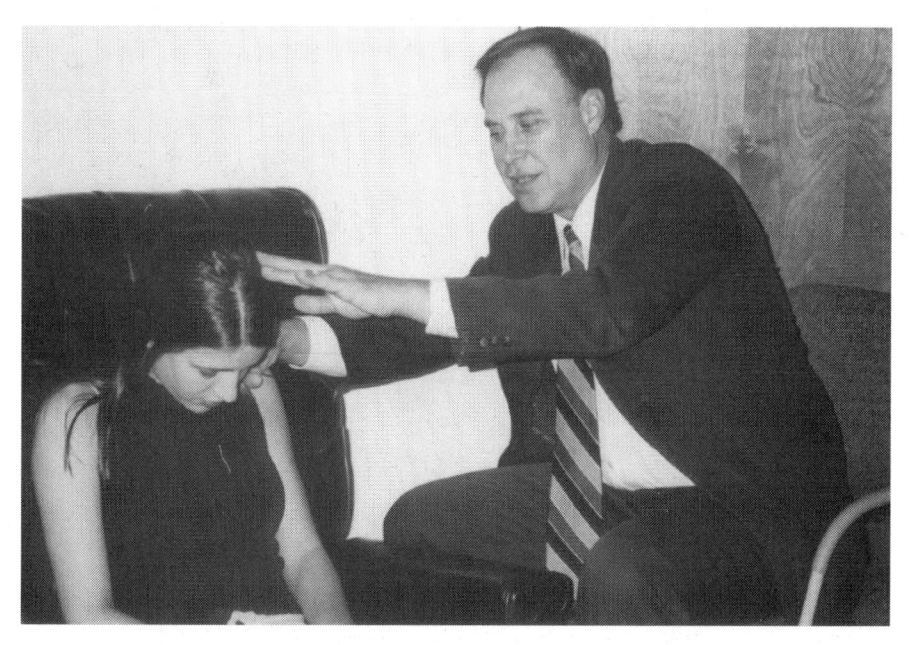

PHOTO FOUR
THE HYPNOTIST PUSHES DOWN ON THE SUBJECTS SHOULDER AND DOWN ON THE BACK TOP OF THE SUBJECTS HEAD AND SAYS "SLEEP" THE SUBJECT IS INSTANTLY HYPNOTIZED AS THEIR BODY RELAXES THEIR HANDS WILL DROP DOWN ONTO THEIR LAP INSTANTLY!

SWINGING PENDULUM INDUCTION
RAPID HYPNOSIS INDUCTION METHOD

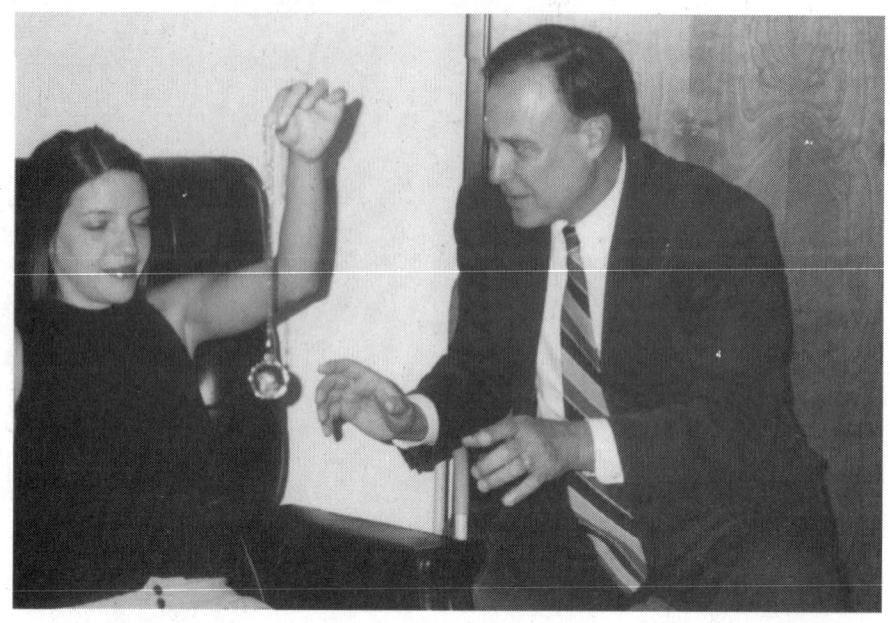

THE HYPNOTIST ASKS THE SUBJECT TO IMAGINE THAT THE PENDULUM IS STARTING TO SWING AND MOVE

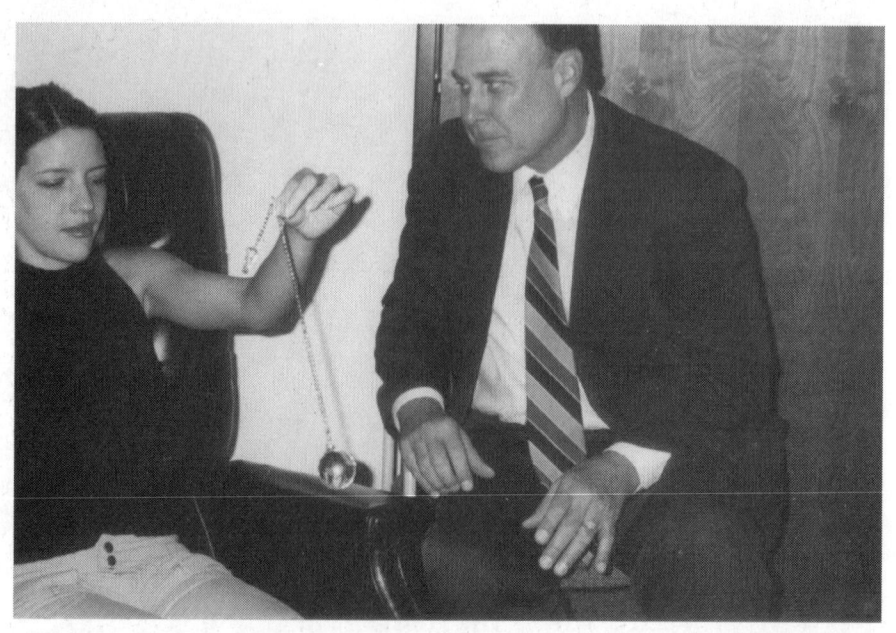

HYPNOTIST SAYS THAT THE PENDULUM IS NOW SWINGING AND MOVING BIGGER AND WIDER AND MORE AND MORE

SWINGING PENDULUM INDUCTION
RAPID HYPNOSIS INDUCTION METHOD

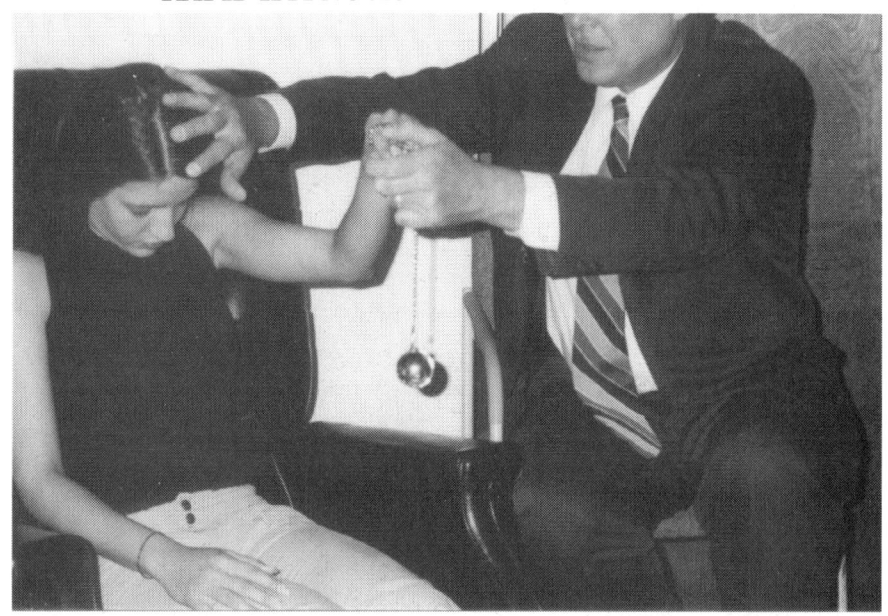

THE HYPNOTIST PULLS THE PENDULUM OUT OF SUBJECTS
HAND AND WITH OTHER HAND TOUCHES TOP OF HEAD

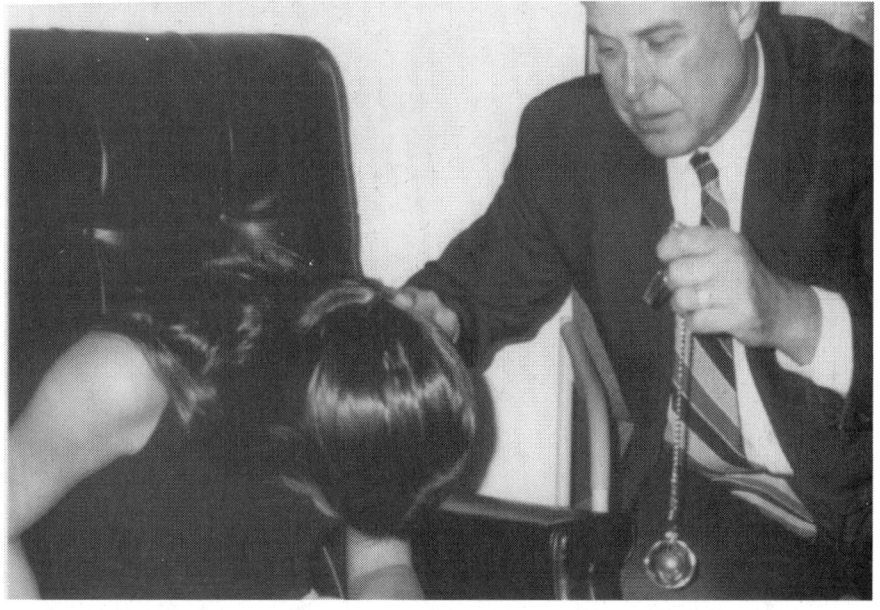

HYPNOTIST SAYS "SLEEP" AND PUSHES DOWN ON SUBJECTS
SHOULDERS AS HE HOLDS THE PENDULUM IN OTHER HAND

INHALE AND EXHALE RAPID HYPNOSIS INDUCTION METHOD

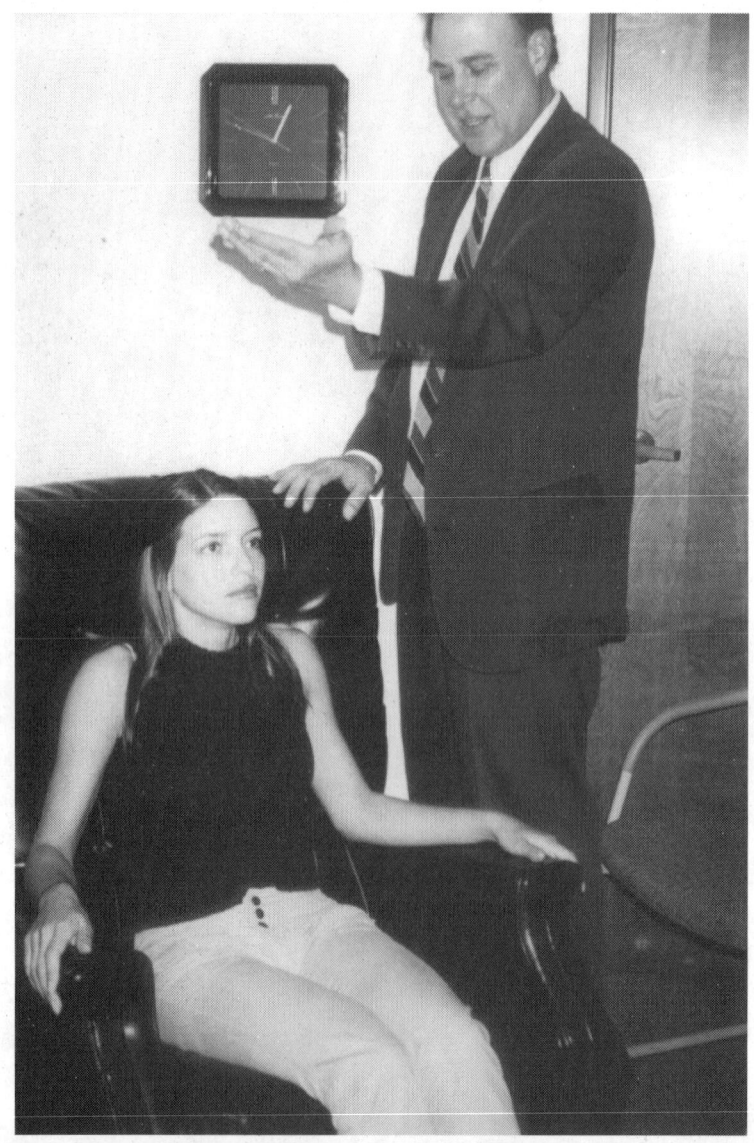

THE HYPNOTIST SAYS TO THE SUBJECT:
"WHEN I ASK YOU TO CLOSE YOUR EYES AND I SAY THE WORD "SLEEP"
YOUR EYES WILL CLOSE AND YOU WILL INSTANTLY BECOME HYPNOTIZED"

THE SUBJECT IS THEN TOLD TO INHALE EVERYTIME THE HYPNOTIST LIFT'S HIS
HAND UP IN THE AIR AND TO EXHALE EVERYTIME THE HYPNOTIST BRINGS HIS
HAND AND ARM BACK DOWN IN FRONT OF THE SUBJECT

CHAPTER TWENTY-THREE

HYPNOSIS DEVICES AND TOOLS

HYPNOTIZING BY FASCINATION

Have subject seated directly in front of you and tell him to lay his hands on his knees, which should be in contact with yours. Lay your own hands on top of his firmly. Now ask him to look you in the eyes steadily without blinking and to think of going to sleep. Keep gazing at his eyes until they close. Through your eyes as you stare at him, express the command of your thought, i.e. "SLEEP".

The subject will drop into deep hypnosis by this eye fascination method. The look of resignation seen in the subject's eyes just before going to sleep is striking.

Deaf people can use this method with advantage. They should be given to understand, before hypnotizing, that by your given signal (like touching the neck twice or something similar) they will awaken.

MUSIC AS AN AID TO HYPNOSIS

Using music as a background to your hypnotic induction process will be found effective. Just as the singing of a lullaby by the mother puts the child to sleep, so does soft music lull adults. Use a soft, meditative sort of music such as the kind easily obtained in cassette form from esoteric bookstores. Keep the music soft so it does not intrude upon your verbal "suggestion formula". Used subtly, it aids the induction of trance.

An interesting experiment with music that you can try is to give a subject a posthypnotic suggestion that when a certain piece is played, he will immediately drop down deep in hypnosis.

MECHANICAL DEVICES FOR INDUCING HYPNOSIS

There are various devices available for inducing hypnosis such as revolving spiral discs, strobe lights, whirling mirrors, etc. These are used as the "fixation object" upon which the subject is requested to concentrate attention.

The subject is requested to be seated in front of the device, which is illuminated in a darkened room, and to concentrate on the device. The principle is the tiring of the optic nerve. After five minutes or so of concentrating attention on the effective instrument, the eyes close and sleep ensues. Tell the subject what is expected and his imagination will do the rest.

Mechanical devices for inducing hypnosis are effective when working with several people at the same time, however for most purposes they are not necessary. As a hypnotist, come to rely on your own personality, not mechanical devices.

HYPNOTIZING WITH A CANDLE

In a sense, hypnotizing using a candle is a "mechanical device" but it is a very subtle one, as candles have long been associated with transcendental and religious ceremonies.

Seat the subject in a chair in a darkened room. Light a candle and set it within two feet of the person's eyes. Set it up high enough so he has to look upward to the flame. Now, make a mark about a half an inch (or less) from the top of the candle and tell the subject positively that when the candle has melted down to the mark indicated he will be sound asleep. Impress on him the necessity of watching the flame with both eyes steadily. If he does not close them of his own accord by the time the candle has burned down to the mark, close them for him gently with your thumbs and suggest that they stay closed and he cannot open them, that he is ASLEEP.

Then present a "sleep formula" and make passes without contact over the body of the subject. Hypnosis is soon induced.

Hypnotizing by candlelight will be found an effective method to hypnotize people who find it difficult to concentrate. The flickering flame seems to exert a fascination that is hard to resist.

TIMOTHY * TOM * ORMOND MCGILL
N.G.H. Conference Banquet Dinner 2002

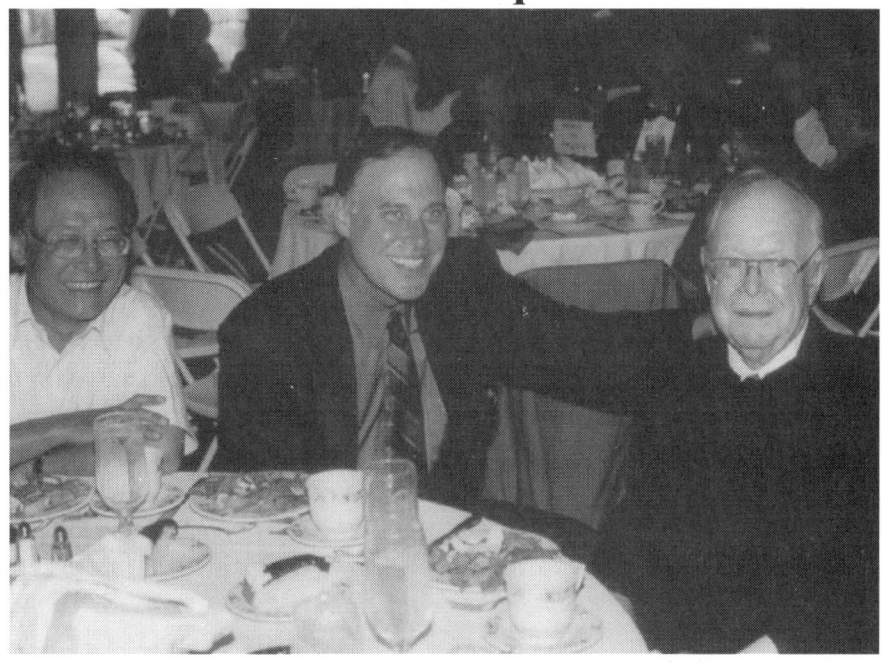

ORMOND MCGILL TEACHING
HYPNOSIS INDUCTIONS

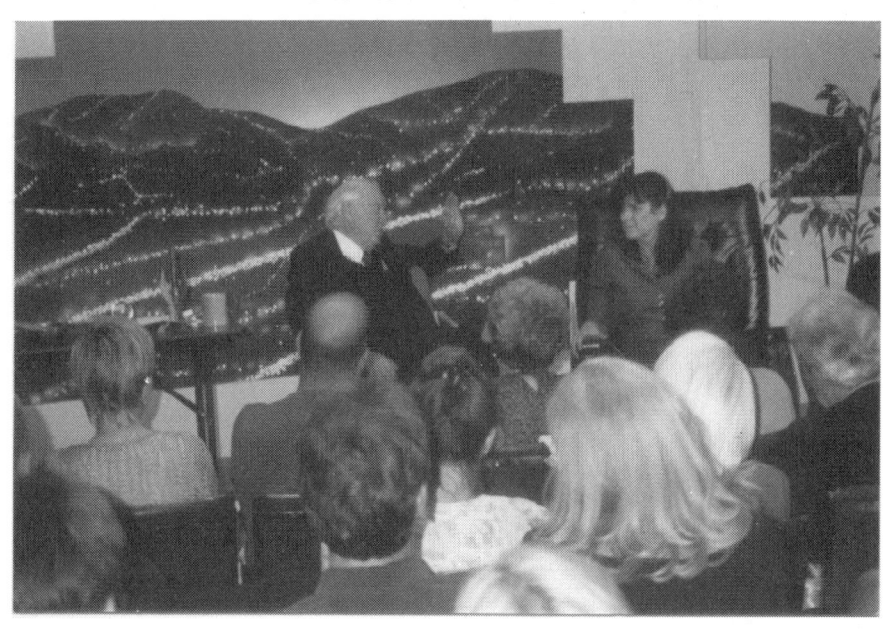

CHAPTER TWENTY-FOUR

HYPNOTIC INDUCTIONS FOR GROUP HYPNOSIS

Especially in presenting stage demonstrations of hypnotism will group hypnosis be employed. Here are three methods of hypnotizing any number of persons at the same time:

METHOD ONE

Seat subjects in a semicircle. Give each one a bright coin to hold and tell them to look at it without moving their eyes from the shiny coin for even an instant. Then stand to one side and after a few minutes say:

"As .. you .. stare .. at .. the .. shiny .. coin .. your .. eyes .. are .. getting .. heavy .. you .. cannot .. keep .. them .. open .. any .. longer ... they .. are .. closing .. closing .. now .. and .. you .. are .. becoming .. so .. drowsy .. and .. sleepy. Go .. to .. sleep .. now, .. etc."

Give sleep formula until they are all in hypnotic sleep.

METHOD TWO

Have the subjects seated in a semicircle. Stand in the center before them. Now say:

"Look me straight in the eyes and think of sleep".

(Look from one to another and then straight ahead and it will seem to each you are looking straight at him.)

"Now .. close .. your .. eyes .. and .. as .. I .. count .. up .. to .. ten .. you .. find .. your .. heads .. are .. getting .. heavy .. and .. you .. will .. be .. sound .. asleep. One .. two .. three .. four .. five .. six .. seven .. eight .. nine .. TEN. Fast .. asleep .. sound .. asleep .. sleepy drowsy .. fast .. asleep. Your .. heads .. are .. so .. heavy .. you .. cannot .. hold .. them .. up .. any .. longer. You .. are .. fast .. asleep."

Continue these suggestions until all heads of persons in the group fall over and rest on chests. Go to each person in turn and place your hand on top of his or her head as you exclaim, *"SLEEP!"* You have hypnotized the group. Some may even fall off their chair. Each will act according to their nature.

METHOD THREE

Have your subjects all seated in a chair with their feet on the floor and their hands on their lap. Tell them that you are going to hypnotize them instantly and to do everything you say. We discussed this method earlier in this textbook on a one on one application. This method works great also with groups of people all at the same time. Here it is.

"Look down at your hands and on the count of three, close your eyes. One...Two...Three...eyes...closed. With your eyes closed hold both of your hands straight out in front of you with the palms of your hands facing the sky. On the count of three imagine that there is a heavy steel ball in the palm of your left hand...on the count of three...instantly drop your left hand down on your lap...one...two...three...steel ball in the palm of your left hand left hand dropped onto your lap...on...the...count...of three...imagine that your right hand is attached to a bouquet of helium balloons and on the count of three...your right hand and arm will lift all the way up into the air...imagine it...and let it happen when I reach three...One...Two...Three...right hand and arm floats all the way up into the air...now in a moment...I am going to go up to you and touch you on your shoulder...when I touch you on your shoulder...you right hand and arm will instantly drop down onto your lap and you will go into a deep hypnotic sleep... When I touch you on your shoulder...and say the word...sleep...you hand will drop down...you head will drop down...and you will enter into a deep hypnotic sleep"...

You then simply go up to each person and push down on their shoulder saying the word "sleep" forcefully and watch your subjects instantly drop down into profound hypnosis. A group induction that will hypnotize a large percentage of everybody there is what can be accomplished through this group induction method.

METHOD FOUR

The mechanical device of the revolving mirror or hypno-disc is used in this method. Place the device on a stand in the center of a group seated in a semicircle. Start it going and tell them to watch it and never to remove their eyes from it. In a few minutes, give suggestions for closing of the eyes; then proceed into "sleep formula". After they are in trance, remove the mirror and you are ready to give performance suggestions. A revolving hypno-disc will also work well as a mechanical device. These types of devices have been known to make some people feel dizzy or even sick and should be used with caution.

HOW TO DEEPEN THE HYPNOTIC SLEEP

Having hypnotized the group, with all heads resting forward on chests, you can deepen the hypnotic sleep by these methods:

"Breathe .. in .. deeply .. now. Inhale (pause) *.. Exhale* (pause) *.. Breathe .. in .. deep .. and .. free .. and .. every .. breath .. you .. take .. will .. cause .. you .. to .. go .. deeper .. and .. deeper .. into .. hypnosis. Deep .. deep .. to .. sleep. Fast .. asleep."*

Go to each subject in turn and lift up his or her right hand as you state:

"When .. I .. release .. your .. hand .. it .. will .. fall .. directly .. to .. your .. lap .. and .. when .. it .. falls .. into .. your .. lap .. you .. will .. be .. fast .. asleep .. in .. deep .. hypnosis."

Go to each subject in turn and lift up his or her hand by gripping the thumb. Let their hand dangle for a moment from the thumb and then release the thumb so that their hand drops into their lap. The moment it hits their lap, state forcefully:
"SLEEP! YOU ARE DEEP ASLEEP!"

Another method of deepening hypnosis is to go to each subject in turn and start revolving his or her head around and around as you state:

"Each .. revolution .. of .. your .. head .. sends .. you .. down .. deeper .. and .. deeper .. into .. hypnotic .. sleep. SLEEP .. DEEP. You .. are .. in .. profound .. hypnosis."

CHAPTER TWENTY-FIVE
By Tom Silver Hypnotherapist

HYPNOTHERAPY SUGGESTIONS FOR CLIENTS

CONFIDENCE

Put the client in as deep a state of hypnosis as you can. Now say to him:

"You are now becoming more confident in yourself because you are learning to use your mind and to control your mind to work for you more every day. You are the master of your mind and your confidence in yourself is becoming strong and powerful because you love and respect yourself more than every before. You realize that you are now allowing one hundred percent of your mind to work for you. All fears of the past are gone and replaced with a peaceful feeling of inner real confidence in everything that you say and do. You are 100% confident in yourself from now on and no one including your old self or negative suggestions from others can ever lower your confidence."

Breathe in a feeling a feeling really good and allow a smile of confidence to grow on your face and lips right now. Every time that you smile from now on, it will increase your confidence in yourself. You are the master of your life and now a true believer in yourself because both of your minds are now working for you. Just as the waves break on the shore, your confidence will simply continue to grow and your confidence is now with you all the time. You feel good about yourself now and the past is over. Everyday you love and respect yourself more and more and enjoy being the leader of your life. Think to your self right now, "I am a person who loves being confident and happy". "My confidence now makes life worth living and I feel really good". "Every-time that you smile from now on, your smile will increase you confidence and love for life"...

Repeating of positive suggestions has a compounding effect on mastering the disease. In hypnotherapy, always repeat suggestions eight or ten times in a positive, earnest, convincing manner. Put your heart and soul into the work. A strong will and desire will accomplish wonders. Believe as a hypnotherapist that you can indeed increase your client's confidence, and you will.

RELAXATION FROM STRESS

Put the client as deeply into hypnosis as possible and suggest the following:

"You are now in a deep relaxed hypnotic sleep, and all the stress and tensions of the day are now gone. Melted off your mind and body, just like wax melts off a candle. From now on, you will now be a calm and relaxed person. Imagine right now that your body was like one hundred lose and limp rubber bands and you feel a feeling of calmness from the top of your head, all the way down to the tips of your toes. Every muscle, nerve, fiber and tissue in your body is now totally relaxed. You enjoy this feeling of total relaxation and no one or anything can ever bother you again because you do not let things get to you. Feel a feeling as though you are floating on a cloud of relaxation.

"You also know that as you are in control of your mind and body now, you will not allow your mind to play tricks on you ever again. Stress and worry are a waste of your time and enjoy being the person you have always wanted to be, calm and relaxed, calm and relaxed. Imagine yourself looking at a calm beautiful lake in your mind and notice how calm the water is, and that calmness is now you everyday, calmer and more relaxed of a person. Yesterdays gone and tomorrows a thousand miles away, and all that matters now is to enjoy life and to enjoy your new happier and healthier self, relaxed, calm and happy and becoming a healthy person. Think you yourself right now".

"I love this feeling of being relaxed". "Little things will not upset me anymore". "Every time I think the word "Relaxed", I relax instantly". "I am now a more relaxed and healthy person who enjoys life as a miracle and the greatest miracle now is that I am in-tune with feeling relaxed, healthy and happy. Everyday and in every way I am learning to control my mind and body and to be a person who can block stress, tension and worry's out of my life". You are now becoming more of a calm and relaxed person with your mind sharp and clear and with lots of positive energy. And now go deeper asleep".

SLEEP DEPREVATION

Induce as deep a hypnotic state as possible. Then say to the client:

"You are now bathed in a deep relaxation and your conscious mind is now resting and quiet and silent. As you go deeper asleep with each exhale, your entire body relaxes from the top of your head, all the way down to the tips of your toes. Imagine yourself in your mind seeing yourself lying in your bed at night sleeping deeply and peacefully. Deeply and restfully. See how calm you look, and how your entire body is bathed in relaxation. Sleeping deeply and peacefully the whole night. Every time that you are now ready to go to sleep, all you have to do is to simply close your eyes and imagine a gentle wave of relaxation moving from the tips of your toes all the way up to the top of your head. Your entire body and mind will relax with each exhale that you take and you will drift into a wonderful deep and peaceful sleep, sleeping deeply the entire night, unless you need to wake up".

"You are in control of your mind now, and you can tell it what to think and when to think. You can also tell it when to stop thinking and simply relax. Imagine right now in your mind, that you are watching a television show. See in your mind, that you are watching a television show, and imagine that the show represents your over- active conscious mind at night. I want you right now to go over to that television show and simply shut it off. Shut it off right now, and nod your head. Good.

From now on when you are ready for bed and close your eyes, simply think of turning off that chattering television set, and as soon as you imagine yourself pushing the off button, or pushing the off button of your remote control, your conscious mind will instantly become silent, quiet and will stop thinking thoughts and every exhale you then take will send you into a deep, peaceful, restful sleep. Every night when you sleep, you will sleep, deeper and better. Deeper and more restful and in the morning, you will awaken with lot's of energy."

FOCUS AND CONCENTRATION

Induce as deep a hypnotic state as possible. Now say something like this to the client.

"You are now becoming more and more relaxed with every exhale you take and your subconscious mind hears and accepts every word that I am saying to you. Your focus and concentration on the words that I am saying is perfect and because you can concentrate on my words so well, you will find that your focus and concentration during the day is now also becoming better and better, because you are in control of your minds to work for you. During the day, at work, you have perfect focus and concentration and your mind is sharp and clear. Whenever you are involved in a project at home, or at work (or school), you can concentrate now on that project with 100% of mental focused concentration. Your concentration and focus is now 9 times stronger and more powerful".

"Think of a magnifying glass and how powerful that is. Think about how a microscope or a telescope can see things very clearly, and how strong and powerful they are. Imagine that your focus and concentration is now like a microscope and is sharp and clear".

"You now can stop your mind from wondering, or from thinking to much while you concentrate. You can stop your mind from thinking thoughts and allow complete focus and concentration at once from both of your minds. Your conscious mind and your subconscious mind. During the day your mind is sharp and clear and your focus and concentration is perfect".

MEMORY RETENTION

Have client deeply hypnotized and then present the following suggestions:

"You are acquiring a strong and power mind and memory and everyday, your memory is becoming stronger and powerful. Just as a sponge absorbs water, your mind and memory absorbs knowledge. Whenever you want to retain information, you simply think of your mind as a powerful computer and everything that you see, read, or study can be instantly accessed into your long-term memory. Imagine sitting down on a chair in front of a powerful computer on the table or desk and imagine that this powerful computer is your long-term memory. Imagine that there is a dial on the computer and above the dial, is the word memory. As you look at the dial, you notice that there are numbers from one up to one hundred. These numbers represent your memory retention ability".

"Your dial is set right now at the number ten. As you are looking at this memory dial, I want you to now turn this dial all the way up to one hundred. Turn the dial up now to one hundred now. As you are turning it up now to one hundred, you are turning up your memory and retention ability up to one hundred. Every time you study or want to learn information that is important to you, your mind is sharp and clear and your memory is strong and powerful. Every time you want to bring up the knowledge and information, you now have instant access to your long-term memory, just like accessing information from you computer. You are in control of your mind and your memory is becoming stronger and more powerful each and every day".

WEIGHT LOSS

As a hypnotherapist, you will find that many clients will be coming in to see you to help them lose weight. The key to being healthy is not only losing weight, but in being fit. A thin person might not be a fit person. Being fit, means that your inner body is healthy. You heart is strong. Your arteries are free from fat, grease and being clogged up. Your circulation within your body is functioning properly. You have a chemical balance within your body. Being fit does not depend on how thin and malnourished you are.

There are people that appear to look overweight or physically challenged, and these people might be more fit and healthy on the inside, than the person who is underweight. If you look at body builders or competitive heavy weight lifters, these athletes are totally fit, but they have big powerful bodies also.

You want your client to get in shape and have a good balance in their weight, body and bone structure. And most of all, the key again is to be healthy and fit. Most people have emotional weight issues and if you separate the emotions from food, sometimes that's all it takes. There are three different types of eaters. These types are emotional eaters, subconscious eaters, and conditioned eaters. An emotional eater eats food because of emotions such as stress, frustration worry, loneliness, boredom, pain, as a reward, as a punishment, to fill a relationship void. Over seventy percent of all weight related issues are based on repressed emotions or frustrations.

The next type of eater is a subconscious eater who eats food and does not even know how much they are eating. These subconscious eaters may eat a whole half a gallon of Ice Cream while watching a movie or snacking on a whole bag of potato chips watching television, or may be putting food in their mouths at work during the day, without even being aware that they are shoving food in their mouths. The operation is subconscious and not conscious.

The third type of eater is a conditioned eater who was programmed from early childhood to finish everything over on their plate because people are starving in other countries. In the past, some people had difficulty acquiring food and food was scarce, so these parents made their children feel guilty if they left food over, or even insisted on their children not leaving the dinner table until every piece of food on their plate was eaten. This type of eater feels guilt, if they leave any food over on their plate.

Here are some hypnotherapy suggestions that you can give your clients to help them lose weight.

"You are now taking healthy control of your life and the foods that you eat. You realize that fatty, greasy foods and foods with sugars and chemicals are harmful to your body. You also realize that you are now going to allow yourself to eat good healthy foods that now taste better than ever and more natural to you".

"Foods with vitamins, nutrients, and minerals are more appealing to you than ever before. Your body is the place that your mind worships in, and you now want your body to become healthy and free from the old fat and weight that has been stored in it".

"Think to yourself now, I will now separate all emotions from food, and I am taking control of the foods I eat and what I put into my mouth. I am now fuller with smaller portions of food. I love drinking lots of water. I chew my food slowly. I love eating fruits and vegetables. I will never again eat unhealthy food without thinking. I am now aware of every piece of food I put into my mouth. Everyday and in everyway, I am becoming the person that I always knew that you I was. Free from fat and in control of the foods that I eat. When you sit down to eat a meal from now on, you will choose to eat healthy foods, smaller portions of food, and you will become fuller, faster with smaller portions of food. You enjoy drinking fresh water, and the taste of fresh water, tastes better and sweeter".

"During the day, you have more energy and you can burn up the old food that has been stored up in your body as fuel and energy, just as wax melts off a candle. Every day you are feeling lighter and

healthier. Think to yourself now, my motivation to exercise or walk is also now becoming stronger and I just don't think of exercising, I now enjoy exercising and feeling healthy".

"No more putting off my health till tomorrow or creating excuses that are only fooling myself. I am making a commitment to trade weight, sickness and death, for health, vitality, energy and happiness. Nothing and no food is going to stand in the way of me looking and feeling the way that I always have known I would look and feel".

"Anything, or emotion that has stood in the way of you losing weight is now gone, just as the ocean moves out to the sea. You have control over your mind and you have control of what you put into your mouth and body and you feel proud that you are now one hundred committed to letting all of the old weight go".

"You have more love and respect for your body than ever before and you know that you are now creating a new healthy relationship with eating healthy foods which now taste better than ever before".

"When you sit down to eat a meal, you will choose healthy food to eat, enjoying the taste of fruits and vegetables and good healthy foods. You will take you time to chew your food slowly, enjoying the taste of healthy foods, and when you have had enough food, you can simply stop eating feeling nothing for any food that is left over on your plate. You simply can stop eating now when you have had enough food to eat and not when you feel stuffed or sick. You are in control of what you put in your mouth and the thoughts you think. You enjoy being your true thinner, healthier, happier self".

I am giving you some of the suggestive techniques that I have created and found useful in my private practice. You should also be aware of the way I turn my suggestions from second person into first person. From you are, to I am. Most hypnotherapists give hypnosis suggestions in the second person and I feel that suggestions that are used in combination from second person to first person really help to make the subconscious respond more. It is good to say to your hypnotized client,

You love to exercise and you enjoy eating healthy foods. But think about how powerful it is when you have your client repeat after you silently to him or herself while they are hypnotized. That suggestion is increased to its effectiveness. Now imagine the impact if you now said to your client while they are relaxed and hypnotized, repeat the following to yourself silently after me "I love to exercise and I enjoy eating healthy foods. My mind is sharp and clear. I have lots of energy.

I am in control of the food that I eat. I love myself". This technique works real well and will give you more success with your results. Think about how powerful conscious affirmations are and how they are used in so many areas of life to stimulate conscious motivation and desire. Now think about those conscious affirmations being 90% more powerful and effective because under hypnosis, they are going directly in the action part of our mind, which of course is your subconscious mind. This is turning suggestions into action by activating the positive emotions and desires of your client.

MOTIVATION TO EXCERCISE

Induce as deep a state of hypnosis as possible, then suggest:

"You will find that you love to exercise your body and enjoy exercising more and more every day. Anytime you know think of exercising, your thoughts turn into action and you are more motivated to become healthy and you really feel good every time that you walk, or go to the gym".

"There is no more resistance towards being healthy because you know that you want your body to work well and to be strong and powerful and all sabotage is gone. You will not create excuses any more or put off your health till tomorrow or next week, or next year".

"You are creating a positive healthy pattern of exercising and you feel great about your decision to have your body and mind in tip top shape. Imagine yourself right now at the gym, or walking, or exercising at home. See a big smile on your face. See you looking happy, confident and feeling great. Repeat silently to yourself after me. I love to exercise. I am in control of the foods that I eat and my body is now becoming more healthy and fit. I have lots of energy when I exercise. No one is going to stand in the way of my health. I fell great every time I exercise (ride my bike, walk, work out, etc)".

"Your imagination will now become reality and you will allow yourself the freedom to exercise more and more. You also find that your energy level is now becoming better, with more and more energy every day".

"Breath is a feeling of feeling proud of your decision to really love exercising and allow a smile to grow on your face right now. That smile represents that you are creating a positive healthy habit and exercising now is fun, exciting and enjoyable and you will create a

positive routine of exercising at least three or four times a week. Nothing and no one, including your old lazy self of the past, is going to stand in the way of you having a great looking body that is fit, healthy and strong."

SPORTS ENCHANCEMENT

Induce as deep a state of hypnosis as you can and suggest:

"Now you realize that your enjoying for playing (whatever their sport is) "golf" is because you are enjoying the game of golf more and more. Each time you play golf or practice, your focus and concentration on the game is becoming perfect. You are more confident in your abilities and your body moves freely every time you swing and hit the ball. During a game or competition, you are calm and relaxed with a happy and positive attitude, and all distractions during your game are gone, because the sounds and noises around will not disturb you in any way, in fact, it will increase your focus and concentration".

"Think to yourself right now, I love playing golf (sport). My body moves easily when I hit the ball. My mind is completely focused on my game. My concentration is sharp and clear. I give myself permission to simply do the best I can. I now have more enjoyment when I play golf (my sport). All fear or worry about winning is now gone. I am successful at playing well. When I play golf (sport), I am always in the zone. I enjoy playing "golf"(sport) more and more every day. You are elevating your level of successful sports up to 100% and letting go of all stress and self-doubts. You now enjoy and love playing "golf"(your sport) more and more and your performance and pleasure of the game allow you the freedom to simply do the best you can".

"With your eyes closed, see yourself in your mind, getting ready to hit the golf ball, and see you swinging and hitting the ball exactly where you want to hit it...now see the ball landing, and nod your head yes. Good".

"You will now elevate your level of sports success and consistency, because both of your minds are working for you now and all mental blocks have disappeared, just like ice that melts into water. Every time you smile, it will increase your focus, concentration and confidence in playing "Golf"(your sport)".

"When I count to five, you will awaken with a smile of confidence on your face, and that smiles represents that you have elevated your level of success and enjoyment in playing golf and every other sport that you perform and play".

SUCCESS MOTIVATION

Hypnosis is a great tool to help increase a person's motivation to accomplish a goal. How many people belong to a health gym but never seem to have the motivation to go and work out? Many people lack motivation and without motivation, which is a subconscious driving force, many people fail. Think of Motivation, as an emotional driving force.

Most peoples motivation are directed though negative habits and patterns. Procrastination is the opposite of motivation. Thinking of excuses why you can't ask for that raise or start your own business may simply relate to you not being motivated towards success. If our subconscious mind is not programmed to work for you, it is conditioned to work against us.

This is called a limited life program. Most people have limited life programs because their minds are not working together as one. Your subconscious mind identifies and associates with your conscious thoughts. How many silently give themselves negative suggestions. "I can't do that". "She won't like me, so why even try". "What if I fail or lose?" etc.

Deeply hypnotize a client and use suggestions such as the following.

"You are now very deeply relaxed. Your subconscious mind is becoming responsive to my positive suggestions. You are now allowing a new and healthy motivation to come into your life which will help you to take positive and healthy control of your mind and thoughts and you know that you are not going to let your mind play anymore tricks on you. A motivation to be successful is starting to grow inside you and is now going to drive you and allow you the freedom to have the motivation and confidence that you need to be successful in everything you do and in every area of your life. You love and respect yourself more and more every day and no one even your old lazy fearful self is going to stand in the way of you getting what you deserve which is the best of everything".

"Think to yourself silently after me, I love myself. I am a success in everything I do. I have complete confidence in myself. My motivation drives me to succeed. I love being more successful everyday. Every time I smile, it increases my confidence in myself. I am becoming more successful everyday. All my fears of the past are gone and can't come back. I enjoy my game of life. I am master of my mind and my mind works for me. I am a witness to my thoughts and the operator of my mind. My mind works clear and sharp. Fear and worry is a waste of my time. I love being and feeling successful in everything that I do, in every area of my life, and in every thought that I think".

"Picture in your mind something that you have been putting off doing or a goal that you set but never reached. Now I want you to see the thing that stood in the way of you reaching your goal...now whatever was standing in the way of you reaching your goals, see it simply disappear and vanish. It's gone and can't come back even if you wanted it to but you don't want it to come back. Your old self is gone and you can accept the fact that your new healthy motivated and successful self who you really are is now here forever".

"Take a deep breath in right now and feel a feeling of being motivated. Every time that you take a breath in a feeling of feeling confident now in every thing that you do. You are now a person who is successful and happy in every thing that you do. When you are positive and simply do the best you can do, you will continuously increase your level of success. Everyday your motivation and positive energy increases and you continue to elevate your level of success up to 100%."

PAIN CONTROL

Pain can be real and pain can be imagined. There are many different types of aches and pains that people feel and the intensities of these pains vary in degree. Medical doctors prescribe many different types of painkillers to help people deal these physical discomforts. Doctors say that some of our pains are mental and are not even related to physical problems or injuries.

Hypnosis has been used for years for pain control and management. These pain relievers are called neuro peptides or mind opiates. They are pain-releasing chemicals that can be activated in the hypnotic state. Our mind and imagination can magnify pain up to levels, which might feel unbearable. There has been lots of wonderful research currently being conducted with hypnosis for pain control and some really good books out on the field of study and research. Here is a little example of the suggestions to help reduce discomfort from pain.

After inducing hypnosis, suggest:

"Your entire body is now becoming deeply and peacefully relaxed and with each exhale. You are drifting deeper and deeper asleep. Imagine a coolness surrounding your entire body, as though every muscle, nerve, fiber and tissue is your body is cooling and calming down. Imagine yourself looking at a gentle stream trickling down a small mountain, and that you are resting on a blanket right near the cool clear water".

"Imagine looking at the water, and seeing the gentle rocks with the water splashing over them as though keeping them cool, and clean and fresh and imagine that the cool water moving gently over the rocks represent yourself being cooled and relaxed throughout your entire body... and with each exhale, all the stress and discomfort is being released and replaced with a cool calming peaceful feeling as you imagine yourself still looking at the cool clear stream, imagine an area of your body, that you felt discomfort or pain in, and imagine that this cool water is gently moving over that area and cooling that area down, cool. Calm...relaxed...feeling peaceful...just as though you have instantly switched off all discomfort and replaced it with feeling cool, calm, relaxed, good and peaceful"...

"Every day, your body becomes healthier and works better...and ...all...discomforts...will leave more and more...

STOP SMOKING SUGGESTIONS

To get a person to stop smoking is very difficult because many people who smoke really do not want to stop smoking and may fail with hypnotherapy because they are fighting your suggestions. Cigarettes are a duo chemical addition of sugar and nicotine. Each cigarette contains about eight grams of sugar, which is about a half of a teaspoon. To get a person off of cigarettes involves removing the two chemical addictions and the emotions and habits of the addiction. There are two different types of smokers and they are identification smokers, and replacement smokers. An Identification smoker started smoking because they identified with someone in their life who smoked. It might be a parent, friends at school, watching commercials on television and so forth. The second type of smoker is a replacement smoker. A replacement smoker is a person who started smoking to fill a void in their life. A relationship breakup or a death in the family for example may be the cause of someone starting to smoke. Many people gain weight after they have stopped smoking because they have never let go of the sugar addiction and need to replenish the sugar that they have smoked for years by eating foods with sugars such as sweets. Smokers need to wean themselves off the sugar after they have stopped smoking by using a hard candy supplement for a few weeks. Each week reducing their sugar intake for about four weeks to completely wean themselves off of the sugar addiction that was created by smoking cigarettes. Most people do not know that they are smoking and breathing in sugar.

Hypnotize your client and give them some positive suggestions of stopping smoking:

"You have made a decision to stop smoking poisonous cigarettes and you feel proud of your decision to trade sickness and death, for live, health and happiness and everyday the old habit and patterns towards smoking leaves and you are becoming free from the smoke and poison. Smoking poisonous cigarettes is just like putting your mouth over a dirty exhaust pipe of a car and breathing in poison smoke and you would never do that. Cigarettes are poison and you don't take poison anymore. Your desire is to be healthy and to put healthy things in your body. You love to now eat healthy foods and you have motivation to exercise. Everyday now your lungs enjoy breathing in fresh air. Imagine and see yourself in your mind, going through every routine in your life now without a poison cigarette because the habit, craving, addition, and desire to smoking poison cigarettes is leaving you now and it is in your past and you are no longer the person you were in the past. You are in control of your mind and you have made a decision to stop poisoning and killing yourself. You will not create any more excuses to put off your health anymore".

"You want to live a long and healthy life and no paper or tobacco is going to stand in your way anymore. No more games of Russian roulette. See yourself standing near the ocean and see that last pack of poison in your hand...now through that last pack a poison away and out into the sea...as the pack of poison splashes in the water and

moves out to sea...it is gone...it has disappeared...and the habit and addition is now gone and can't come back...think of how great is feels now, not having to smoke...and think about how healthy you are now becoming...and wiser...and more confident and happy...and breath in a feeling a feeling healthy and free of that poison forever...your smile is your confidence to never, ever go back to breathing in poison and congratulations of your healthy decision to be a non smoker forever".

COOPERATION WITH THE PHYSICIAN

As a hypnotherapist, remember your place is to be an adjunct to the physician. You do not replace the doctor. Cooperate and work with the physician. He has his ways of curing and you have yours. Together, remarkable results in curing human ills can be achieved.

NOTE: Most cases in working with physical ailments by the hypnotherapist are in response to physician recommendation as supplemental treatment or via direct referral.

CERTIFICATE OF COMMITMENT

CERTIFICATE OF COMMITMENT AND DECISION TO *STOP SMOKING FOREVER !*

I _____

ON THIS DAY _____

MAKE THE COMMITMENT AND DECISION TO MYSELF AND MY HEALTH TO <u>STOP SMOKING</u> POISON <u>CIGARETTES FOREVER</u> !

<u>I WILL STOP SMOKING NOW !</u>

THE DECISION I WILL MAKE TODAY <u>TO BE AND STAY</u> A NON SMOKER FOREVER WILL SAVE MY LIFE AND HELP KEEP ME FREE FROM THE SICKNESS, PAIN, DISEASE AND DEATH FROM CIGARETTE POISON !

I MAKE THE DECISION TO BE A NON SMOKER BY KEEPING MY COMMITMENT TO MYSELF NOT TO SMOKE POSION CIGARETTES ANYMORE

<u>I PROMISE THAT I WILL LISTEN TO MY SUBCONSCIOUS PROGRAM AND GIVE MYSELF POSITIVE CONSCIOUS AFFIRMATIONS EVERY DAY FOR AT LEAST 20 DAYS OR MORE IN A ROW</u>

_____
SIGNATURE

_____
DATE

TOM SILVER'S "CONTRACT WITH CLIENT
STOP SMOKING FOREVER!

THIS CERTIFICATE WILL HELP TO MOTIVATE A CLIENT TO STICK TO THEIR COMMITMENT TO BE AND STAY A NON-SMOKER FOREVER!
"THE CLIENT SIGNS THIS AGREEMENT AFTER THEIR HYPNOTHERAPY SESSION"

CHAPTER TWENTY-SIX

MASTERING UNWANTED HABITS

Habits can be good or bad. We want the good ones and are better off without the bad ones. Habits are usually based in bringing some kind of pleasure to the user. Once habits become solidly established as a way of behavior for the individual, they enter the realm of the subconscious and operate beyond critical thought. Hence, since hypnosis provides a direct means of controlling the subconscious, it provides an excellent means of getting rid of unwanted habits. And since habits are mainly based on a pleasure response for the individual all that is needed to get rid of these habits is to reverse pleasure for displeasure. With this understanding, here are suggestion formulas for the control of habits that you can use with your clients in hypnotherapy.

In treating habits, suggestions related to the particular habit must be used. The essential thing is to repeat each suggestion many times to produce a counter "mental set" to the habit. Positive habits are effectively obtained by the repeating of the anti-habit suggestions over and over until the habit changes occur. Patience and not haste is the essential requirement for successful treatments of unwanted (often vicious) habits.

For any form of unwanted habit to be removed, its removal must commence on the conscious desire of the one who has the habit to have it removed. The person with the habit must to change that habit.

MASTERING THE DRINKING HABIT

Before hypnotizing the client to master the drinking habit, find out the quantity of liquor he daily consumes. This done, hypnotize him and suggest:

"From now on you will only drink half of what you have been used to drinking. If you try to drink one glass more than that, it will taste like vinegar to you. You cannot drink any more than that. Every day you will care less for whisky, beer, wine and liquor of any kind. Any drink with alcohol in it is losing its appeal to you. You will learn to hate it. It will make you sick to drink it. All craving for alcoholic

drinks of any kind is leaving you. You have no desire for it anymore and the habit is leaving you. You will sleep well nights and you have no desire at all for liquor in the morning."

Repeat to the hypnotized client these suggestions for twenty minutes. Do not tell him to stop at once altogether. Reduce his allowance every day for three or four days and then tell him positively he does not care to drink anymore! Then stress how proud he is that he has kicked his drinking habit and how happy it has made everyone he loves. Tell him what a credit he will be to his family, friends and all those for and with whom he works. Spread a bright future before him as a nondrinker and appeal to his pride and ambition. Use this method when working with any client who wants to master his drinking habit.

MASTERING THE HABIT OF TAKING DRUGS (MARIJUANA, COCAINE & HEROIN)

Deeply hypnotize the client who wishes to stop drugs and directly suggest:

"When I awaken you from deep hypnosis, you will say NO to drugs forever. All dangerous drugs such as marijuana, cocaine and heroin you positively can't stand anymore. All craving is completely gone. It is easy for you to stop the habit of taking any kind of vicious drugs and you are so proud you have."

Repeat these suggestions over and over to the hypnotized person. His attitude towards taking drugs will drastically change. Sometimes the habit becomes mastered immediately. With other suggestions, a gradual cutting down until there is no more habit left works best. As a hypnotherapist, you must use your intuition as to how best to handle things. You might also require the client to seek medical consultation.

ALL HABITS CAN BE CURED BY HYPNOSIS

As habits are seated in the subconscious, hypnosis provides the perfect therapy. Drug habits, worry, melancholia, phobias and neurosis all yield to hypnotic suggestion. The list of habits that can be corrected goes on and on: kleptomania, lying, bragging, perversion, nervous difficulties, bedwetting, swearing, gambling, bashfulness, stubbornness, etc. All these and more are readily cured through hypnotherapy. The untold benefits are almost beyond comprehension, as long as the client truly desires to be cured. Desire causes the "will" to act and, if the latter is properly directed, nothing can resist the influence.

THE DRIPPING CANDLE
VISUALIZATION TECHNIQUE AND IMAGERY
BY HYPNOTHERAPIST TOM SILVER

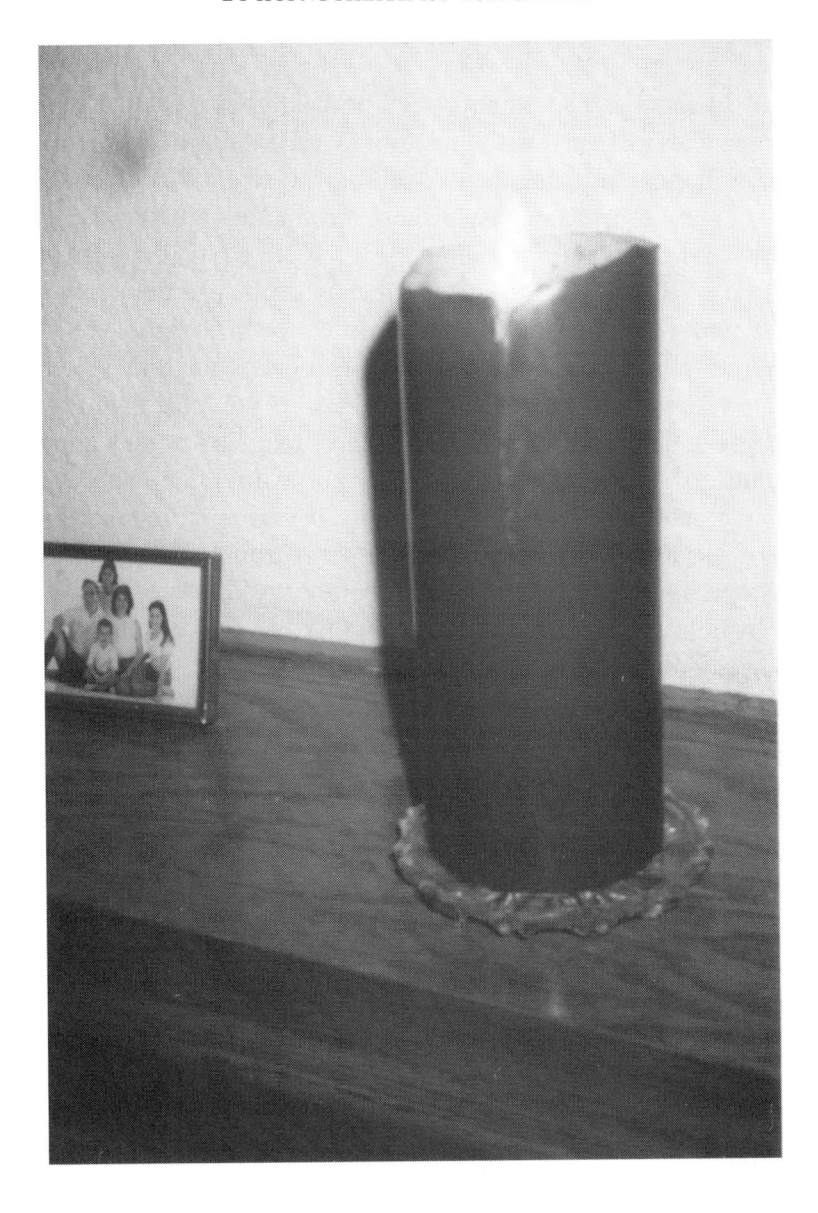

THE SUBJECT GAZES THEIR ATTENTION AT THE WAX MELTING OFF THE CANDLE AS THE HYPNOTISTS SUGGESTS THAT THE MELTING WAX REPRESENTS STRESS, TENSIONS AND WORRIES MELTING AWAY, OR THE MELTING AWAY OF NEGATIVE HABITS

CHAPTER TWENTY-SEVEN
By: Tom Silver

VISUAL IMAGERY SUGGESTIONS AND TECHNIQUES

Visual Imagery is becoming a very popular tool to help people over come obstacles in their lives. This tool is a mental tool that is based on a persons hopes and dreams, as well as the operation of imagination through creative or inner visualization techniques to activate positive emotions and motivation to help a client create a positive change, habit or pattern. We find that visualization can also be used in every day life by each and every one of us, but in order to do it right, you have to control the self-talk or suggestions that you give yourself.

If you wake up in the morning and say to yourself, I am going to have a great day, and you use your inner imagination and imagery by imagining to yourself, what a great day would feel like, you will probably create that "great day" for you. If you reinforce that image of having a great day, by saying to yourself throughout the day, "I am having a great day"; it will be an ever better day.

The trouble we have in the world is that people's visual imagery of themselves is sometimes very negative, which can be based on negative experiences in life. Most people who have a negative habit or emotion, can not use positive creative visualization by themselves, because they are to close to the situation. As a Hypnotherapist, visual imagery techniques can be very useful when working with a client. You can even create a visualization imagery suggestion when you are writing your "mental prescriptions" during the conscious cognitive part of your session. Here a few imagery techniques that I find very useful.

BLACK BOARD OF NEGATIVITY IMAGERY

With this visual imagery technique, I have a hypnotized client imagine that they are opening up a door and walking into a classroom and up to a chalkboard in the front of the classroom. I tell my client that on this chalkboard is some words written on the board that represent their old self. Here is how I would present this image to my hypnotized client:

"Imagine with your eyes closed, that you are in school and that you are going up to a classroom door and opening the door and walking in the classroom. You may even see yourself back in your classroom when you were in school. As you look in the classroom, you see a chalkboard in front of the class. Its kind of chalkboard that teachers write on. You see the eraser and a piece of chalk right next to the chalkboard.

As you walk up to the blackboard, you see that there are some different words that are written on the blackboard. These are words that represented your old negative self. See the word Loser, see the word, Lazy. See the word...fear...sad...angry...(Any words that represent the negative) and see every negative word or emotion that you have given yourself, or that others have given you. These words do not represent you, they are not you, they are just words that mean nothing to you anymore.

I want you to take that eraser next to the chalkboard and pick it up right now and erase every word on the board. Erase every negative word, thought or suggestion that you have given yourself, or that others have given you in the past. Erase Angry. Erase the word Lazy. Erase the word sad and erase the entire board right now. "Nod your head yes, if you have erased every word on the board"...*(wait for response)* "Good ...Now pick up that white piece of chalk now and I want you to write the following words down now on the chalkboard.*

Write the word...CONFIDENT (Therapist Spells the word slowly out loud), CONFIDENT, C...O...N...F...I...D...E...N...T...CONFIDENT. "You are now more confident than ever before and are becoming more and more confident, each and every day with each breath in and out in every way and because you are becoming more confident in yourself, you find that you now have more positive motivation than ever before...*

Write down on the chalkboard right now the word MOTIVATED". "M...O...T...I...V...A...T...E...D MOTIVATED.... You are more motivated to be happy and successful, motivated to be healthy and eat healthy foods...You are more motivated to stop dwelling on the past or worrying about the future...because your motivation is to live every day as a miracle and this brings in to you a new happiness that is real and powerful.*

Write the word HAPPY now on that chalkboard. H...A...P...P...Y. Because you are now a happy, healthy more confident person who enjoys every day as an adventure with more love and respect for yourself and your life, you find a new healthy motivation to be more productive and more successful in every area of your life.

Write the word SUCCESSFUL right now on the chalkboard. S...U...C...C...E...S...S...F...U...L...L. You are now becoming more successful in every thing that you do. Everyday, your confidence and motivation increases your success, making you a very happy person who can now get what you deserve in life, which is the best of everything. These words that you have written down on this imagery chalkboard represent who you real are and your true self which is CONFIDENT...MOTIVATED...HAPPY...AND MORE SUCCESSFUL IN EVERY THING THAT YOU NOW DO".

This visual imagery is wonderful for removing negative emotions and habits from the past and for re-writing a person's life script programming. This mental cleansing of negativity helps a person consciously and subconsciously reprogram emotional behavior.

DRIPPING CANDLE TECHNIQUE AND IMAGERY

This visual imagery technique involves hypnotizing your client and having them visualize that they are walking into a room where there is a melting candle in the middle of the room on a table. The candle is in a candleholder and the wax is slowly melting off and dripping off the candle. You then give the positive suggestions that relate to letting go of negative emotions, or stress and tension, or even a fear being released, by using suggestions like this:

"As you look at the candle on the table with it's wax slowly dripping down off the candle, imagine that your stress, tensions and worries, (Fear or negative habits etc.) Are now melting away, melting away, just as the wax melts off the candle...and you notice that the candle is disappearing, melting away until it completely disappears. All of your stress, tensions, and worries (Fear etc.) are now disappearing and melting away...Now you notice that the candle has now completely melted away and has dissolved and disappeared...and all of your old useless, stress, tensions and worries (Fears or negative habits), have now disappeared, dissolved, and are gone and can never come back, even if you wanted it to, but you don't and it is gone, just like the wax that has melted off the candle and the candle that is now gone, dissolved, and disappeared."

OCEAN AND WAVES "REMOVAL OF NEGATIVE EMOTIONS" VISUAL IMAGERY TECHNIQUE

This visual imagery involves hypnotizing a person and under hypnosis having them imagine that they are lying on a beautiful beach, on a blanket or towel on the sand and watching the waves breaking gently on the shore. It goes something like this:

"Imagine in your mind, that you are lying on a beautiful beach. Just imagine any beach that you can imagine or even maybe a beautiful beach that you have been to in the past. Use your imagination and imagine yourself lying on a blanket or towel on the warm soft sand...Feeling the warmth of the sun, the smell of the salt in the air, even the singing of the sea gulls as they fly by...A beautiful private beach...and as you look up at the sky, you notice there are some little black clouds in the sky.

These black clouds represent your old fears and self doubts, or negative habits or emotions...and imagine now that there is a gentle breeze now simply blowing those black clouds of negative habits or emotions right out of the sky...until they have now disappeared and they are gone...and as you notice the clear blue sky, you realize that your mind and body is now clear and free of negative emotions, or habits and the clear sky represents your clear sharp mind.

Now imagine yourself looking at the waves and the ocean and notice the beautiful waves breaking gently on the shore...The waves breaking gently on the shore are washing away all of your old negative thoughts, habits and emotions...and as each wave breaks now onto the shore, the waves are relaxing and recharging you and rejuvenating you, just as though the waves are cleaning your mind and body...the waves breaking gently on the show are now increasing your confidence and trust in yourself...more confidence each and every day...and as you notice the waves breaking onto the shore...you are becoming more calm, peaceful and happy...just as though you have now been cleansed of all negative thoughts and habits...and as you notice the ocean now as it moves out to the sea, it takes with it, all of your negative habits and emotions...because now you feel as though you are now refreshed and recharged with a new and exciting desire to live life to the fullest and to get what you deserve, which is the best of everything...and now go deeper asleep".

THE LOST GRAIN OF SAND NEUTRALIZING OF HABIT, FEAR AND NEGATIVE EMOTION VISUAL IMAGERY

This is a way of releasing a negative habit and even a compulsive behavior. I (Tom Silver) call it the "lost grain of sand" technique. Here's what you do. Hypnotize your client and say something like this:

"You are now deeply hypnotized...and I want you now to tap into your inner creative imagination. Imagine that you are taking a lovely walk on the beach and it's a beautiful day. See and picture yourself in your mind...taking a really nice walk on the sand...and as you look at the sand ...you see that there are millions or even billions of grains of sand on the beach...what I would like you to know do...is to imagine and even pretend...that you are bending down and picking up just one little grain of sand...pick up one little piece or grain of sand and hold it is hand with your finger and thumb. You can hardly see the sand pebble, but you can feel it in between your first finger and your thumb. Imagine that this sand pebble represents your old negative habit of picking your finger nails (Or any other negative habit)...this grain of sand...represents the old uncontrollable compulsive habit that you are letting go of".

"I want you to take the grain of sand now...and throw it onto the beach right now...throw it onto the sand...and as you through it away...you are also throwing away and letting go of all compulsive negative habits...you have thrown the sand grain onto the beach and as you look to see where the grain of sand is, you can not see it because it has disappeared onto the beach and into the billions of sand grains on the beach...and it is gone...disappeared...and so has the habit of picking your nails (or whatever habit or emotion) has now vanished, disappeared as though it has been thrown out of your life, thoughts and actions and it to has disappeared and is gone just like the little grain of sand has now disappeared on the beach...and you are now taking healthy control of your life and actions, because the old habit is gone and you can't find it again...just like you can not find that one piece of sand again, because it too has now disappeared and vanished onto the sandy beach."

THE DRIPPING FAUCET HABIT OR EMOTION REMOVAL VISUAL IMAGERY TECHNIQUE

This method involves the client releasing the habit from the mind using a method I call the "Dripping Faucet Technique". Here's what I do. I hypnotize a client and give suggestions such as:

"Just imagine that right now...you are going to let your negative habit or emotion go...nod your head yes to give me permission to help you now...good...imagine that you are standing in a kitchen in a house...any kitchen that you can imagine...maybe when you were young...or in your current house. Imagine that you are standing next to the kitchen sink and that you are seeing water dripping out of the sink faucet. Imagine that the water which is dripping out of the faucet represents you letting go of your negative habit (or emotion) and that each drip down into the sink, let's your habit become less and less...less... and ...less. Now as you look at the water dripping down and out of the facet, you see that the water is dripping less and less now and is starting to slow down. Your habit is slowing down and becoming less and less now and as you look at the facet, you see that the water has stopped dripping and that there is a drop hanging on the facet ready to drop off and disappear into the sick below. That one last drip...is the last of your habit (emotion) leaving you ...leaving you...and as you watch it now...it drops off...and disappears into the drain at the bottom of the sink ...and there is no more water dripping out of the facet and the habit is now also gone and disappeared...and even it you went over the handles to try to turn on the water to drip out, you can not because the handles are turned to off and the dripping water is gone and so is the habit gone...and you feel so much better each and every day"...

EMPTYING OF THE GARBAGE REMOVAL OF NEGATIVE HABIT VISUAL IMAGERY

You can take a negative habit or emotion and throw it away into the garbage can.

"Imagine that you are taking out the garbage in your house and before you dump it, I want you to take the negative habit of eating fried foods (or any negative habit) and I want you to imagine yourself

throwing that negative habit into the trash right now...see the habit of eating fried, greasy foods and imagine that you are taking this habit and simply throwing it into the trash bag because that old useless habit is garbage and you are throwing that habit away. You can now take this trash bag and imagine yourself walking it out of your house and placing it on the street for the garbage man to take away". "Place it on the sidewalk and back up from it and now imagine that the garbage man and the garbage truck is pulling up in front of the garbage and picking it up and dumping it into the truck and it all disappears away as the truck now drives away and now the useless negative habit of eating unhealthy fried and greasy foods (or any negative habit) is now gone.

TOLIET FLUSHING AND EMPTYING VISUAL IMAGERY

You can use the same concept of emptying the trash or garbage just by having your client under hypnosis visualize him or herself taking their negative emotions or behavior and simply flushing it down the toilet and away from their life. As the toilet bowl empties, all of their negative thoughts, habits or feelings leave.

"VISUAL IMAGERY TECHNIQUES THAT WORK"

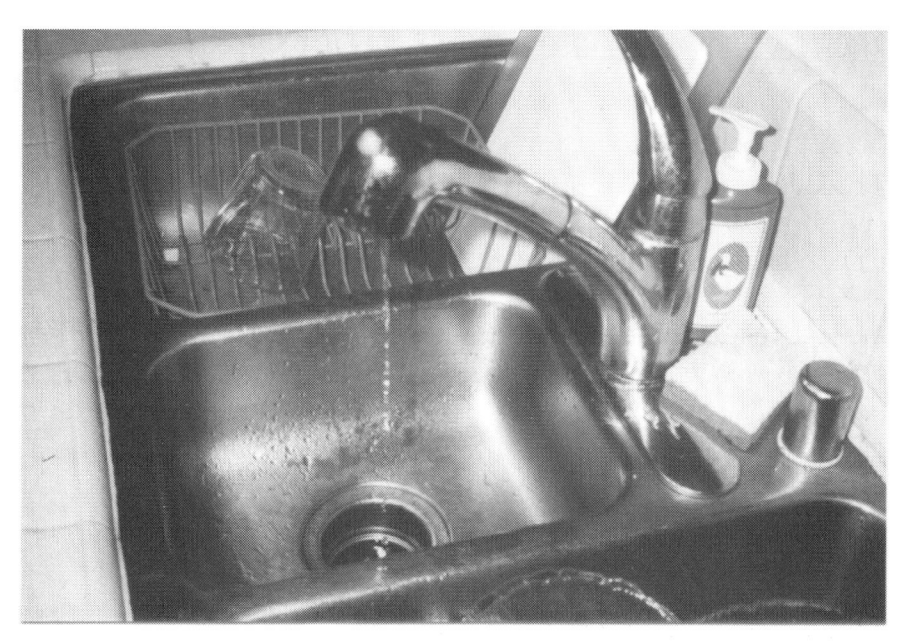

THE DRIPPING FAUCET HABIT OR EMOTION REMOVAL VISUAL IMAGERY TECHNIQUE

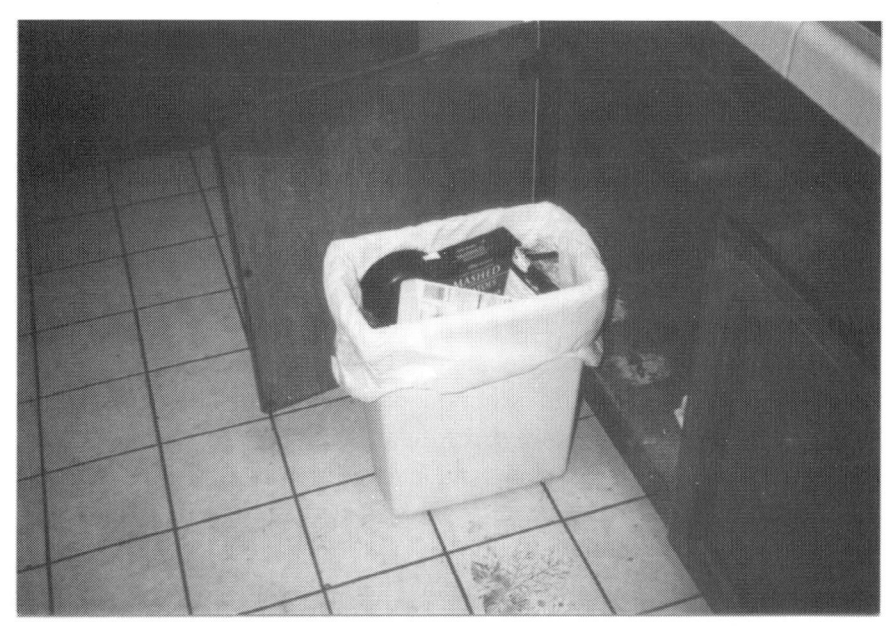

EMPTYING OF THE TRASH VISUAL IMAGERY TO RELEASE NEGATIVE HABITS OR EMOTIONS

CHAPTER TWENTY-EIGHT

HYPNOTHEAPY PROCESSES
Created By: Hypnotherapist Tom Silver

The following hypnosis processes I (Tom Silver) have been developing and formulating for over a period of twenty years of practice as a clinical hypnotherapist. They are based on my experimenting, research and practice of creating new faster and more successful hypnotherapy methods and processes in America and in Taiwan. There are many hypnosis techniques and methods that have been pioneered over the past two hundred and fifty years and have been very beneficial to the hypnotherapy field. You might find that the following techniques add to your own library of hypnosis knowledge.

EMOTION REPLACEMENT THERAPY (E. R. T.)

Emotion Replacement Therapy (E.R.T.) works best in the hypnotic depth, which we call somnambulism, or in scientific terms (EEG) low theta or delta. The deeper the depth of hypnotic trance, the less interference from the subject's conscious mind. This therapy is based on replacing and exchanging a negative emotion or anxiety with a positive emotion.

E.R.T. can be utilized for removal of fears and phobic emotional anxieties. Specific Fears and Social fears and phobias have both been successfully removed through this therapy method. In the fears and phobias chapter of this training manual, I will give you a full hypnotherapy script to remove fears through my Emotional Replacement Therapy.

This therapy can also help clients reduce and resolve stress, tension, anger, sadness, worry and other negative emotions that disturb the balance of our "autonomic nervous system" which regulates our respiratory, circulatory system and even our metabolism. I am 80% successful in removing fears and phobias with this technique and it is the first method that I use to remove fears.

"Regression" Emotion Replacement Therapy involves the reactivation of positive emotions from our past or childhood which again become activated through age regression. The emotions that are again felt and experienced during the regression are progressed (brought up) up to the subject's current life and this newly remembered positive emotion and feeling replaces the useless, destructive current negative emotion. I can actually regress a person who feels sad and unhappy in their current life situations, and regress them back to a very happy memory and time in their past (provided they had a happy past) and under deep hypnosis, I can have them relive that memory and emotion and even bring up that positive happy emotion and feeling to their current life. I have been also able to replace emotions by utilizing "Past Life Regression Emotion Replacement Therapy. Bringing up positive emotions from one's past life. Emotion Replacement Therapy creates a new Subconscious Reconditioned Emotional Response. We will talk a little about what that mean in this a few moments.

PASSIVE RECEPTIVENESS

Where your conscious mind is resting or in a state of inactiveness such as induced by hypnosis. Your conscious brain wave activity is in theta or delta, and your subconscious mind is a complete open receptor to positive transmitted suggestions, emotions, pictures and words.

MISDIRECTED CONSCIOUS MIND BYPASS

This brain science term is the term used when you purposely misdirect a persons conscious mind by giving it various directions to follow while at the same giving positive suggestions to the subconscious mind creating confusion and misdirection in the conscious mind in order to bypass critical mind thought and thereby being able to direct positive suggestions, emotions, pictures and words. Counting silently backwards from 100 trying to get down to zero, with each exhale thinking the words "deep asleep" before you reach 37 the numbers will disappear and vanish as though they are erased from you conscious mind and you will go deeper into hypnosis. Giving the conscious mind "busy work" during the session in order to by pass conscious resistance and transmit directly into the subconscious without interference.

SUBCONSCIOUS RECONDITIONED RESPONSE METHOD
(S. R. R.METHOD)

Subconscious reconditioned response is really what hypnosis is all about. You want to recondition the way a person thinks and acts. Changing bad habits into good habits. This method I call the (S.R.R. Method) really involves teaching your client how to get their mind to respond to them and not to the old habit. Conscious Affirmations play an important role in this process working as it is vital that the client is taught how to control his or her conscious mind and to exercise their mind to think only positive thoughts and suggestions. This process is based on educating and teaching the client how to create the positive conscious thoughts, suggestions and words that will automatically trigger the response of the positive emotions to surface up to the conscious mind creating a perfect balance of conscious mind process "analytical" mind and subconscious mind process which emotions, habits, patterns".

In this process you are teaching your client to recondition and reprogram their mental bio computers to automatically respond to each other in harmony and balance so that your client can get whatever in life they may desire.

POSITIVE SUBCONSCIOUS EMOTION
IDEO MUSCLE RESPONSE

A Positive Subconscious emotional ideo muscle response is an emotion that is tied into something physical that you may do well. Such as speak in public, play a musical instrument, take a test and be successful with your memory and concentration, play a specific sports well every time, such as baseball, basketball etc.

A positive subconscious emotion ideo muscle response can create consistency, more accuracy, higher achievement levels, and the peak of total performance every time. It is simply tying a positive emotion into any physical action that the client my do.

A NEGATIVE SUBCONSCIOUS EMOTION
IDEO MUSCLE RESPONSE

A Negative Subconscious emotional response is a negative or destruction emotions that is tied into something in life that you may do poorly, inconsistently or something that you might always fail at. This could range from one specific area of performance of in total dysfunction created by emotional negativity or insecurity. This could be a baseball pitcher who one day throws a bad ball and at the same time thought a negative emotion that became embedded in the subconscious area and now is triggered off simply by the conscious mind thinking a fear full conscious thought of doom or failure. This physical negative emotion or habit mental block needs to be replaced with the Positive Emotion Subconscious Physical Ideo Motor Muscle Response.

EMOTIONAL SUBCONSCIOUS BLOCK

An emotional block is when there is a subconscious emotional wall or emotional barrier preventing a person from achieving a specific goal. Emotional blocks appear to exist in most people and vary in degree of intensity.

RECEPTIVE BIO COMPUTER

The Receptive Bio Computer is another name for the subconscious mind. The reason it is called the receptive mind is because what's transmitted into it directly without conscious resistance is accepted automatically every time and it is the purest of mind receptors because it does not analyze information, it is simple acceptance.

CYBERSUGGESTION

The cyber universal mind method to attach all your brain electrical neurons into perfect function and harmony though subconscious and conscious suggestion processes and visualization multi sensory attachment to link your bio mental computers together to run is series with each for full 100 % mind energy power. Cyber Mental linking and anchoring. To combine mind computer power with a physical link or anchor. A person who has a fear of animals simply puts his first finger and thumb together and the fear is gone. Anchor a positive emotional stimulant. Suggestions triggered into physical body movements.

CHAPTER TWENTY-NINE

HOW TO PRODUCE HYPNOTIC ANESTHESIA

Pain in the body can be controlled by the mind. Hypnosis provides the means to numb pain using direct suggestions. The brain under hypnotic suggestion via the "hypothalamus" (a small organ in the lower part of the brain that acts as a type of transceiver between the brain, body and the autonomic nervous system) can produce "neuro peptides" (natural opiates) which can reduce and remove pain throughout different areas of body allowing some people to be able to have total surgical procedures without the need for a chemical anesthesia. The American Medical Association recognized the science of hypnotism back in 1957, for it use in pain control.

They also recommended that students of medicine should all study the science of hypnotism. In the early 1900s, the Mayo Brothers tested the use of hypnotic anesthesia by hypnotizing patients and producing natural "mind chemical" anesthesia and also reducing the amount of chemical anesthesia that was normally given during an operation down to 10% to15% of it's normal dosage. In thousands of major surgical procedures including abdominal operations, not one of the patients died because of the chemical anesthesia. During those days, statistics show that one out of four hundred people died from anesthesia administered for surgical procedures.

There are many various hypnotic techniques, suggestions and visualizations that you can use to help reduce or remove pain. The deeper into hypnosis you can your client, the better your results for obtaining "mental anesthesia".

Always when working with a client, as a hypnotherapist, you will always want to talk to them about where their pains are located, and what triggers them to react. Remember pain can be real and pain can also be created and imagined by the mind. Emotional pain can and does create physical pain. Look at what stress, tension and worry does to people. Some Doctors say that about 60% or our physical problems are mental.

Here are a few methods to reduce or remove pain. Before you hypnotize your client, ask them to describe to you what would be a place of tranquility or peace. You can tell them that it might be the beach, in a park, by a stream or lake, in the mountain, the desert or anywhere to them that represents a pace of peace and relaxation. Now place your client into deep hypnosis. This might happen on your first session, or upon repeated sessions. You want to get them so relaxed that their conscious mind stops focusing on you or their pain.

Now have them imagine themselves in their place of peacefulness and relaxation. Now say to your hypnotized client,

"Imagine yourself in a very peaceful restful place of beauty and relaxation. Imagine that you are now there feeling so peaceful, calm and relaxed. Maybe it's at the beach lying on a blanket in the sand, or in a park on the grass, or near a little stream trickling down a mountain, or near a lake. What ever is a place of peace and beauty to you. You are now seeing and feeling this peaceful place of relaxation and you feel so cool, calm and peaceful. Feel your entire body feeling cool, calm and relaxed".

"Let this relaxation move into every muscle, nerve and fiber of your body allowing you to feel as though all cares and discomforts are now leaving just as the cool ocean moves out to the see".

"Any time you feel discomfort in any area of your body, you can close your eyes and imagine your self in this peaceful, soothing, and cooling place of relaxation".

A method that Ormond uses is to put the subject in as deep a state of hypnosis as possible. Now make a few passes over the spot and then press your hands firmly on the spot in the body where the pain is felt. Press on the area lightly, then release the pressure, but still allow your hands to rest on that spot while you give these direct suggestions:

"The .. place .. upon .. your .. body .. on .. which .. my .. hand .. is .. resting .. is .. becoming .. numb. All .. sensation .. in .. that .. spot .. is .. becoming .. numb. All .. sensation .. in .. that .. spot .. even .. when .. I .. pinch .. your .. skin .. you .. feel .. nothing .. at .. all. It .. is .. insensible. It .. is .. anesthetized."

Repeat these suggestions in a forceful manner three times. Then give the subject's skin (over the spot which pains) a sharp pinch. If nothing is felt, anesthesia has set in.

When possible, do not mention the word "pain" when giving suggestions to remove pain. Center your suggestions on numbness and insensibility.

FOR DENTAL WORK

Hypnotherapy for dental work was very popular in the 1950s. Hypnotherapy was also wonderful for relaxing the patient before, during and after the procedures were performed.

It appears that fear and sound in a dental office can create major emotional anxiety in a large percentage of the population. In my private hypnotherapy practice over the years, I have found hypnosis to be very effective in removing worries and fears about going to the dentist.

A post hypnotic suggestion is always useful to your clients so that when they sit in the dental chair, they can feel relaxed and calm.

Hypnotize subject a few times (each induction following the other rapidly) before the dentist starts operating. This handling is known as pyramiding. It produces a deep state of hypnosis. When you know the subject is deeply entranced, suggest:

"You .. will .. do .. everything .. your .. dentist .. tells .. you .. to .. do .. perfectly. Your .. mouth .. is .. insensible. It .. feels .. absolutely .. numb. Just .. have .. a .. peaceful .. sleep .. while .. your .. dentist .. fixes .. your .. teeth."

Occasionally during the dental session, suggest to the patient:

"You .. are .. having .. a .. pleasant .. snooze .. while .. your .. dentist .. works .. on .. your .. teeth. You .. feel .. nothing .. in .. your .. mouth. You .. will .. just .. sleep .. on .. until .. I .. tell .. you .. it .. is .. time .. to .. awaken."

When the dental operation is complete, tell the patient he will feel fine when he awakens and will recall nothing whatsoever of the dental session.

COMPLETE BODY ANESTHESIA

After a deep state of hypnosis has been produced, take each part of the body and suggest anesthesia separately to them. Do not simply tell the subject that his whole body is without feeling, as that is too general. Make passes over each part and press in with your hand when suggesting insensibility in each part until arms, legs, head, shoulders, chest, torso and lower limbs are included in the anesthesia.

ANESTHESIA IN THE WAKING STATE

Hypnotic sleep is not always necessary to produce a condition of analgesia in a subject. Absence of pain can be suggested very often in the waking state. Physicians can use this method in trifling operations performed in the office. A placebo method is applied using indirect suggestions. In such instances, the doctor may say to the subject:

"Mr. Jones (subject's name), I .. have .. here .. a .. new .. form .. of .. anesthetic .. which .. has .. recently .. been .. developed. It .. works .. very .. rapidly .. and .. will .. completely .. remove .. any .. sense .. from .. the .. area .. upon .. which .. I .. will .. perform .. this .. very .. minor .. operation. You .. will .. find .. it .. will .. make .. the .. area .. absolutely .. numb."

A little of the imaginary anesthetic is then rubbed on the spot. A few moments of waiting and then the physician proceeds. Remarkably, the patient feels nothing.

To successfully use this process, the physician must have knowledge of how to give positive suggestions. Three essentials must work in harmony: the voice should be even toned and positive, the suggestions must be positive and definite, and the physician must have the confidence of knowing what he says will be believed. As an example, suppose it is desired to induce analgesia in the hand of a patient; go about it in this manner:

Take the patient's hand in your left hand. Look him squarely in the eyes. Do not blink and hold his attention on the eyes. Stroke his hand with your right hand a few times.
Now say to him:

"Your .. hand .. has .. no .. feeling .. in .. it .. at .. all. It .. is .. numb .. and .. insensible. See, .. even .. when .. I .. pinch .. the .. skin .. you .. feel .. nothing .. at .. all."

The whole secret is positive suggestions and concentration of will on what is being done. Even the flow of blood can often be controlled, as a few suggestions will verify. Repeat suggestions a few times.

CHAPTER THIRTY
By Ormond McGill

GAINING LOVE AND RESPECT

Put the subject back into deep hypnosis and give the following suggestions in a positive and forceful manner as you place your hands on his head with your thumb at the root of his nose:

"A strong bond of friendship is developing between us. We love and respect each other. You will have confidence in me as I have in you. You love and respect me. You will strongly sense this bond of love, respect and friendship flowing between us when you awaken from hypnosis."

Repeat these suggestions three times. Then let him remain silently in hypnosis for about five minutes before arousing. The harmonizing effects between people of such positive suggestion functioning on the posthypnotic level are remarkable.

ALTERATION OF CHARACTER

Hypnosis provides a wonderful way to motivate and improve the character of a person. For example, if a person is inclined to be lazy and restless to succeed in life, you can alter that disposition remarkably by the use of posthypnotic suggestions. Secure the subject's consent to improve his character and send him into deep hypnosis.
Then give these suggestions a half dozen times or so:

"From now on, you will work steadily, you will not care to change positions every few days, and you will be filled with the ambition to succeed. It will be a pleasure for you to work every day, earn your own way and be a success in business and your life. By doing this, you will become a credit to your community and your country and everyone will like you and speak of you highly. When I arouse you from this hypnotic trance, you will not remember that I have given you these suggestions but you will do exactly as I have told you, and you will imagine that it is your own impulse and idea. You are headed towards success, now and forever more."

WOMAN HYPNOTIZED!
TO OVERCOME HER "FEARS" OF
GIANT SPIDERS!

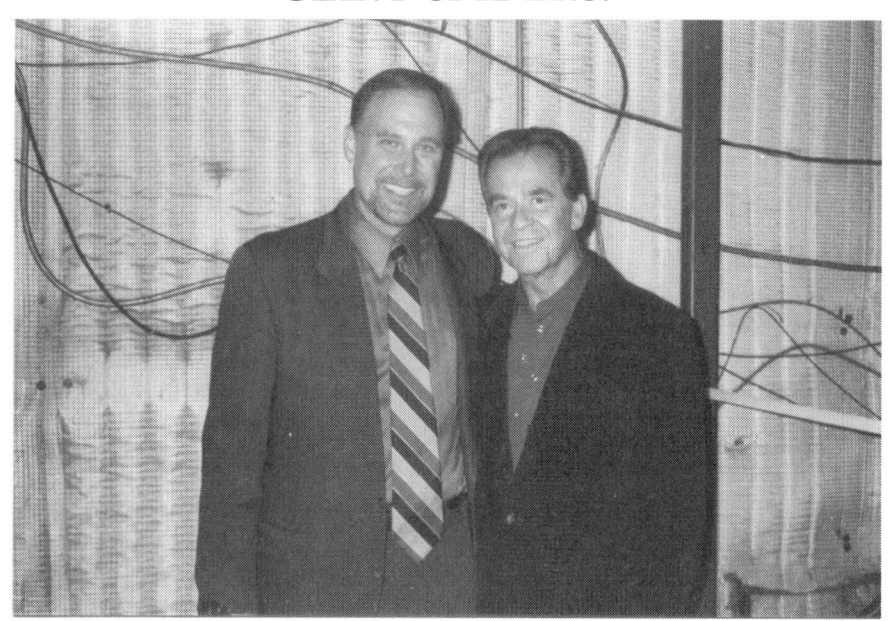

HYPNOTHERAPIST TOM SILVER WITH HOST OF "THE OTHER HALF" NBC NATIONAL TELEVISION SHOW STAR AND ALL AMERICAN CELEBRITY STAR MR. DICK CLARK DICK TELLS TOM ABOUT HIS EARLY ADVENTURES AS A PERFORMING HYPNOTIST!

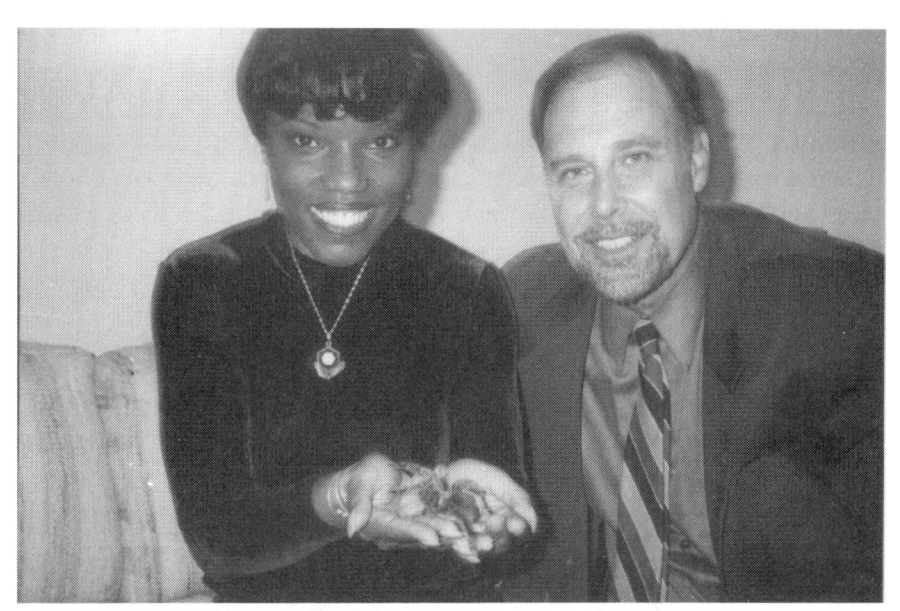

WANDA THOMAS "HOLDING" A GIANT SPIDER! * AFTER HYPNOTIST TOM SILVER HYPNOTIZED HER TO RELEASE HER LIFE LONG FEARS OF SPIDERS

CHAPTER THIRTY-ONE
By Tom Silver

FEARS AND PHOBIAS

WHAT IS A FEAR AND PHOBIA?

Fears and Phobias are extreme anxieties.
A manic Fear that terrorizes a persons mind and body.

When the phobia occurs and the person losses it and has an emotional explosion. Their heart beats fast, they can perspire, sometimes their throats tighten up and constrict to a point where you might feel as though you can't breath and you are gasping for air. It creates a shock to our central nervous system and what we call our autonomic nervous system.

You may also have an uncontrollable desire to run away which is the primitive area of your subconscious mind wanting to escape from the emotional pain. You might have an urge to just run away from the fear as fast as you can.

This is our primitive area of mind and primal instinct to run away from danger. This area of our brain is called our "Para limbic region" it is where are primal responses are triggered. The fear or Phobia is activated by your conscious mind by thinking about the fear, or seeing the actual physical thing that creates the fear.

An example of this would be a person who has a fear of "ants" and then all of a sudden that person sees an ant on the ground. The conscious mind using logic and reason sees the ant and computes that visual information. The fear instantly comes up from the subconscious mind like a title wave breaking onto the sea and an emotional and physical Volcano erupts. A firecracker of physical shock waves hitting many areas of the body and throwing an internal overdose of adrenalins into the body creating an over stimulation of the entire nervous system. A person who has a Fear or Phobia will spend lots of time figuring out ways to avoid the situations that create Phobic responses, sometimes becoming obsessed. What we call avoidance. I knew a business man that instead of having to deal with his fear of flying, he would simply just drive everywhere, even hundreds of miles to a destination. This is called avoidance. The harder a person works to avoid the things they fear, the more the brain grows convinced that the fear is real. This is called the law of reverse reaction. Most things that people do to reduce fears and phobias just makes it worse.

There are over 500 labeled fears that people experience every day. All extreme phobic behavior is extreme emotions or fears.

WHAT ARE PEOPLE AFRAID OF?

People are afraid of almost anything including: Bathing - itching - sourness - darkness - noise - heights - drafts - air - pain - open spaces - Wild animals - crossing the street - needles and pointed objects - cats - chickens - garlic - opinions - dust - riding in a car - walking - being scratched - colors - days of the week - books - toads - meat - hair - punishment - satin - stars - clouds - snakes - spiders - wines - rain - kissing - beards - fire - puppets and here are some official phobic terms to name a small few out of the over 500 labeled fears.

Pediophobia:	Fears of Dolls
Doraphobia:	Fear of animal fur or skins
Testiophobia:	Fear of Tests
Erotophobia:	Fear of sexual love
Iophobia:	Fear of Poison
Ergophobia:	Fear of going to work
Hydrophobia:	Fear of Water
Heterophobia:	Fear of the opposite sex
Logophobia:	Fear of words
Dentophobia:	Fear of Dentists
Claustrophobia:	Fear of confined spaces

Other fears include: paper - smells - wines - dirt - the moon - wasps - relatives - bulls - the sea - shellfish - ghosts - mice - Childbirth - sermons - feeling pleasure - empty spaces - cooking - germs - mushrooms - night - hospitals - death - pain - surgery - looking up - how about "Liticaphobia" Fear of Lawsuits!

DIFFERENT TYPES OF PHOBIAS

Most Psychologists now assign phobias to three different categories.

CATEGORY ONE

SOCIAL PHOBIAS

A Social Phobia is a paralyzing fear of social, intimate, or professional encounters. Examples of social phobias are fears of dating, boss at work, failure, going to social events or large parties, fears of business meetings, going shopping, fear of sex, fear of rejection, being in a group of people, fear of public speaking and so fourth.

Social Phobias sufferers grow increasingly more isolated, closing themselves off from areas of their life. They grow increasingly hopeless and can develop conditions as depression, alcoholism and drug addiction. 35 million people suffer from social phobias.

CATEGORY TWO

SPECIFIC PHOBIAS

SPECIFIC PHOBIAS ARE BROKEN DOWN INTO FOUR DIFFERENT GROUPS

Fact: Woman experience 90% of all Specific Phobias

Fact: 40% percent of all people suffering from Specific Phobias have at least one phobic parent!

GROUP ONE:
THE FEAR OF INSECTS AND ANIMALS:
Bugs, flies, Bees, spiders, wasps, beetles, ants, Fleas, snakes, dogs, cats, bears "Equinophobia is the fear of horses. Alextorophobia "Fear of Chickens".

GROUP TWO:
FEAR OF NATURAL ENVIRONMENTS:
Heights, water, darkness, fear of thunder, Fear of mountains, ocean, lakes, Daylight, rain, rocky cliffs etc.

GROUP THREE:
FEARS OF BLOOD AND INJURY:
Fears of pain, dying, doctors, needles, hospitals, surgery, cuts, injury Accident, bleeding, seeing blood, falling, fear of getting killed, medicine, getting needle shots.

GROUP FOUR:
FEARS OF DANGEROUS SITUATIONS:
Being trapped in a small space, elevators, amusement ride, tall buildings driving a car in a snowstorm, airplane flights in storms, trains, floods, earthquakes, tornadoes, title waves.

CATEGORY THREE

PANIC DISORDERS

A person for no apparent reason is blindsided by an overwhelming Fear. Panic disorders can eventually grow and mutate into full-blown Agoraphobia, which is the fear of going out of the house or even a room in a house.

The most disabling of all phobias, Panic attacks are to anxiety conditions what a tornado is to weather conditions. A devastating sneak attack that appears from nowhere wreaks havoc and then simply vanishes, unlike the specific phobia or social phobia where one usually knows what will trigger it. A person might get a panic attack just walking in a Supermarket one day.

The modern therapy treatment for agoraphobia is much the same as it is for social phobias, which usually is cognitive-behavioral therapy and drugs. These types of programs usually run once a week for 10 to 12 or more weeks and are usually conducted as private therapy.

PERCENTAGES OF PEOPLE SUFFERING FROM PHOBIAS

Social Phobias: Up to 55% of all social phobias occur in woman.

Specific Phobias: Up to 90% of all specific phobias occur usually in woman.

This percentage may be because women tend to own up to the condition more than men do.

Over 50 Million Americans suffer from Phobias and 35 million of those 50 million Americans suffer from "SOCIAL PHOBIAS"

WHAT CREATES A FEAR, PHOBIA, OR PANIC DISORDER?

Fears and Phobias can be learned. Phobias can be created by a traumatic event in a person's life. A small child left in the dark, a car accident, a house-fire, a dog running up to a small child, watching a scary movie, physical abuse, mental abuses, parents having fears and the child seeing and recording the fear.

Young children appear to be inherently fearful until they grow up and figure things out. Also some people seem to have a generalized sense of danger and fear and sometimes it may be therapeutic for them to deposit all that unformed fear into a single object such as a fear of rats or spiders. Sometimes a specific phobia might be a backfire for a generalized fear. Kind of like a controlled blaze that may prevent other fears from cropping up.

SECOND HAND FEARS:

Some people suffer from what is called "Second Hand Fears". If you have a fear of cockroaches and you acquired it because you saw your mom scream when she saw one when you were young. This is called a "second hand fear" Mom's fear of cockroaches is now your fear of cockroaches. Fears can be learned from childhood. Some Doctors believe that Fears and Phobias can be genetically influenced. Doctors are saying that they have even found a Phobic gene meaning that a Phobia might be passed down in a family.

A PERSONS TERMPERAMENT:

Temperament and emotional control may also play a role in creating a Phobia. Two people go through the same exact traumatic event but the high-strung person or the more emotional person may be more prone to having a Phobic Attack or episode. An earthquake might trigger a major Phobic Behavior in someone and another person going through the same Earthquake may not be affected at all.

How many times do we hear about someone having a heart attack and dying from being in a natural disaster?

In test studies at fear centers, subjects told to expect an electrical shock; neurological reactions to the anticipated jolt of electricity were as powerful as fears based on actual experience. The thought and emotional wave of fear was as strong as the fear from the actual experience.

DOCTORS AND PSYCHOLOGISTS METHODS TO TREAT FEARS AND PHOBIAS

Cognitive therapy, which is conscious therapy involving the method of "gradual exposure" or what one might call graduated exposure. Stripping off the fear slowly from the outside and lightest to the inner or most intense phobic anxiety. Quieting the alarm slowly and each time increasing the intensity. Doctors use Graduated Exposure for both Social Fears and Phobias and Specific Fears Phobias. Psychologists tend to treat people with social phobias in groups because it provides more of a support system. The very act of gathering with other people can serve as a first critical rebellion against the disorder. Social Phobia standard approaches are usually done in a series of 12 or more sessions, although Psychologists have been able to resolve some specific phobias in one long intensive exposure session like the work which is being done by psychologists at Stockholm University in Sweden. Panic disorder sufferers standard therapy practices are usually done on a one on one type of sessions like I mentioned earier.

This method is a gradual exposure to the fear or anxiety and to slowly get over the emotions or anxiety one level at a time starting with the least exposure first and then progressing it in intensity. An example of this would be a person who has a fear of blood. This phobia is called a hemophobia.

The psychologists will first introduce to the client just words such as cut, injured, blood, vile, or thought of someone having a cut or bruise, and bleeding. He might show a person a picture a person holding an empty vile in a hospital. Maybe the next visit he might talk about the word blood or show a picture now of a person holding a vile of blood.

He might try to get the client to hold the picture of the blood in the vile. After that maybe on another visit, he brings in an actual vial of blood for the client to look at. Then the next session maybe he gets the client to actually hold the vile of blood. The exposure to the trauma is increased until the client can tolerate the fear.

Also Virtual Reality devices are used more these days to desensitize the fears by having the client interact with the fear on a virtual reactor, which simulates the real fear experience. An example would be a person who has a Panic attack when driving a car. The simulator might produce the effect of the actual fear created when driving a real car. Then through a graduated approach method the speed and challenges are increased in intensity along with the fear being increased and hopefully controlled.

Or a person who might have a fear of flying using a virtual reality simulator to give them the same physical feeling as though they are really going onto an airplane and they feel and experience the plane taking off, flying and even landing. The intensity of the movements and feelings are slowly increased as though they are experiencing turbulence and weather conditions.

Doctors and psychologists like to prescribe drugs to use as an antidepressant to block out some of the anxiety or to repress the anxiety. That is like putting a bandage over a wound and never really healing the wound. Paxil is the number one most prescribed drug for social anxiety disorder phobias including agoraphobia. Other prescription drugs used for fear and phobias repressors are Luvox, Prozac and Celexa and a host of many more.

These are all antidepressants or mood blockers. They do not cure the person from the emotional nightmares they just temporary bury the emotional scare. In diagnosing Phobias, Doctors and Psychologists can sometimes make mistakes. An example of this might be a person who feels compelled to wash their hands all the time might have a fear of germs and the clinician might peg the problem as obsessive-compulsive disorder and not a specific phobia. The survivor of a plane crash may exhibit a phobic panic at even a picture of a plane, but likely as not, the fear is one component of a larger case of "Post Traumatic Stress Disorder. Different conditions require different treatments.

Phobias can beat a person down mentally and physically because the feeling they feel seems so real, and the dangers they warn of so great. Most of the time, however the dangers are just over reactive imaginations which are not even based in reality and only created by an overactive negative imagination. To the person having it, fears are real.

Let me give you an example of how strong of an impact imagination can play on our life. If I was to lie a 2/4 piece of wood down on the floor and ask you to walk on it from one end of the room to the other, you could do it easily. You would not think or imagine any danger at all and you would easily walk on it.

If I was to take that same long piece of wood and place it between to tall buildings or between to 40 foot ladders and I asked you to walk on it from one end to the other. Once you stepped onto the wood and looked down, your imagination would color that safe easy feeling with fear, danger, death and falling. Your body would start to shake, your heart would beat faster and you would start to perspire.

Your imagination would create such fear that as soon as you started to walk on that wood, the thought of falling would be so great that within a few seconds you would indeed fall off that wood and down to the depths below. Because your imagination would convince you that you would fall, you will fall. Most Phobias are due to a very overactive negative imagination.

WHAT IS THE HYPOTHALAMUS? (A Small Organ in the Medulla)

The brain conveys "tranduces" (technical term) information and instructions to the nerves, muscles, circulatory and decease fighting systems of the body through the Hypothalamus.

All brain sensory images and messengers including, conscious mental images and pictures and self induced suggestions and hypnosis suggestions are transmitted from the brain down to the hypothalamus which is the a small organ in the medulla or inner part of your brain which is located close to you brain stem.

The hypothalamus is a modulation box or transmitter/receiver that registers information from the brain. It then transmits that information to the body through the hypothalamic limbic system.

The first hypothalamic limbic system in called the autonomic nervous system. The hypothalamic limbic system also controls your immune system and activates neuropeptides (natural opiates) and also body energy source. There is a brain to body connection through the hypothalamus and hypnotism taps into that connection.

THE AUTONOMIC NERVOUS SYSTEM

"Autonomic nervous system" is the sympathetic and parasympathetic nervous system" through the adrenal glands and spleen. The "autonomic nervous system" if not working properly because of extreme emotions such as fear, terror, extreme anxiety or any other extreme emotional feeling including anger, rage, extreme depression, worry and so fourth will affect your health and may shut down completely.

Fears and Phobic attacks can negatively affect your nervous system. This emotional explosion to your nervous system throwing it off balance will create physical shocks to the body and a real breakdown of the body resulting in a psychosomatic illness or medical illness and even death. The "autonomic nervous system" controls our circulatory system, respiratory system and our metabolism.

Sensory images, visual images, and verbal suggestions can be transmitted directly to the hypothalamus by using and utilizing hypnotherapy to create the direct link to the subconscious mind.

AUTONOMIC NERVOUS SYSTEM
THE HYPOTHALAMIC LIMBIC SYSTEM

HYPNOTIC SUGGESTIONS ARE TRANMITTED VIA THE HYPOTHALAMUS

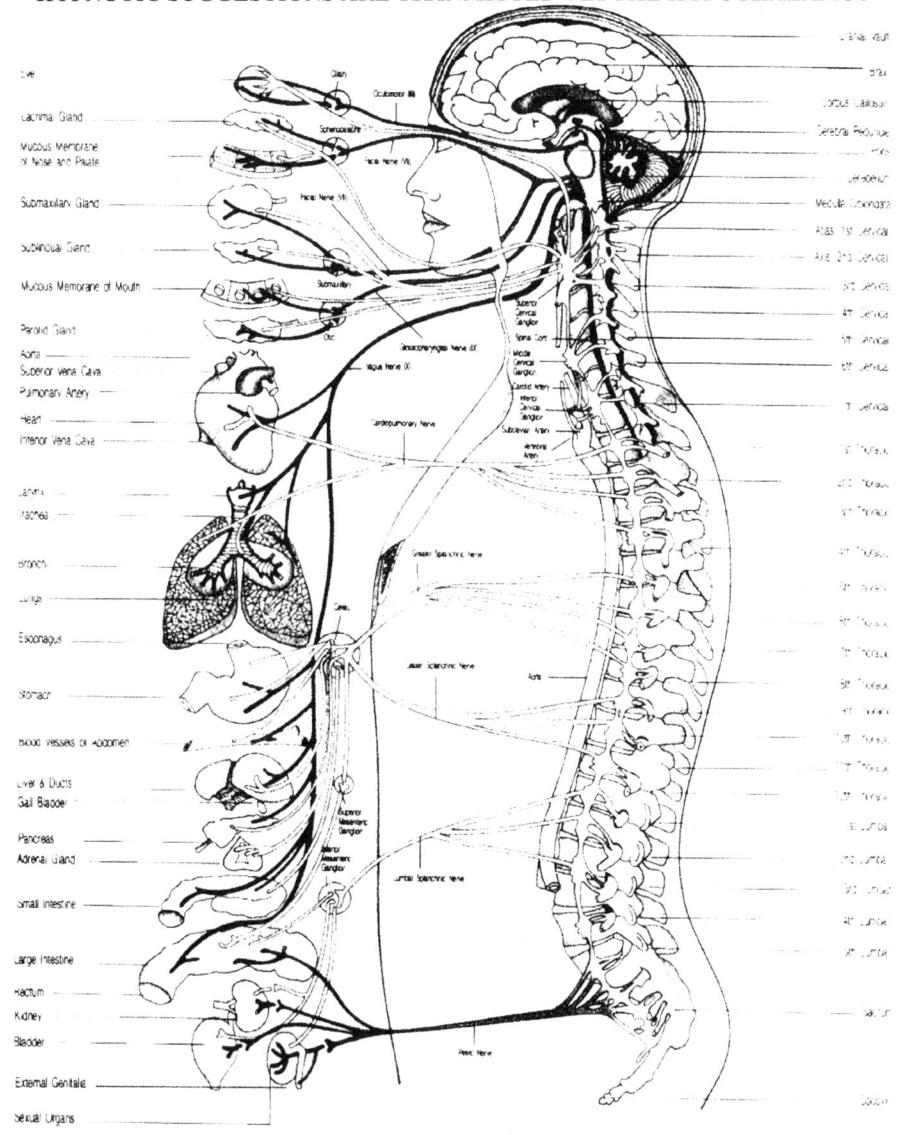

HYPNOSIS HELPS TO BALANCE A PERSON'S AUTONOMIC NERVOUS SYSTEM WHICH INCLUDES OUR RESPIRATORY SYSTEM CIRCULATORY SYSTEM AND OUR BODY METABOLISM

CHAPTER THIRTY-TWO
By Tom Silver

HYPNOTHERAPY TECHNIQUES TO REMOVE FEARS

Always Start With Your Personal Agreement With Your Client

You will start off each hypnosis induction by saying:

"I am here to hypnotize you and to help you. I promise to take good care of you. You are safe and secure and want me to hypnotize you. I want you to do exactly everything that I ask you to do without instantly without thinking, and I will help you to overcome this obstacle that is standing in the way of your health and happiness. Do you understand and agree to allow me to hypnotize you"?

The client will say: "Yes".
Then say to the client:

"We now have a contract with each other. I will hypnotize you to overcome your obstacle in your life, and you will instantly and without thinking, do everything that I ask you to do and you will enter into a very deep hypnotic relaxation".

This is the hypnotic agreement by therapist and client.

HYPNOTHERAPY TECHNIQUES THAT REALLY WORK TO REMOVE FEARS AND PHOBIC ANXIETIES

LITERAL DIRECT SUGGESTIONS:

Literal suggestions that the fear and anxiety is completely gone. The subconscious mind is a simple child like mind that accepts simple literal suggestions the best. The subconscious mind does not distinguish reality from fantasy. The conscious mind does. Hypnotize the subject and say under hypnosis that you can now feel calm and safe and secure in any situation. Here is an example of a literal direct suggestion:

"When you go onto the plane to fly, you will feel calm and happy. All the fears of now gone, replaced with a feeling of being safe and secure, secure and calm, calm and happy. Imagine yourself now and see yourself sitting in the plane. See a smile on your face because you are now feeling happy and peaceful".

"As the plane takes off, you are calm and peaceful. See you looking and feeling comfortable and very relaxed. Even being able to fall asleep while you are sitting safely in your seat on the plane. As the plane is flying you feel a warm feeling of calmness in your mind and body". "Thinking happy thoughts. As the plane is about to land you still have this calm, peaceful feeling and a smile of "freedom". Your smile is increasing your feeling of well-being and even excitement because you can now fly anywhere and anytime feeling safe, in control and very peaceful. See yourself in your minds eye now releasing the safety belt and feeling so good about now being able to fly anywhere, anytime feeling peaceful, safe and secure".

The Post Hypnotic Suggestion

"Every time you now fly in a airplane you will feel calm, safe, secure and happy. When you sit down in your seat in an airplane, you will feel this feeling of calm peacefulness and you will now and forever be able to fly anywhere, anytime feeling this peaceful feeling. Feel a smile on your face right now that represents your new freedom in your life. Feeling really good and happy. Now when I count to three you will awaken feeling good happy and now free to fly anywhere feeling safe and secure".

EMOTION REPLACMENT THERAPY (E.R.T.)

This process involves replacing a phobic anxiety with a non-phobic emotion. This works well with specific phobias as well as with social phobias. Replacing a negative emotion with a positive emotion.

FEAR OF SNAKES:

Hypnotize the client into a very deep state of hypnosis. Theta, Delta or what we call somnambulism is the most effective. Before the hypnosis, find out what type of animal the client likes and feels comfortable with. Maybe the client likes a puppy dog or cat as an example. After the client is deeply hypnotized, ask them to imagine that they are petting a little puppy or kitten on their lap. Bring up the positive emotions of feeling so happy and good. Actually have them pet their favorite little pet and even talk to it.

FEAR OF DARKNESS:

Hypnotize the client and have them imagine the feeling of how calm and happy and safe they feel during the day and then transfer that same feeling to having them imagine that it is now night time, but they still are feeling the same positive emotions just as if it was day light. Outside. Get a physical response from the client.

"You will now feel safe, calm, and peaceful every night, just as you feel safe, calm and peaceful during the day. Nod your head yes"

THE NEXT PROCESS IS TO RECONDITION A PERSON'S SUBCONSCIOUS MIND TO RESPOND TO POSITIVE EMOTIONS. THIS PROCESS IS CALLED

<u>"THE SUBCONSCIOUS RECONDITIONED RESPONSE METHOD"</u>

This method to remove the phobic anxiety from a person's subconscious mind involves the utilization of Ideo Muscle Motor Response to release the anxiety. It also involves the processes of "Negative Subconscious Emotion Ideo Muscle Response" and "Positive Subconscious Emotion Ideo Muscle Response. Hypnotize the client into a very deep state of hypnosis. Theta or delta depth in required to perform this therapy. Once the person is very deeply hypnotized. Tell them the following:

"In a moment I will have you imagine that you going to get into a airplane to fly somewhere. When I do, I want you to bring up with anxiety and fear of flying. When I count to three, you will imagine that you are really there, feeling this fear and anxiety. I will transfer this fear into your left hand and arm and when I count to three, your left hand and arm will lift all the way into the air. You will not feel the fear but it will be transferred into your hand and arm, which will lift

up all the way into the air. Now one, imagine that you are now going to get into the plane (or car etc) two, feeling fear now going into your left hand and arm, now three, your hand and arm now lifts all the way into the air". (The client's hand and arm will lift right up into the air.)

Now say

"When I pull down on your hand and arm, you will release 50% of the fear out of your mind and body. (Then pull down and jerk the client's hand and arm down and as it drops onto their lap say, "Sleep"). Say to the client "We have now removed 50% of that useless fear and anxiety, that overactive imagination. And even if you wanted to bring back that fear and anxiety, you can't and you won't because now 50% of the fear in now gone." "In a moment, I will ask you to imagine again in your mind that you are going into an airplane to fly and as you bring up that fear and anxiety when I count to three your left hand and arm will lift up into the air, but your hand and arm will only go halfway up in the air because 50% of that old useless anxiety in now gone and can't come back even if you wanted it to, but you don't want it to".

"Now when I count to three your left hand and arm will only go halfway up into the air because 50% of the anxiety is now gone. One, imagine yourself in the airplane two, bring up that anxiety and fear, now three, your left hand and arm now lifts halfway up into the air and can not go any higher no matter how hard you try".

The client's hand and arm will go up halfway in the air and stop

This is your way of monitoring the subconscious anxiety. If the clients arm goes all the way into the way, repeat the first procedure again as many times as it might take, until the clients arm goes only half way up in the air.

Then say to the client

"When I pull on your hand and arm, your hand and arm will drop instantly onto your lap and 80% of that useless over imagination and negative anxiety will leave your mind and body and you will go deeper into the hypnotic sleep".

Grab the client's hand and jerk and throw it down onto the subjects lap and say

"80% percent of this useless negative fear and over imagination is now gone. Deep asleep. Now 80% of your old fear and anxiety is now gone and can't come back even if you wanted it to, but you don't want it to. There is only 20% of that useless fear and anxiety left in your mind and body because 80% of it is now gone and can not come back even if you wanted it to, but you don't want it to. In a moment, when I count to three, I want you to bring up that fear again". (Fear of flying, insects, heights, darkness etc.)

"When I count to three, you will bring up that fear of "Flying" But now 80% percent of that fear is now gone from your subconscious mind and can't come back. When I count to three, your left hand and arm will now only lift just a few inches up in the air and can not go any higher no matter how hard you try because 80% is now gone forever and can not come back. One, Two, Bring up that fear now, Three and your hand and arm now only lifts just a few inches into the air".

The client's hand and arm will only lift from maybe 1 to 10 inches off their lap.

Now Say

"Now 80% of that useless negative imagination is now gone and can not come back even if you wanted it to, but you do not want it to. It was just an overactive imagination. When I pull down on your hand and arm, 90% percent of that useless negative fear will now leave your mind and body forever".

Pull down on the client's hand and arm and say, "Sleep" as the clients hand and arm drops onto their lap. Then say:

"Now 90% percent of that useless negative fear and false imagination is now gone and can never come back even if you wanted it to, but you don't want it to."

"Now there is only 10% of that useless negative imagination

because 90% of it is now gone, replaced with a feeling of being safe, calm and secure. When I count to three. You will try to lift up your left and your left hand and arm will only lift up just a inch or so off your lap because 90% of that useless negative over imagination and fear is now gone and can't come back no matter how hard you try, because 90% of it is gone out of your mind and body. When I count to three you will try to bring up that fear or anxiety of flying, but 90% of the fear is now gone and your hand and arm will only lift a inch of two off your lap".

"One, Two, Three, try to bring up that fear and your hand and arm only lifts a inch or so off your lap. The client's arm and hand will only lift an inch off their lap. Then go up to the client and say in a moment, I will pull on your hand and your hand and arm will drop instantly onto your lap and you will let go of that last 10% of useless anxiety and false imagination, replacing it will a feeling a feeling safe, calm, happy, and secure to fly anywhere".

Pull down of the client's hand and say

"Sleep". Now 100% of that false imagination and useless fear and anxiety towards (Flying, insects, etc.) if now gone forever and can not come back no matter how hard you try, because the fear of flying in now gone forever. When I count to three, you will try to lift up your left hand and arm, but will not be able to. Your hand and arm will remain on your lap as though it is stuck to your lap because the fear of _(whatever)_ is now gone forever, replaced with a feeling of being happy, calm, safe and peaceful".

"When I count to three, you will test yourself by trying to bring up that negative anxiety, that false imagination and your hand and arm will now move or lift into the air no matter how hard you try, because the anxiety is now gone forever and can not come back even if you wanted it to, but you don't want it to".

"When I count to three your hand and arm will not move, and you will feel a smile on your face because you feel so good and happy. Now on the count of three imagine that you are sitting in your seat on a airplane with a big smile on your face feeling happy, safe and in control".

"One Two Three, your hand and arm will not move because the

anxiety and negative over imagination is now gone forever. That useless negative over imagination is now gone forever, replaced by a new happy freedom, feeling very good and safe".

"Breath in a feeling of feeling happy now because the anxiety is now gone. You are now giving yourself a new and wonderful freedom in your life and you feel happy".

"No matter how hard you try to bring back the old fear, you can't because it is gone forever, replaced with a wonderful new happy feeling of feeling peaceful, happy, safe and secure. Deep asleep now. When I count to three you will awaken feeling refreshed, safe, happy and now free to do anything in life".

(Then awaken the subject out of hypnosis).

FEAR OF PUBLIC SPEAKING

Use the same process as I described above. Have the client in a deep state of hypnosis. Tell the client that when you count to three, you want them to imagine that they are standing in front of a group of people ready to speak to the group.

You want them to bring up the fear and anxiety that they normally feel. Say that they won't physically feel the anxiety but that their hand and arm will lift all the way up into air because you are transferring their anxiety and fear into the hand and arm.

"When I count to three, your left or right hand and arm will lift all the way up into the air. Then say now imagine that you are now standing in front of the group of people and bring up the fear on the count of three. One, Two, Three, "your hand now lifts all the way into the air." Etc.

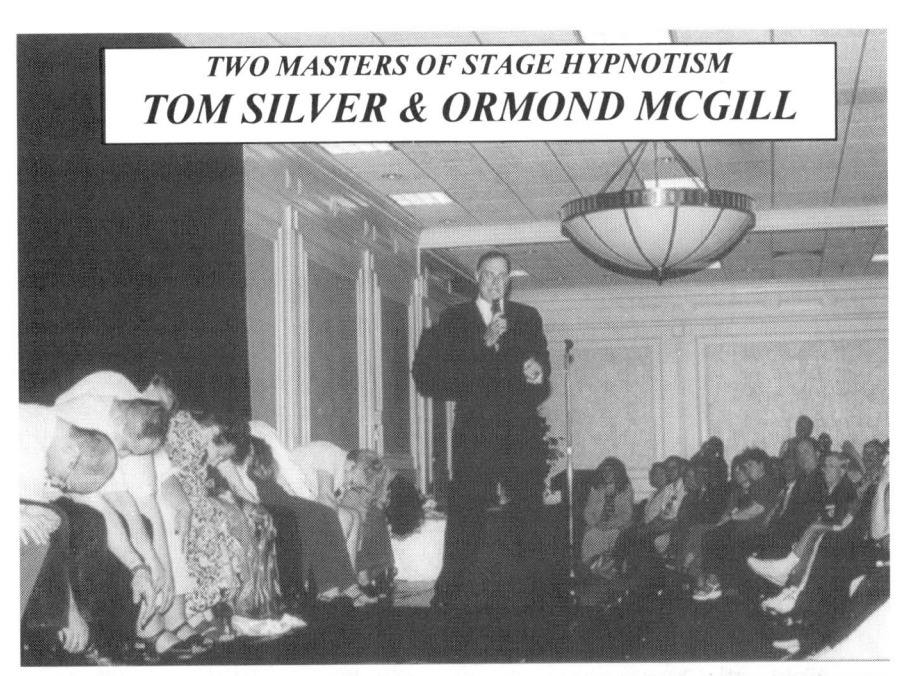

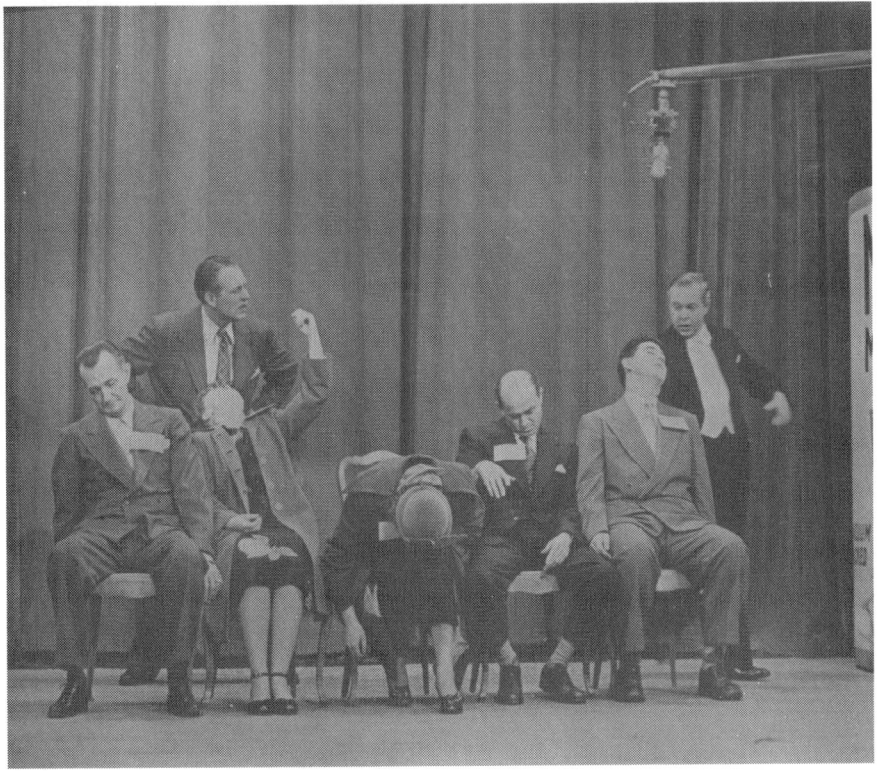

TWO MASTERS OF STAGE HYPNOTISM
TOM SILVER & ORMOND MCGILL

ORMOND MCGILL ON THE ART LINKLETTER SHOW IN THE 1950s

CHAPTER THIRTY-THREE

DEVELOPING YOUR PERSONAL MAGNETISM

Charisma is a synonym for personal magnetism. It is charm. It is exerting your personality to influence. In that sense, it is a form of hypnotism. It might be interpreted to mean exerting a hypnotic influence over others without arousing the least bit apprehension. People obey your commands through this mental influence. The more you develop your personal magnetism, in direct ratio, the better hypnotist you will be.

Personal magnetism has been the means of success for top ranking people. John F. Kennedy is an excellent example of personality in action. His personality influenced all of America and an entire generation. A great entertainer like Elvis Presley is another example. His personality was so powerful that the entire world followed his life and career, on and off the stage. Let's boil it down to the personality of you.

Some people are naturally endowed with personal magnetism; others acquire it by persistent practice. One may win success in some degree without personal magnetism, but the person will never attain great heights without it in the way of living a truly successful life. Whether you are a businessman, physician, politician, actor, lawyer or salesman, it is a gift to acquire. For the hypnotist, it is the becoming of a really GREAT hypnotist.

The man or woman who has developed this mighty power need never lack friends, for everybody wants the magnetic personality. There is something irresistibly fascinating about a magnetic personality that is difficult to describe in words. It is felt, invisible-like, and compels admiration. A man may carry his magnetism in his voice. It may be carried in his eyes. Others manifest it in their gestures, smiles and self-confidence of bearing. Some will develop it in one direction and others in another, but everyone can become magnetic to a greater extent by following the instructions given you in this chapter. You can use your personal knowledge of self-hypnosis for the development of this power.

CULTIVATING SELF-CONTROL

You cannot expect to control others unless you can control yourself.

Remember this. Learn to know yourself. Find your faults and correct them. Find your good qualities and amplify them. What you will learn here will help you become magnetic. In other words, it will increase your charisma. It will increase your charm. So it can be said that the first essential for developing a magnetic personality is your personal self-control.

The second essential is confidence in yourself and in your ability to develop a magnetic personality. This is a matter of Will Power. You must have the necessary willpower to carry out your desire. You must be strong and firm in the mastery of yourself. To be strong and firm does not mean you should be egotistical. An egotist is usually stubborn. Stubbornness is a sign of a weak will. A person who will not be amenable to others from pure stubbornness denies everything and is anything but strong willed.

The man with magnetic personality can always master the man who is stubborn. If you would influence such a person, never argue with him. Remember, "Where ignorance is bliss, it is folly to be wise". Try to lead him with something that interests him and side with him. Play on his ego and you will accomplish your purpose. By way of an example, if you are a salesman, lead with a smile. Many an important business transaction has been successfully accomplished by a winning smile.

Cultivate the faculty of giving quick decisions and sticking to them. Do not change them until you are absolutely convinced you are wrong. A vacillating, unsteady disposition is anti-personality.

Become a master of anger within yourself. If you feel anger arousing within you, right in the middle STOP AND TAKE THREE DEEP BREATHS so that you become rational and deal with it, not allowing it to undermine your personality. Anger takes away your vitality and weakens your well-being. Conversely, cheerful thoughts are infecting, and there radiation produces corresponding actions in the minds of others. A magnetic personality radiates sunshine and good will, and these thoughts are contagious.

If you are in company and there is discussion of things on which you are not especially well informed, do not force your views. Just be a good listener. Avoid debate unless you are absolutely sure of your ground. Some people like to talk just to hear them-selves talk, without really saying anything. These people are a bore, and boredom is anti-personality.

Some people are magnetic to some extent, but their use of language destroys their influence. Use tact and study the characteristics of the person you wish to influence. Gain confidence in yourself because "confidence begets confidence".

All persons are magnetic to some degree and the power can definitely be developed. The basic principle of personal magnetism is strong Willpower. Personal magnetism is a Nerve force that is produced and directed by the Will of the producer. Exercising it can strengthen the Will. You cannot expect the will to be strong without training. Hypnosis (self-hypnosis), used upon your-self provides a remarkable way to exercise the Will and develop WILLPOWER.

THE TECHNIQUE OF SELF-HYPNOSIS

This technique employs the ideomoter response idea that every thought held is the mind produces an accompanying subjective response in the body. That is to say, if we consciously think an idea, we subconsciously tend to move in that direction. This is the process you can effectively use to increase your personal magnetism.

Take a seat and THINK about yawning and actually yawn. As you do this, you will find yourself really yawning and yawning is very relaxing to the body, moving in the direction of sleep and deliberately thinking of going to sleep moves you into hypnotic sleep, wherein mind becomes activated to accept suggestions, as you know. Now, close your eyes and THINK of how you are becoming relaxed all over. THINK of how receptive your subconscious mind is becoming to accept and act upon the suggestions you are going to implant in it that will increase your personal magnetism. Continue on, relaxing, and THINK sleep. THINK GOING TO SLEEP. THINK sleep. You will find yourself becoming very sleepy, but just let your mind drift and don't allow yourself to actually go to sleep. You are close to sleep, yet still not asleep. You have placed yourself into self-hypnosis.

In this receptive and passive condition of mind, place the palms of your hands over your ears and press in a little. Now, SPEAKING OUT LOUD OR TO YOURSELF, present these suggestions which, by this process, will seem to "ring" inside your head:

FOR CULTIVATING SELF-CONFIDENCE

"I .. am .. a .. man (or woman, as the case may be). I .. have .. strong .. willpower. My .. will .. is .. powerful. I .. believe .. in .. myself .. and .. my .. ability .. to .. succeed. My .. personality .. is .. becoming ..

magnetic .. and .. nothing .. can .. prevent .. me .. from .. succeeding. My .. will .. is .. strong. My .. confidence .. in .. myself .. is .. unlimited. I .. will .. rely .. absolutely .. on .. myself. My .. confidence .. cannot .. be .. shaken."

Repeat these suggestions to yourself in this special mental state three times. Then, drop your hands from pressing on your ears to relax into your lap and go to sleep, if you wish. Awaken when you will.

These are enough self-suggestions for the first session. The next day, you can try another. Apply the same method to induce self-hypnosis in yourself and present to yourself these suggestions:

FOR CULTIVATING DETERMINATION

"I .. am .. developing .. a .. magnetic .. personality. I .. am .. determined .. to .. succeed. I .. will .. complete .. successfully .. everything .. I .. start .. out .. to .. do. I .. have .. the .. ability .. to .. influence .. people. People .. respond .. to .. the .. influence .. of .. my .. personal .. magnetism. People .. respond .. to .. the .. power .. of .. my .. will. I .. am .. determined .. to .. radiate .. cheerfulness .. at .. all .. times. I .. have .. powerful .. determination .. to .. do .. whatever .. I .. set .. out .. to .. do. Nothing .. can .. deter .. me. The .. power .. of .. self-confidence .. is .. mine. The .. power .. of .. determination .. is .. mine .. as .. well. It .. is .. the .. case."

Repeat these suggestions to yourself three times while in the state of self-hypnosis you have induced, and then go to sleep. Awaken when you will. End of session for this day.

FOR CULTIVATING SELF-CONTROL

Induce the self-hypnosis state in yourself and proceed as before. With palms of hands pressing against your ears, repeat out loud or to yourself these suggestions:

"I .. have .. full .. control .. of .. myself .. at .. all .. time. I .. will .. never .. lose .. my .. temper. No .. one .. can .. ruffle .. me. I .. will .. always .. have .. a .. smile .. when .. needed. I .. will .. never .. be .. discouraged. I .. will .. never .. be .. nervous. I .. am .. the .. controller. I .. am .. master .. of .. myself .. and .. master .. of .. others *at .. all .. times. I .. do .. not .. needlessly .. worry. I .. am .. cheerful .. and .. happy. My .. WILLPOWER .. is .. vast .. and .. supreme .. and .. I .. have .. a .. magnetic .. personality .. that .. will .. influence .. others .. as .. it .. is .. my .. will .. to .. cause. My .. eyes .. exert .. this .. power. My .. entire .. BEING .. exerts .. this .. power. I .. have .. developed .. a .. MAGNETIC PERSONALITY."*

Repeat three times and conclude the session the same as always. Awaken when you will. Use this process daily for a few weeks. The results will amaze you in the qualities of personal magnetism it will cultivate in your personality.

REINFORCING SELF-HYPNOTIC SUGGESTIONS

Write the suggestions you have given yourself on paper. Write each exercise on a separate sheet so you are prepared.

In your private room, just before going to bed, darken the room and place a lit candle on a table before a comfortable chair in which you seat yourself. Have the candle positioned high enough so that you have to open your eyes wide in looking at the flame. Now study the paper containing one of the willpower exercises you have written. As you read its message, speak out loud to yourself what you are reading. Read it and speak it thus several times, committing it more or less to memory. Then relax in the chair, stare directly at the candle flame and as you stare at it, repeat verbally what you have memorized. When your eyes get tired, close them and relax even more. Now, mentally review what you have been speaking. Continue to do this until you can absorb no more and just want to go to sleep. Go to bed and have a good night's sleep.

Use only one setting of the willpower exercises at each of these reinforcement sessions. Sometimes, after looking at the candle flame for awhile, it will seem as if it were becoming very large and you will seem to see the suggestions written in the flame. When this illusion happens, it means your self-suggestions have very much become your own.

Personal magnetism is essential to your outstanding success as a hypnotist. Follow these instructions and develop your WILL and you will achieve your highest ambitions for success in life. Persevere; practice and you will cultivate PERSONAL MAGNETISM.

CHAPTER THIRTY-FOUR

PERSONAL MAGNETISM FOR THE PROFESSIONALS

Personal magnetism and hypnotism are invaluable to the various professions. No great professional success can be attained without the practical employment of this wonderful power. Its use will benefit you in every way.

FOR THE LAWYER

Every successful lawyer pleading his case before a jury uses hypnotic suggestion, especially criminal lawyers. The judge's and the jury's attention is skillfully drawn towards him and every ounce of will power and magnetism is directed toward them to get their minds to accept his view of the case. No lawyer can hope to attain full use of the Power of Suggestion without combining it with Personal Magnetism.

FOR THE PHYSICIAN

No profession can use the power of personal magnetism more importantly than that of the physician. In connection with his medical knowledge, the use of hypnotism and magnetism will make him paramount in his profession. In addition to being a doctor, he will become a healer. By using these processes, he will be able to affect cures that would be otherwise impossible. The physician who uses what has been instructed in this text will have gained the full confidence of his patients for his ability to make them well. Therein lies a great secret for the healing of the sick and that is in suggestions.

FOR THE MINISTER

The minister has a wonderful opportunity to use the power of suggestion and personal magnetism. The minister who has personal magnetism is the one who fills his church. Such a minister knows how to keep and attract the attention of the congregation. He is magnetic.

He emanates forceful and powerful thought waves each time he delivers a sermon. His personal magnetism attracts people to his pews like bits of iron are attracted to a magnet.

FOR THE SALESMAN

The most far sweeping field for the use of personal magnetism and hypnotic influence is in the profession of salesmanship. The "knight of the grip", the insurance solicitor, the canvasser, the clerk behind the counter, the merchandise salesman, the real estate broker, everyone connected with the profession of salesmanship, the list goes on and on, could easily double their sales by the use of hypnotic suggestion combined with his cultivated personal magnetism. All persons engaged in the business of selling to the public would do well to study this text thoroughly and master what it tells.

SELF-HYPNOSIS FOR THE USE OF ALL PROFESSIONS

As you have learned the technique of self-hypnosis, let each professional design his own suggestion formula, which apply especially to his work. Then put such formulae into operation exactly as has been described in the obtaining of personal magnetism for the individual. A bit of thought, a little effort, and the professional results achieved are excellent.

CHAPTER THIRTY-FIVE

SELF HYPNOSIS FOR PERSONAL USE

SELF-INDUCED ANESTHESIA

All people have the power to render their own body immune to pain, but few of them have ever mastered this gift. Some people seem to develop this power spontaneously, but most have need to practice. Self-confidence, willpower, concentration of direct thought and patient practice are required. Some children have been able to acquire this power as part of their nature. Such a child can be spanked severely and yet feels nothing in the way of pain.

Stage hypnotists are frequently seen to pass a needle through a subject's cheek or the flesh of the arm, and no pain at all is experienced as a result of the anesthetic suggestions given prior to the penetration. Stories are often told of how the fakirs of India pass pins through most any part of their body without experiencing the slightest discomfort.

Developing the ability to establish anesthesia takes practice, but you can acquire it if you wish. Use the same general technique of inducing hypnosis in yourself that you have learned and direct into your mind, in precisely the same way, suggestions for the abolishment of pain sensations. It will seem startling, even to your-self the results that are obtained with surprisingly little practice in that direction.

The mastering of pain, i.e. producing self-induced anesthesia is but the beginning of the remarkable things you can do to benefit yourself using this power.

Whatever you have learned to do for others when you hypnotize them, you can equally do for yourself when you hypnotize yourself.

HYPNOTIC INFLUENCE FOR SUPER-LEARNING

The use of hypnotism for increasing learning ability is outstanding. Most learning is largely a matter of retaining the information taught and recalling it readily when it is required. The subconscious mind operates like the memory banks of a computer and all information stored therein can be recalled when you press the right buttons, as it were. Self-hypnosis can give you that ability.

The night before the examination takes place, instead of staying up all night trying to cram, place yourself in a hypnotic state and give your inner mind the suggestion that all the answers will pop out and appear on your "screen of mind". Write down what appears and there you are. Learn how to do this and you will come out 100% each and every time.

When you study and when you receive instructions from a teacher, just relax and listen. Allow the information to sink in. Even taking notes is not necessary, unless one is in the habit of taking notes. Actually, the information given you is all there for the taking.

If you want to recall something you have been taught and cannot seem to recall it, just relax and stop trying so hard. Just let your mind drift, while holding onto the thought as to where you want it to drift. Answers will seem to float in all by themselves.

The secret is to make the effort to recall without trying hard to recall. In other words, make the effort without the effort.

Many examinations given these days are based on knowing whether a question asked is right or wrong and the examination requires that the student place a plus (+) for right before the question asked if it is correct and a minus (-) if it is wrong. In self-hypnosis, tell your subconscious the correct symbol will appear for each question asked in the exam. If you seem to hallucinate in seeing the symbols, so much the better. Try this and see how it comes out.

Basically it is the job of the teacher to teach and the job of the student to learn. Yet, far too often, education becomes a challenge between the teacher and the student. It is almost as though the instructors were saying, "I dare you to learn what I have to teach you." Such is the challenge and a challenge invariably sends a message of stress to the mind. Instead of a challenge, education should be presented as a game to be played and enjoyed between teacher and student. Games are fun and relaxing to the mind. Mind functions best when it is relaxed.

More and more, as the educational system begins to apply these principles of how the mind operates (many of which you have learned in this book), more and more geniuses will be produced.

CHAPTER THIRTY-SIX

MORE FOR YOUR HYPNOTIC "KNOW-HOW"

HYPNOTISM IS SAFE AND SANE

The hue and cry occasionally set up by ill informed people that hypnotism is harmful to the mind is ridiculous. Hypnosis is a perfectly natural function of the mind. Millions of cases of hypnotism have been conducted all over the world and not a single, harmful result has been reported.

However, everything has both a positive and a negative aspect. The mind can take on harmful suggestions just as well as it can take on helpful ones. As an example, look at how Hitler hypnotized the whole nation of Germany. But by and large, hypnotists are highly principled people who are out to help humanity, not harm it. In stage demonstrations of hypnotism, the entire audience is there to witness that no harmful suggestions are presented. Furthermore, in hypnotherapy, usually a third party is present to witness the procedure with the client.

Hypnotism can be looked upon as a rapid way of changing the mind. It is an effective way to produce both physical and mental changes in the body and mind of the hypnotized individual. Mind affects body and body affects mind. Correctly used, hypnosis provides a wonderful tool for mental training. If there is ever any harm, it is never from the hypnosis. Any harm must rest entirely on the scruples of the hypnotist. However, it can equally be said that the physician is in the same boat, in relation to standards.

HYPNOTIC INFLUENCE AND CRIME

A study of hypnotic suggestion may offer some useful ideas to the penal code that are worthy of thought. Someone or something influences everybody to a greater or lesser degree consciously or subconsciously, or by the environment to which they are exposed. Environment greatly enhances suggestive influence. If a man is continuously exposed to a criminal side of life and commences to feel that such is the best way to get along, he is likely to become a criminal. On the other hand, if he lives in an environment that goes along with the accepted protocol of society, he is most likely to so conform. He becomes a good citizen.

Beyond question, there are some persons that seem to have rebellious, antisocial instincts in them that lead to criminal behavior. However, even in such persons, there seems to be a countering trait of goodness that can often be developed.

For example, as has often happened if a criminal is placed in the company of, shall we say, sensible and honest people who seem to be getting along okay in life, he will often revert to ways of good behavior rather than bad behavior for, basically, good in humanity predominates over bad. If such a man is removed from the environment of criminality and placed in an environment of usefulness to his fellow man, often a remarkable shift in attitude will occur. On the other hand, if he is sent to jail on his first offense and placed among others far more criminally minded than him-self, he is very likely to sink yet deeper into attitudes of crime. In this is seen the obvious operation of hypnotic suggestion which we have learned so well, which operates so powerfully within the mind of the individual.

By removing him from the criminal influence so often found in the penitentiary and placing him in a different environment, his mentality will, hopefully, head towards reform for the better.

Physical punishment will never reform a criminal and on the contrary, it fills his mind with hatred and malice towards mankind, and at the first chance he gets, he seeks to avenge himself. On the other hand, if the appeal is made to the subliminal self via the hypnotic suggestions and example, the spark of good that is within him may be kindled.

As was mentioned, in actual experience, good seems to predominate over bad in most people. For example, a good man, even when deeply hypnotized, will not obey a suggestion against his ingrained moral nature. The instinct of self-preservation steps in and says, "No." In the same manner, a moral woman cannot be induced to perform an immoral act, and if such is insisted upon by the operator, will awaken from the hypnosis, frequently with a shock.

A dramatic experiment to induce criminal behavior in hypnotized individuals was tried in psychological laboratories, in which a deeply hypnotized person was told that his worse enemy was before him and the suggestion made that he would kill him. The subject was then handed a length of paper suggested to be a knife and told to stab his enemy in the back.

Invariably, the subject would plunge the imaginary knife in the back of his enemy. But when the same subject was handed a real knife and told to kill the enemy, the suggestion was never carried out. Some would drop the knife. Others would tremble violently when the suggestion was insisted upon. Most subjects would simply awaken immediately from the hypnosis spontaneously of their own volition.

A rule of thumb in relation to hypnotic suggestions is that the subject will carry out all suggestions given by the operator providing they do not conflict with his moral nature, personal characteristics, or produce serious consequences to him-self. In a nutshell, it can be said that the subconscious mind of a person is basically protective of the individual.

When told by the hypnotist that they are great movie stars, sports personalities, singers, or politicians, they impersonate the characters suggested to the best of their ability. Often the acting out of the character is truly first rate. As a politician he will give a speech you suggest. As a singer he will sing a popular song he knows. Put the proper music behind him and you'll get a performance.

Any person can be cured of bashfulness or stage fright immediately while hypnotized. Incorrigible children can be made very pleasant by the use of posthypnotic suggestion.

NO WEAKENING OF THE WILL

Some people claim that hypnotism weakens the will. This is absolutely untrue. A subject is naturally more responsive to the hypnotist because of a deep-rooted idea that he must follow the operator's suggestions on command. But no weakening of the will occurs. In fact, hypnosis can make the person stronger willed!

If you are working with a subject who feels that he is too susceptible to hypnotic influence, put the person into hypnosis and suggest that he can only be hypnotized upon his own request. Tell him that the one he has most confidence in is himself, and that he is the personal director of all he does, as is his wish.

AWAKENING SOMEONE ELSE'S SUBJECT

If you should ever be called upon to awaken a subject someone else has hypnotized but failed to arouse, go about it in this way. Re-hypnotize the subject while he is still in trance until you reach a stage where he will answer your questions or respond to performing some action you suggest. In this way, you will get in rapport with him and it will be an easy manner to arouse him.

The only reason a subject sometimes refuses to come out of hypnosis at the moment suggested is because he enjoys being in the stress free state of hypnosis so much that he is loath to come back to the outside world. Tell such a subject that unless he snaps out of it quickly now, he will never again be able to enter hypnosis. He will awaken instantly.

FINALLY ...

Here are two, great "suggestion formulas" for you to use. One formula that increases hypnotic responsiveness and another formula for appreciating living life to the hilt. Use #1 after hypnotizing a subject and before you commence any hypnotherapy suggestions.

Number One:

"Everything .. we .. do .. together .. is .. in .. perfect .. harmony .. between .. us, .. and .. it .. gives .. you .. the .. greatest .. pleasure .. to .. go .. into .. profound .. hypnosis, .. and .. perform .. to .. perfection .. everything .. that .. I .. suggest .. you .. perform."

This harmonizing suggestion forms a background for all hypnotic proceedings the subject will experience, motivating him towards profound hypnosis.

And before arousing a subject from hypnosis, use formula #2. Suggest:

Number Two:

"When .. you .. awaken .. from .. hypnosis .. and .. come .. back .. to .. the .. here .. and .. now, .. you .. will .. be .. in .. love .. with .. the .. total .. of .. Existence .. and .. will .. appreciate .. the .. miracle .. that .. you .. are."

Awakening from hypnosis with that suggestion embedded in the subconscious is truly miraculous.

TALKING ABOUT FUTURE PLANS
"TAKING OUR TWO-MAN HYPNOTISM SHOW ON THE ROAD"

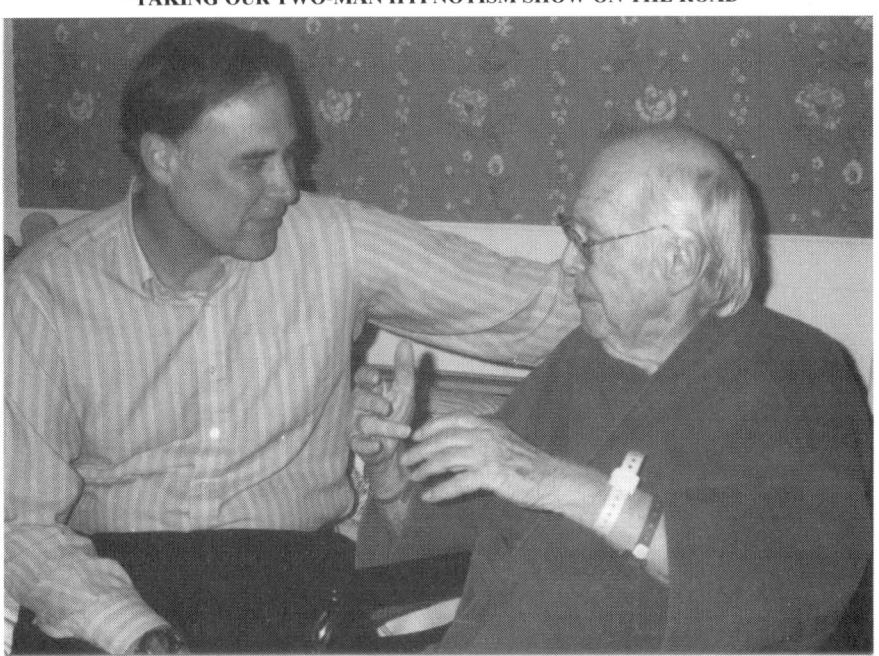

ORMOND TALKING TO TOM ABOUT THEIR PLANS TO PERFORM HYPNOTISM SHOW "FUND-RAISERS" FOR UNIVERSITIES IN CALIFORNIA

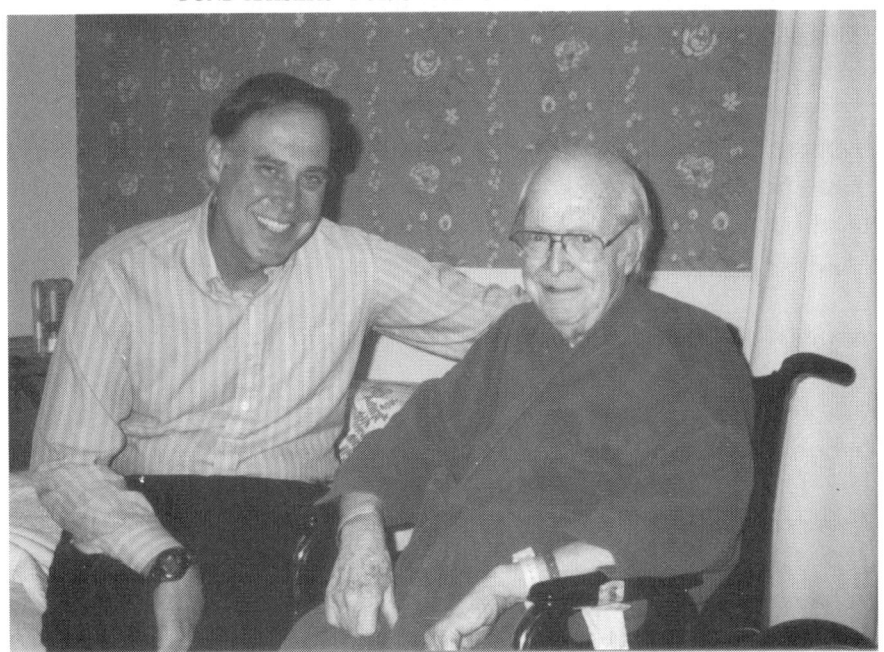

TOM SILVER AND ORMOND MCGILL TALKING ABOUT FUTURE PLANS WHILE ORMOND RECOVERS FROM SURGERY IN NORTHERN CALIFORNIA *JANUARY 2002

CHAPTER THIRTY-SEVEN

THE RELAXATION METHOD OF HYPNOTIZING

This method is performed entirely without suggestions of sleep. In fact, there is no need to mention hypnotism at all, the subject's attention being entirely directed towards relaxation. First, consider these two important aspects related to entrancement:

1. Consent:
The consent of the subject (willingness) to be hypnotized is basic to the successful induction of hypnosis. This can be either a conscious acceptance or an unconscious acceptance that can be summed up in the idea of EXPECTANCY (expectancy of being hypnotized).

2. Communication:
There must be an avenue of communication between the operator and the subject. In the case of interlingual hypnosis, our working via an interpreter provides an avenue of communication to the subject, as he translates our words into the appropriate language. If an understanding of the expected hypnotic occurrence can be conveyed to the subject, either through an interpreter or by the subject watching other persons hypnotized, the hypnotizing technique can be successful even in pantomime. We always handle this method of hypnotizing without mentioning the idea of going to sleep in close association with our interpreter providing a personal communication with the subject.

Application of the Relaxation Method of Hypnotizing

You and the person you are going to hypnotize by this method sit opposite each other, and have a chat about relaxation.

You comment:
"I will show you a pleasant way of relaxing that will make you feel very good. Doctors to relieve tension often use this method. The physician would probably define it as concentrated relaxation of mind and body. It will make you relax and feel good all over. Would you like to try the experience"?

Obtain the subject's verbal consent that he (or she) would very much like to. You continue:

"Okay then. As you sit in your chair right now, make yourself comfortable and relax. Let me take your hand for just a moment. Now, relax the hand I am holding as much as you can. Relax it so it becomes completely loose and limp. (Subject does as requested) That's fine. You are doing excellently".

BY NOTING THE SUBJECT'S RESPONSE IN RELAXING HIS HAND, AS IT RESTS IN YOURS, YOU CAN IMMEDIATELY DETERMINE HIS STATE OF MIND IN RELATION TO FOLLOWING YOUR SUGGESTIONS. INSIST THAT HE BECOME COMPLETELY RELAXED. WHEN YOU SENSE THAT HIS HAND IS ENTIRELY RELAXED, PROCEED ON.

"Now, take a deep breath. Breath in slowly and deeply. Hold your breath for a moment now let it out slowly. (Subject does as instructed.) Very good. Now, once again take a deep breath, hold it, and let it out. It relaxes you"

"Now, let your eyes close and think of relaxing all tension from your body. (Subject does as instructed.) Fine. You are doing fine. Feels better already, doesn't it! Now, relax the muscles around your eyes; relax them so completely that they feel loose and limp. When you are sure your eye muscles are so relaxed that the muscles won't work, try to make them work, and you will find that they will not work at all, and you cannot open your eyes because the muscles of your eyes have become so relaxed. You are now obtaining real deep relaxation".

AT THIS POINT IN THIS INDUCTION PROCESS, THE SUBJECT HAS BYPASSED HIS SENSE OF JUDGEMENT, WHICH IS HIS CONSCIOUS MIND TELLING HIM THAT HE CAN CLOSE AND OPEN HIS EYES AT WILL. IF HE SHOULD OPEN HIS EYES, TELL HIM THAT HE HAS JUST PROVED THAT HE HAS NOT COMPLETELY RELAXED HIS EYE MUSCLES AS YET, AS THEY STILL OPERATE. REQUEST HIM TO CONCENTRATE FURTHER ON THE RELAXATION OF THOSE MUSCLES SO THEY BECOME COMPLETELY RELAXED AND WILL NO LONGER FUNCTION. HAVE HIM TEST HIS EYES, AND IF THEY REMAIN CLOSED PROCEED WITH THESE FURTHER

SUGGESTIONS OF RELAXATION.

"Now that your eyes are closed and the muscles of your eyes are completely relaxed, you will find that you can now relax your whole body much deeper than ever, and you feel wonderful. So extend that same feeling of your eyes relaxing down over your whole body relaxing. Just let the relaxation of your eyes flow down over your whole body. Extend that same feeling of complete relaxation right down from your eyes to the very tips of your toes. What a nice feeling it is to relax like this. You enjoy it".

"Now, here is something very interesting. When I ask you to, I want you to gently open and close your eyes. You can do this easily, and you will find that it will make you more relaxed than ever. In fact, it will make you ten times as relaxed as you are right now. All the other muscles of your body will continue being completely relaxed, only your eyes will open and close gently when I tell them to".

"All ready, one, two, three ... open your eyes gently ... now close them ... and relax ten times as much as you were before. Notice what a wonderful surge of relaxation this brings over you. Now, when you do that again, just double your relaxation this time, and you will feel like you have a blanket of relaxation covering you from head to toes".

"Ready again ... one, two, three ... now open your eyes and now close them, and double the relaxation you had, and you will feel that blanket of relaxation covering you from head to toes".

THROUGHOUT THIS INITIAL PROCEDURE, YOU HAVE BEEN HOLDING TIE SUBJECT'S HAND IN YOURS. FOLLOW WITH THESE SUGGESTIONS:

"Now, when I release your hand, it will drop like a limp rag into your lap, and you will be completely relaxed".

RELEASE HIS HAND AND LET IT FALL INTO HIS LAP. YOU HAVE INDUCED HYPNOSIS, AND ARE NOW READY TO DEEPEN THE STATE BY THIS TECHNIQUE. SUGGEST TO THE SUBJECT:

"You have achieved a splendid state of physical relaxation, but if you can relax mentally as well, you will find it will make your feel a hundred times as good as you do right now.

Here is how you can do it".

"When I tell you to, I want you to start counting backward, beginning with the number one hundred, and each time you say a number double your relaxation, and by the time you get to number ninety-seven, the numbers will have been relaxed right out of your mind. They will simply fade out and disappear, and you will not be able to find any more numbers. Now, relax deeply, say that first number, double your relaxation, and watch what happens".

(SUBJECT SAYS THE FIRST NUMBER.)

One hundred.

YOU INSTRUCT

"That's fine! Now double your relaxation and they will commence to fade away. Say the second number now".

(SUBJECT SAYS THE SECOND NUMBER.)

"Ninety-nine".

CONTINUE ON IN THIS MANNER UP UNTIL NUMBER NINETY-SEVEN.

AT THIS POINT YOU INSTRUCT.

"And now they'll all be gone. All gone! You can't see any more numbers in your mind. You can't find any more numbers. They are all gone. That's fine. Now relax more and more with every breath you take, and notice how relaxed and wonderful you feel".

IF THE SUBJECT CONTINUES TO COUNT ON BACKWARD FROM ONE HUNDRED AT THIS POINT, STOP HIM WITH THE SUGGESTION:

"You are doing fine, but stop now saying any more numbers. Relax in between the numbers. Relaxation will make them disappear.

Now, I will pick up your right hand and drop it, and as I drop it let those numbers drop right out of your wind at the same time".

PICK UP HIS HAND AND DROP IT IN HIS LAP, AS YOU SUGGEST:

"There, the numbers are all gone. The numbers have dropped right out of your mind. They are all gone and you can't find any more numbers. The numbers are all gone from your mind, and your mind as well as your body is now relaxed".

THIS PROCESS HAS PLACED THE SUBJECT IN DEEP HYPNOSIS, AND HAS COMMENCED ANMESIA, AS EXEMPLIFIED IN THE FORGOTTEN NUMBERS SEQUENCE. NOTE THAT YOU HAVE NOT STATED THAT THE SUBJECT COULD NOT REMEMBER ANY NUMBERS. YOU HAVE STATED THAT HE CANNOT FIND ANY MORE NUMBERS. THE FINE USE OF LANGUAGE IS THE KEY TO EFFECTIVE SUGGESTION. CONTINUE THE INDUCTION PROCESS FURTHER BY TESTING FOR INCREASED AMNESIA, AS YOU SUGGEST:

"Now you are relaxed so completely both physically and mentally, that if I asked your phone number you wouldn't be able to find it to tell me ... would you"?

SUBJECT RESPONDS WITH A SHAKE OF HIS HEAD OR A WHISPERED NO. YOU HAVE INDUCED AMNESIA RESPONSE IN THIS GENTLE WAY, WHICH IS CHARACTERISTIC OF A DEEP SOMNAMBULISTIC LEVEL OF HYPNOSIS. YOU ARE NOW READY TO PRESENT TO SUBJECT' S SUBCONSCIOUS WHATEVER SUGGESTION FORMULA WHICH IS DESIRED, AS THE CENTRAL PURPOSE FOR WHICH THE SUBJECT HAS BE HYPNOTIZED TO ACHIEVE.

IN RELATION TO PURPOSEFUL SUGGESTION FORMULAS I AM GOING TO GIVE YOU A WONDERFUL GIFT IN GIVING YOU A SERIES OF THESE TELLING HOW TO BECOME MASTER OF ONE'S MIND. IT IS THEN THAT ONE BECOMES A MASTERMIND. YOU CAN PRESENT THESE FORMULAS TO

THE SUBCONSIOUSNESS OF A SUBJECT USING HETERO-HYPNOSIS, OR TO YOURSELF USING SELF-HYPNOSIS.

NOTE TO HYPNOTIST:

In this method of hypnotizing the entire attention of the subject is centered on the idea of achieving physical and mental relaxation. Hypnosis can be induced very effectively this way, and with some persons who object to the idea of going to sleep, which infers a loss of consciousness, the method will be found excellent.

CHAPTER THIRTY-EIGHT

OPERATING YOUR BIO SUBCONSCIOUS COMPUTER

TEACHING YOUR CLIENTS HOW TO BE THE OPERATOR OF THEIR MIND?

This is a question asked by great many and in fact, very few succeeded. You can most effectively control the mind of others when you learn how to control your own mind. When you learn how to control your own mind, then you can show others how to control their mind. And, as a hypnotist, you can hypnotically induce that control. That is the process here suggested. The power of the process of mind has potential beyond our wildest dreams. Controlled it can lift one to the heights of genius. Uncontrolled it can plunge one into the depths of insanity. Most people are in-between.

When a client seeks your service as a hypnotherapist, it is usually because something in the mind is out of control. They hope that through hypnosis they can regain control. Let's begin by considering how you can best control your own mind.

To really control your mind you must recognize that you are not your mind. That is to say, you use your mind but that mind is not YOU. You are your SELF -- a consciousness that uses your mind as a means of producing thoughts. That realization is your first step in controlling your mind. Follow these three rules and put them into effect as your way of using your mind.

The first rule of mind control is to
Make your mind think what you want it to think.

Mind for so long has had the freedom to think whatever it wants to think, that it is easy to feel that it is in control of you. Reverse this process, and recognize that mind is actually there only as an activity you can engage in, as you wish to use it. To control your mind, you must tighten up on this discipline. Learn to regulate your mind as though it were a mechanism that you can turn on and off at will. Learn to do this for yourself, and then you can help others do it. Remember, a mind out of control is the basis of all mental disturbances.

The second rule of mind control is to
Make your mind think when you want it to think
And stop thinking when you do not want it to think.

For many, mind for so long has been allowed to bring in thoughts unbidden, that it seems that it does your thinking for you. That way thoughts can be a confusing shambles without organization, and often disturbing. To correct this, you must become master of your mind instead of it being master of you. Use mind when you want to use it and do not use it when you do not want to use it. In other words, you must learn to make your mind become silent when you want it to become silent.

The third rule of mind control is to
Become a witness to the thoughts you think.

The more proficient you can become at witnessing your thoughts (as though from a distance viewing) the more control you will develop over your mind. Allow this witnessing perspective to thinking apply to all forms of mental activity. Make it your habitual way of thinking In doing this, you will find it will greatly alter your sense of perception, and it will not be long before the recognition will come that it is your SELF that is doing the actual thinking, and not your mind that is doing the thinking.

Let us now consider a little deeper how these rules apply to controlling your mind:

Rule Number One:

Be willing to accept the fact that up to this point in your life (and that goes for your client's life as well) the operation of your mind has been pretty much hit-or-miss. Sometimes your thinking has been reliable but just as often it has been unreliable. Sometimes your thinking has produced thoughts of truth, but just as often it has produced untrue thoughts. And, you have had little means of knowing what is true and what it not true.

Rule Number Two:

Become able to regulate your mind is to be able to turn it on when you wish to use it, and to turn it off when you do not wish to use it. For this purpose, look upon your mind as a mechanism that you use to think with; and, you can make it think because you want it to think, not because it makes you think. Looking upon your mind in this manner brings in awareness that you can operate it precisely as you wish.

To be able to turn off your mind seems a paradox, as the word mind conveys everything you feel is important to your life. How then can you turn it off without losing your mind? To turn off your mind does not mean you will lose your mind, as you cannot exist without your mind. But you can learn to control it to stop thinking when you want to become quiet inside, as mind is just an activity. Possibly it can be explained through an analogy. You talk and you say you are talking. What is talking? If you stop talking, where is the talking? Talking is nothing tangible. It is just an activity. Mind is precisely like that, and just as you can control the process of talking so you can control the process of thinking. How can you do this?

In the Orient, there is a proverb which says that mind is like a restless monkey, and the more you try to control the monkey the more restless the monkey gets. To control the monkey, the best way is to just leave the monkey alone and allow it to control itself. Mind is like that; if you wish to control your mind do not try to control it. Just let it be, and let your mind do whatever it is doing, but do not allow yourself to become identified with the thinking it is doing. In other words, just become a witness to whatever your mind conjures up, as though you were watching a motion picture upon a screen, and don't be concerned with what your mind is picturing. This brings us to a consideration of Rule Number three.

Rule Number Three:

Be as unconcerned about what your mind is doing as if it didn't belong to you. Do that and you will soon get your mind under control, for it continues to produce thoughts because you have always helped it produce thoughts. But, if you don't cooperate with it, while the thoughts will continue on for awhile, it will not be long before they stop coming by themselves, and your mind will become quiet.

A quiet mind is a peaceful mind, and a peaceful mind is a mind under control. That is the discipline, and when you learn how to use that mental discipline for yourself you can then pass it along to others. Implanting these controlled methods of using the mind in the subconscious of your-self and other (via self-hypnosis and hetero-hypnosis) where they become conditioned as habit of thinking brings about amazing results. And the amazement is unending.

WHAT IS CONSCIOUSNESS?

Awareness can be another meaning for consciousness. The more aware you are of what is happening around you, the more consciousness you are. In relation to human beings consciousness can be recognized in four main areas or levels:

One:
Unconscious Consciousness. Such as a rock is in this state of consciousness. A rock has no conscious level of thought energy at all.

Two:
Simple Consciousness. Consciousness appears to advance from Unconsciousness, and the next upward level of thought energy can be found in plants, trees, etc. Consciousness is there, but it is a poorly defined consciousness, without a personal awareness of self. It is a simple form of consciousness. The next leap in simple consciousness can be found in animals. Complete recognition of self is not there as yet, but it far more advanced than it is in plants. Because this level of Consciousness has instinct, habit, emotion and more. Self Consciousness is arising.

Three:
Human "Self" Consciousness. Man is the most advanced of any creature on earth having Self Consciousness. Man is aware of himself, as an individual. The degree of this awareness differs with individuals, of course, but it is there. For most, in this stage of consciousness, which took place historically starting around 60,000 years ago, according to the archeological discovery, man recognizes his outer self, but the potential is there to recognize his inner self, as well. Hypnosis provides a definite aid in giving man this recognition.

With this recognition, man makes the next quantum leap in awareness to.

Four:
Advanced "Optima Consciousness. Optima Consciousness or Awareness, which has also been called, Cosmic Consciousness It is the recognition of consciousness being directly related to the consciousness of the Universe. Through Advanced Consciousness comes recognition that the entire Universe has a connection. The more Advanced Consciousness you experience, the more conscious you become of ALL that exists, and appreciate that YOU are an innate part of that All. This concept applies only to those who want to accept it and who believe in it. Most people live in the world "Human "Self" Consciousness".

CHAPTER THIRTY-NINE

LIFE-ENERGY VITALIZING HYPNOSIS
BY ORMOND MCGILL

This is one of the most powerful techniques ever developed for revitalizing your clients. As a hypnotherapist you will recognize that many personal difficulties among people exist from simply not having sufficient vitality to deal with the stress of the many problems they have to face in daily living. When sufficient vitality is there to handle things life becomes a joy instead of a struggle. Using this technique you give your clients a boundless source of vitality. Then, like magic imagined difficulties evaporate away like a drop of water on a hot tin roof. The method can become a specialty of your office practice.

PRELUDE TO THE METHOD:

Hypnotize your client by whatever method you prefer, opening the subconscious to mastery of visualization for bringing vitality into the body via life-energy.

Now, stand beside your entranced client and place your hand in comradeship upon his (or her) shoulder, as you give these suggestions to the opened (via hypnosis) subconscious mind:

AFTER HYPNOSIS THE BEGINNING:
(Suggest to the client while in hypnosis) Visualize (Imagine) a mass of energy the size of a glowing light bulb forming in the base of your spine. See it glowing brightly in your mind. Now feel it also as that area of your body becomes warm from the glowing light. Do you experience it successfully thus?

Note to the Hypnotist: Some subjects do not have the ability of visualization, and then, just use the word Imagine.

Obtain an affirmation before proceeding on. A positive affirmation assures that your client will greatly benefit from this technique.

(Confirm) Good. Feel it strongly. Experience it fully. It brings life-giving vitality into your Being. Now you are ready to move the light throughout your body from organ to organ bringing you wonderful health and strength. All ready, let's start. One, two, three...

(The mind likes to start an operation on a One, Two, Three because it is used to handling constructive activities in that manner.)

STEP ONE:
Now visualize the energy from the base of your spine moving up your spine to the top of your head.

Experience it.
RELAX BETWEEN

STEP TWO:
Now visualize the energy glowing at the top of your head, and move it down between your eyes clear down to the tip of your nose.

Experience it.
RELAX BETWEEN

STEP THIREE:
Now take a deep breath and draw the light into your nose, visualize it going down into your throat and into your lungs. Strongly with your mind see your lungs as alive with light.

Experience it.
RELAX BETWEEN

STEP FOUR:
Imagine the energy permeating your lungs -- filling all space between your armpits. Your lungs are alive with light. Your lungs are filled with energy.

STEP FIVE:
Now with your mind move the energy from your armpits down your arms to the thumbs of your hands. Feel your thumbs become warm and commence to tingle. Then, from your thumbs visualize the energy in your thumbs sparking across to your forefingers, and spark on to other fingers, as a living electrical current, until your hands are alive with energy,

Experience it.
RELAX BETWEEN

STEP SIX:
Now move the energy from your hands on back up your arms to your shoulders. (Pause there a moment) then move across your shoulders to your neck to the points where your jaw meets your cheeks. Feel your cheeks flush and glow with warmth.

Experience it.
RELAX BETWEEN

STEP SEVEN:
Now move the energy from your face down the front of your body to your navel -- to a point in the area of your appendix just right of your navel.

Experience it.
RELAX BETWEEN

STEP EIGHT:
Now move the energy up the right side of your abdomen, and move it into the colon bathing any obstruction therein in the light and healing.

Experience it.
RELAX BETWEEM

STEP NINE:
Now move the energy from your colon on out of the rectum.

Experience it.
RELAX BETWEEN

STEP TEN:
Now imagine the warm tingling energy flowing over your sex organs causing teasing sexual feelings. (Experience it) Now from your sex organs move the energy straight up the front of your body -- up and up until it covers your chin and now let it divide and move over each cheek just below the bottom of each eye.

Experience it.
RELAX BETWEEN

STEP ELEVEN:
Now from your cheeks visualize the energy flowing down your cheeks over the sides of your jaws, and again descending clear down to your stomach. Bath your stomach in the energy, aiding every digestive and assimilation process. Feel your stomach glow while filling the entire center of your Being with vitality.

Experience it.
RELAX BETWEEN

STEP TWELVE:
Now move the energy down either side of your abdomen and on across your groin ... continue on and move it on down the front of your legs letting it find its way to your feet and moving across to the second toe. Take your time there is no hurry.

Experience it fully.
RELAX BETWEEN

STEP THIRTEEN:
Now let the energy leap from toe to toe until, your toes are tingling with the energy. Think it and you will feel it. Finally let the energy leap to your big toe on each foot.

Experience it.
RELAX BETWEEN

STEP FOURTEEN:
Now move the energy up the inside of your feet to your ankles, and on up the inside of each leg.

Experience it.
RELAX BE'IWEEN

STEP FIFTEEN:
Now let the energy move into the inside of your thighs.

Experience it.
RELAX BETWEEN

STEP SIXTEEN:
Now move the energy again across your groins and then divide it so it passes up each side of the center of your body moving on up to reach beneath each armpit.

Experience it.
RELAX BETWEEN

STEP SEVENTEEN:
Now let the energy move to the area of your pancreas, which is located on the left side of your abdomen just below the bottom of the ribcage. Feel this entire area become warm and filled with light. Feel a freedom from all tension in this area of your body.

Experience it.
RELAX BETWEEN

STEP EIGHTEEN:
Now let the energy, which is your life force, move to the center of your body on to your heart. Feel your heart become filled with the energy ... healing the heart in everyway and opening it up to loving emotions for everyone and everything. Let the energy bathe your heart.

Experience it.
RELAX BETWEEN

STEP NINETEEN:
Now move the energy again back into your armpits and then move it on down the inside of each arm and across the palms of your hands to the fingers. Feel your fingers tingle.

Experience it.
RELAX BETWEEN

STEP TWENTY:
Now move the energy up the back of your arms to the outside of your elbows and again on up to the armpits and on across your shoulders.

Experience it.
RELAX BETWEEN

STEP TWENTY ONE:
Now move the energy across your jawbone and bury itself in either cheek. Now imagine the energy manifesting itself deep in the center of each ear.

Experience it.
RELAX BETWEEN

STEP TWENTY TWO:
Now move the energy to your third eye center at a point between the eyebrows. Imagine a glowing in the center like the bursting of a star. Let the glow from that center move on to the top of your head and your entire head become hot with force. Then see it in your mind's eye as sending the generated force as a searchlight of the energy from the top of your head far out into the space of the very Universe itself. Your entire head is aglow with energy. Your brain is filled with energy and the energy brings in KNOWING of truth to you and activates your powers of ESP and intuition.

Experience it.
RELAX BETWEEN

STEP TWENTY THREE:
Now know you have benefited your body in everyway. You have filled it with vitality, and have become master of YOURSELF.

Experience it.
RELAX BETWEEN

STEP TWENTY FOUR:
Now rest. Feeling your entire body being alive with vitality, aglow with energy. Breathe deeply and fully and just relax, as the energy of life itself surges through you from head to toes.

Experience it.
RELAX BETWEEN

STEP TWENTY FIVE:
Gradually allow the energy within yourself to subside now and sink down into rest, from which you will gradually return to full alertness master of your place in life. The process is complete. Come back with me now to THE HERE AND NOW again, as is your wish. Of such nature is the process of Vitality Hypnosis. Nothing further need be done.

On arousal from this trance, your client with leave your office with a bounce to his step happiness in his heart, with a body filled with vitality and a will to do and dare in meeting life's many adventures.

As a professional hypnotherapist you can allow a full hour for the process. Allow full time for each experiencing of the moving of the energy about the body to occur. Then allow client to relax some moments in silence before proceeding on to the next movement. The results are phenomenal.

VITALITY SELF-HYPNOSIS.

You have been shown how to used the process for the benefit of your clients, and in this doing you will have learned it well. Now you can use it equally for the benefit of yourself in the renewing of your personal energy. Just lie down in the comfort of your bed and relax. Breathe deeply and freely and visualize the ball of white light generating at the base of your own spine. Then move it through your own body in precisely the same manner you have instructed your client to do.

Just make the effort of performing the process without undue effort and just drift dreamily through the various processes, and when you finish lie still and become silent both within and without yourself. You will return to your own here and now refreshed in everyway; with vast sources of vitality springing ever anew within yourself.
ARISE AND SHINE!

It will be noted that Vitality Hypnosis is based in imagination in visualized forms of mental picturing. Indeed this is true for imagination is the creative power of the mind. Everything commences in imagination, from which, with energy, it becomes transformed into reality. Of such is the precise operation of Vitality Hypnosis. As a hypnotherapist always knows that mind is that within each one of us that produces thoughts, and those thoughts are things

(Forms of directed energy), for the truth is that
"AS A MAN THINKEST IN HIS HEART SO IS HE".

Hypnosis makes it possible to direct and control the thoughts that make man master of his mind so he can become exactly what is his wish to be.

CHAPTER FOURTY

SUGGESTION-FORMULAS

SUGGESTION FORMULAS FOR ACHIEVING CONTROL OF MIND

In this chapter, you are given four "suggestion formulas" to be used in connection with Mastermind Hypnosis. These do not offer suggestions, which deal with surface things as stopping smoking, eating less to become slim, mastering unwanted habits, and such run-of-the-mill problems. These "suggestion formulas" are basic to strengthening the inner structure of the client's personality, mastery of mind, and advancing consciousness. These are important, as once self-mastery is achieved other behavioral disturbances are easily corrected. When one's true nature is recognized and mind is under control of SELF, a mere flash of thought and it is done!

As you present these "suggestion formulas" to your subjects, at the same time, allow yourself to slip into the hypnotic state, and you will be benefiting yourself while you are benefiting your client.

SUGGESTION FORMULA FOR CONTROLLING MIND

Using Hetero-Hypnosis when working with other persons or Self-Hypnosis when working with yourself induce the inspired subconscious state of mind of hypnosis in as profound a state as possible ... this renders the mind wide open and receptive to these suggestions:

"You are obtaining perfect control over your mind. Your control over your mind lifts you up and up and up to heights of genius".

"You instinctively know that you are not your mind and that you use your mind to work for you. Your mind is your servant and it works for you. You use your mind to produce your thoughts, and your thoughts are filled with wisdom in every way".

"You are becoming instinctively able to make your mind think you want it to think. You have automatic control of your mind and it thinks what you want it to think".

"You are becoming instinctively able to make your mind think when you want it to think, and to stop thinking when you do not want it to

think. You have absolute control over your mind, and you can make it think when you want it to think and to stop thinking when you do not want it to think".

"When you use your mind, it is absolutely under your control and the thoughts you think are orderly and disciplined. You can turn your mind on and off at will".

"You are becoming instinctively a witness to your thoughts. You witness the thoughts as you think them. Your entire sense of perception is that of becoming a witness to your thoughts".

"You are obtaining perfect control over your mind, and this perfect control over your mind is now your very own. Your subconscious makes the way you use your mind become your reality".

Repeat this "suggestion formula" three times, arid awaken the client from hypnosis.

NOTE TO HYPNOTHERAPIST

These suggestions given in hypnosis to your clients will prove of great benefit to them. Be sure, via self-hypnosis, to make them your very own as well. As commented upon, they will prove of equal benefit to yourself, for the truth is that as your subconscious mind directs your thinking such is the way that you will think spontaneously.

SUGGESTION FORMULA FOR FUNCTION OF MIND

Using Hypnosis, induce a deep level of hypnosis, rendering the subconscious mind wide open and receptive to these suggestions:

"Know that your mind has five main functions: right knowledge, wrong knowledge, imagination, sleep, and memory. Remember this always. Remember that your mind has five main functions: right knowledge, wrong knowledge, imagination, sleep and memory. Remember always that your mind has five main functions: right knowledge, wrong knowledge, imagination, sleep, and memory. Always remembering you will use these functions of mind perfectly for benefiting your life".

"You will use your mind automatically always to bring in right knowledge for you.

"You will make the right decisions, you will do the right thing and always you will turn your mind in the direction of right knowledge. Right knowledge is the way you will use your mind".

"And you will turn away from wrong knowledge. You reject your mind's function of wrong knowledge. Wrong knowledge has no place in your life from this moment on. Your new functioning in right knowledge completely overwhelms wrong knowledge, and wrong knowledge vanishes from your mind forever. From this time on you will function from your center of right knowledge".

"And you will use your imagination to create wonderful and beautiful things. Your imagination is very powerful, and it creates a wonderful and bountiful life for you. Your imagination has great power, and you will use it from this time on always to create wonderful and beautiful things. You have perfect control over your imagination, and you use it to benefit your life in every way".

"And you will use the power of sleep to benefit you in every way. You will sleep soundly and well, and sleep will refresh you and revitalize you. Sleep will be healthful in every way. Sleep is beneficial to you in every way, and as you sleep, from this time on, the quality of your sleep will begin to change and you will become a witnessing consciousness while you sleep. Each night when you go into deep sleep, you will become a witnessing consciousness while you sleep. Your body will sleep and benefit from the sleep, making you well, happy, rested, and happy in every way. Your body will sleep in refreshing sleep, and while your body sleeps, your witnessing conscious will remain. It will completely advance your control over your mind. And you will come to use your mind for the superb process it is".

"And you will use your memory accurately. You will remember things and recall things perfectly. Your memory functions perfectly in every way. Your memory functions perfectly. Your memory functions perfectly. Your memory is accurate and precise. And you will always have memory of things as they actually are. You are free from all disturbing memories from out of the past.

"All past memories have completely lost influence over you, and you live your life fully in the here and now. You appreciate fully that you are living in the here and now". "You appreciate fully that you are living in the here and now. You appreciate fully that you are living in the here and now".

"All these five functions of mind are coming completely under your control, and you can use these five main functions of mind to benefit your life in every way. The functions of your mind are at your command".

"The five functions of mind are right knowledge will always be yours; wrong knowledge you will automatically reject and allow it to have no place in your life; your imagination will be creative, and create wonderful and beautiful things. Your sleep will bring you perfect rest and well-being and while your body sleeps your witnessing consciousness will remain, advancing your control over your mind. And your memory will function perfectly, and you use your memories to help you to live life fully in the here and now".

"All of these suggestions go deep into your subconscious and become your reality; they become your way of life. The power over all your five main function of mind is your very own"!

Repeat this "suggestion formula" to your client three times in succession, ending with this suggestion.

"You now have perfect control over using correctly the five main functions of your mind; they will cause you to use your mind correctly, and will benefit you in every way".

Awaken from the hypnosis.

NOTE TO HYPNOTHERAPIST

Your subconscious knows intimately these five main centers of mental functioning. These suggestions presented in hypnosis stimulate them into action, heading mind in the direction of becoming the perfect process for producing thoughts that it is.

SUGGESTION FORMULA FOR MASTERING DESIRES

Using Hypnosis induce a deep level of hypnosis, rendering the subconscious mind wide open and receptive to these suggestions:

"You are becoming the master of your desires, for you know that your true source of happiness originates inside yourself. You still have desires for you are very much alive in the world and are filled with

energy to live life fully to the hilt. But your desires lead to self-betterment and benefit you in every way."

"You have discovered your inner SELF, and you know that your real source of happiness comes from inside yourself. Knowing where your real happiness comes from gives you perfect mastery over all desires. You can have fun with desires; you can play games with desires, but you can play the games or not play the games entirely as you choose, for you have become the master of your desires."

"In having perfect control over your desires you can enjoy whatever you want to desire. It is just a game of fun you play in existence. As master of your desires, happiness flows through you at all times, and you radiate happiness to others."

"You are filled with boundless energy, and your energy makes you complete master of your desires. Whenever you feel a need for desiring something, you witness it as a thing apart; and the decision whether or not to satisfy the desire is entirely under your own control. For you are the master of your desires and in this you have achieved a high state of the consciousness of desirelessness, and desirelessness makes you master of all your desires. In this awareness of your true nature you realize that your real happiness emanates from inside yourself and you know that you have no need to desire anything, as you already have it ALL. And so you can let desires come and go entirely as you please. For in knowing that your inner SELF is your real source of happiness desire for anything has completely lost control over you. For you are the master of all desires. You are the master of your SELF."

"You have discovered your SELF, and know that your true happiness comes from deep inside yourself. Knowing this has given you perfect control over all desires. You have become the master of desires."

"And your mastery over desires has given you control over all your habits. You can enjoy a habit when you want to enjoy it, but you enjoy it because you want to enjoy it not because the habit makes you. When you do not want a habit, you simply let it go. It is easy, for becoming master of desires has given you absolute control over your habits. So you are now also the master of your habits."

"You know from whence your real source of happiness comes, and so you now have perfect control of all desires in the world. You will appreciate and enjoy life to the fullest extent in the world, but you know that your real source of happiness is not to be found in the *outside world but is found within yourself."*

"It feels so good to be master of your desires. It makes your mind free and happy, as you have no need whatsoever to satisfy desires. You are the master of all desires."

"You know your SELF which dwells in your inner world. You know that you are complete in every way, and there is nothing you need to desire. YOU HAVE IT ALL ALREADY!"

"These suggestions of being master of your desires go directly into your subconscious mind and become your very own, making you the master of all desires for your SELF, which is your source of real happiness."

Repeat this "suggestion formula" three times in succession to your client, and then awaken from hypnosis.

NOTE TO HYPNOTERAPIST

Mastering desires and recognizing the source from which real happiness comes produces a quantum leap in awareness. It heads you in the direction of optima consciousness.

SUGGESTION FORMULA FOR ADVANCING CONSCIOUSNESS

Using Hypnosis induce a deep level of hypnosis, rendering the subconscious mind wide open and receptive to these suggestions:

"You know your SELF as an individual consciousness. There is no one else precisely like yourself in the entire universe. You now know your true nature. You are becoming increasingly conscious of your consciousness with every breath you take."

"You are becoming ever more aware of your true nature with every breath you take. You recognize yourself as a consciousness dwelling inside your body. You recognize yourself as consciousness. You recognize yourself as a consciousness. You recognize yourself as a consciousness. And in this becoming conscious of your consciousness you are advancing your consciousness; your consciousness is advancing to become optima consciousness in which you recognize your true nature as the immortal being that you are, in complete harmony with the universe."

"This advancing of consciousness to optima consciousness floods your mind like a bright light, and all things become clear to you. You begin to experience flashes of optima consciousness coming into you. And these flashes of KNOWING the truth about all that IS will come into you more and more from this time forward. Your consciousness is advancing. You are attaining optima consciousness."

"As your consciousness advances, your mind is freed of the chatter of thoughts and becomes silent; and the input of KNOWING WHAT IS comes into you. KNOWING comes into your mind with crystal clarity."

"As your consciousness advances, more and more you recognize your immortality, and you cease to identify so closely with your body in this lifetime or in previous lifetimes."

"Your mind is becoming clear like crystal, and you are beginning to think with crystal clarity. Direct perception of truth of what IS about all things and about what you think flows into you, as your consciousness advances. Your mind is beginning to function to perfection."

"As your consciousness advances the reasoning powers of your mind become positive and optimistic. Your thoughts are filled with energy and produce energy that you direct toward their attainment. And you are attaining to optima consciousness. Your intellect and your ability to think with crystal clarity and to know instinctively what is truth are advancing in leaps and bounds. Your mind is becoming boundless. You can clearly answer all questions for yourself and others through the direct perception that comes through optima consciousness. You are advancing to optima consciousness. You are advancing to optima consciousness. You are advancing to optima consciousness."

"You can use the power of reflection now which brings you in glimpses of truth about the things you reflect upon. This experiencing of truthful reflection advances more and more your consciousness."

"Your mind is becoming silent and you can automatically clear your mind of a ceaseless barrage of thoughts anytime you please. It is easy for you to do, and as your mind becomes silent under your control you advance more and more towards attaining optima consciousness. And you are beginning more and more to KNOW about your true nature. You recognize your true nature, and you understand about your immortal nature, and that you have lived lives upon lives in an ever-increasing expansion of consciousness."

"The memories of your past will more and more begin to flow into your mind, bringing up information that will be valuable to you. And memories will begin to flow up from your subconscious of things that happened in the past, and facing them squarely will remove their influence over your current life, and give you perfect peace of mind."

"As your consciousness advances to optima consciousness you are developing faith in yourself. You are becoming filled with bio-energy. And this energy advances your consciousness ever more and more."

"And you are developing self-remembrance, and in everything you do you will witness yourself doing it, and you KNOW you are the one who is doing whatever you do. Your self-awareness is advancing and is part of your advancing consciousness."

"When you walk you will know it is YOU who are walking. When you eat you will know it is YOU who are eating. When you talk you will know it is YOU who are talking. With everything you do YOU will have self-remembrance that YOU are the doer."

"And as your consciousness advances you will be discriminating in recognizing your true nature. KNOWING will come into you in having an awareness of your SELF. As your conscious advances to optima consciousness your mind concentrates upon whatever you turn your attention. This quality of concentration goes hand-in-hand with your advancing consciousness."

"Your consciousness is advancing to optima consciousness. Your consciousness is advancing to optima consciousness. Your consciousness is advancing to optima consciousness. It is the case!"

Awaken your client from hypnosis now, and the session is complete.

NOTE TO HYPNOTHERAPIST

The four "suggestion formulas" given in this chapter are very powerful. Present them to subconscious mind one at a time. That is one per session. These are the suggestions of a MASTERMIND, and will subconsciously go into action They open up the vistas of mind and a new way of life

CHAPTER FOURTY-ONE

Chinese Special -- Hypnotic Acupressure

We are giving you a method of hypnotizing of special use to all the people of Asia. it is based upon the ancient Chinese art of acupuncture.

Healing by acupuncture, in-which needles are inserted in various meridians (energy centers) to master various forms of illness has been used by the Chinese for centuries. In recent years, interest in acupuncture has swept into the Western World as well.

The use of inserting needles in the meridians requires skillful training, so while the same method is applied in this method of hypnotizing, acupressure on special points of the body is used instead of needles. The method will be found to operate splendidly, and is readily handled. Study it well.

This method of hypnotizing belongs to the Chinese people. It operates by applying pressure directly on the meridian centers of the body. These centers are nerve sensitive, and when depressed automatically command attention and compound with the suggestions of the hypnotists to produce affects upon the body producing deep relaxation, and leading directly to responsive hypnotic sleep. These meridian areas can be felt as little depressions in the body into which the fingertip can be inserted in maintaining pressure. Some areas are quite sensitive and pressure will produce slight sensations of pain. This is beneficial to the process. So as you perform it press in firmly and deeply. The method can be applied to subjects either seated or lying upon a bed. The latter is recommended.

Begin by energizing your hands, as you have been instructed. Now perform the process in the following steps.

STEP ONE:
Have client remove any excess clothing and shoes. Then recline in a comfortable position with hands resting at sides and feet slightly apart. Client is to be absolutely comfortable. Explain to client that in this method of hypnotizing you are going to apply pressure to the various meridian centers of his body, using scientific Acupressure; that the process will cause him to automatically relax, and that he will very likely doze off to sleep. Tell him to just let himself GO!

STEP TWO:
Have client close eyes and take three deep breaths. Then touch center of top of head and instruct him to roll his eyes back under his closed lids as though looking at the point inside his head. Tell him to keep looking at the inside point as you suggest Eyelid Fixation. In this position, the client will find it physically impossible to open his eyes. This successful, tell him to relax his eyes downward now and drift off to sleep, as you stimulate the Meridian Centers of his body, starting at his feet and advancing to his head -- each pressure point sending him down deeper and deeper into hypnosis.

STEP THREE:
Locate point on left foot just behind ball of foot in line with middle toe. Press in deep. Hold for five seconds, while suggesting to client that he will notice how relaxed the pressure on this center causes his foot to become and it feels numb.

Do the same on right foot.

STEP FOUR:
Locate point on left foot just below the bulge of inner ankle. Press in deep. Hold for five seconds. Continue suggestions of how relaxed the pressure is making his feet become.

Do the same on right foot.

STEP FIVE:
Move fingers up left leg about 3" above ankle, and press in on the inner rear edge of shinbone. Hold for five seconds. Suggest that the numbness and relaxation experienced in feet is now beginning to arise on up his legs.

Do the same with right foot.

STEP SIX:
Locate point on left foot just below the outer bulge of outer left ankle. Press in. Hold for five seconds. Continue suggestions of feet relaxing.

Do the same on right foot.
STEP SEVEN:

Locate point on left leg just below level of kneecap. Press in at top of calf muscle. This is a tender spot. Suggest legs becoming relaxed and numb.

Do the same with right leg.

Suggest that legs and feet are now completely relaxed, and the relaxation causing sleep will move on up his body now, as further Acupressure is applied.

STEP EIGHT:
Locate point on front of body midway between pubic hair and navel. Press in firmly. Present suggestions and just let your-self GO now and drift away to pleasant sleep, as the pressures on the meridians, continue on up the body.

RELAX BETWEEN

STEP NINE:
Locate point on front of body just below end of breastbone. Press in firmly. Suggest, Let yourself go completely now, and just drift away into sleep.

STEP TEN:
Locate point on body 3" up from last point depressed, and press in thus upon center of breastbone. Press in firmly. Suggest, Sleep, go deeply to sleep now.

STEP ELEVEN:
Perform pressure together using both thumbs at points located in depression end of shoulder bones where the arms and shoulders meet. Continue suggestions of Sleep. Deep sleep. Drift away into sleep, as you feel the pressures. The pressure will melt away as you drift away into sleep. Breathe deep and sleep.

RELAX BETWEEN

STEP TWELVE:
Locate point (called "Joy of Living" point) at inner crease of right elbow. Bend elbow and place tip of thumb in crease.

Then unbend arm and press in. Press on relaxed tissue always. Suggest Sleep. Deep sleep.

Perform the same on left elbow.

STEP THIRTEEN:
Move hand down arm from point twelve, to point located 2" down arm on outside of right arm. Press in. Suggest, Your arms are becoming numb and you are going to sleep. Sleep. Deep sleep.

Perform the same on left arm.

RELAX BETWEEN

STEP FOURTEEN:
Move on down right arm further on outside to point 2" up from wrist, in line with little finger. Press in. Suggest, Sleep. Go to sleep. Deep sleep.

Perform the same on left arm.

RELAX BETWEEN

STEP FIFTEEN:
Locate point on back of right hand between thumb and index finger. Press in deeply. Suggest Sleep. Deep sleep. RELAX PRESSURE. Press in deeply again and suggest, Sleep. Deep sleep. Perform this relaxation and pressure on the point for five consecutive times.

Perform the same on left hand.

RELAX BETWEEN

STEP SIXTEEN:
Locate point on crease inside of right wrist, in line with little finger. Press deeply. Suggest. Sleep. Deep sleep. Breathe deeply now and go deep to sleep. Watch client's breathing in response to these suggestions. If it deepens trance is ensuing.

RELAX BETWEEN

STEP SEVENTEEN:
Locate point top of each shoulder, midway between neck and tip of shoulder. Press deeply with both hands together. Suggest Sound asleep now. Deep sound sleep now. Deep into hypnotic sleep now.
Relax between allowing time for suggestions to sink home.

STEP EIGHTEEN:
Locate point on face and press in on crevasse between upper lip and tip of nose. Suggest, Deep in hypnosis now. Sleep deep in hypnosis now.

RELAX BETWEEN

STEP NINETEEN:
Press in on area between the eyes (3rd eye area). Skull bone structure does not allow depressing on this point surface pressure will suffice. Maintain a steady pressure, as you suggest, You are deep in hypnosis now, and as you sleep your subconscious mind opens wide to receive the beneficial suggestions that will now be given it.

RELAX BETWEEN

STEP TWENTY:
Press on top of head in small depression located there. Continue a steady pressure on top of head, as you suggest. Sleep on deeply now completely undisturbed, but your subconscious mind is fully alert and is receptive to the beneficial suggestions which will be now presented to it. These suggestions are exactly what YOU want and will benefit you in everyway. They will become your very own.

Relax a moment and remove pressure from top of head. Then press in again on this acupressure point, and present whatever positive suggestion formula is desired as requested by the client.

Repeat suggestion formula three times. Then suggest:

"These suggestions go deep into your subconscious and become your habitual way of healthful behavior for yourself. When they have become thus establish as reality in your subconscious, you will automatically arouse yourself from the hypnosis feeling wonderful and fine with a KNOWING that you have successfully accomplished what you desire".

ALLOW THE CLIENT TO SLEEP ON HYPNOSIS UNTIL AWAKENING FROM THE TRANCE ON THEIR OWN DESIRE TO AWAKEN. ACCUPRESSURE HYPNOSIS WILL HAVE BENEFITTED YOUR CLIENT IN EVERYWAY. THIS WILL BE FOUND A SUPERLATIVE METHOD OF HYPNOTIZING, AS THE ACUPRESSURE UPON THE MERIDIAN CENTERS AUTOMATICALLY PRODUCES RELAXATION AND CAUSES A SLEEP RESPONSE. THUS, THIS METHOD EMBODIES BOTH A PHYSICAL CAUSATION COMBINED WITH THE PSYCHOLOGICAL ASPECTS OF SUGGESTIONS PRODUCING A PROFOUND STAGE OF HYPNOSIS, WHICH IS VIRTUOUSLY IRRESISTIBLE.

HYPNOTIST TOM SILVER STANDING INFRONT OF A BUDDHIST TEMPLE IN THE MOUNTAINS OF TAIWAN (1994)

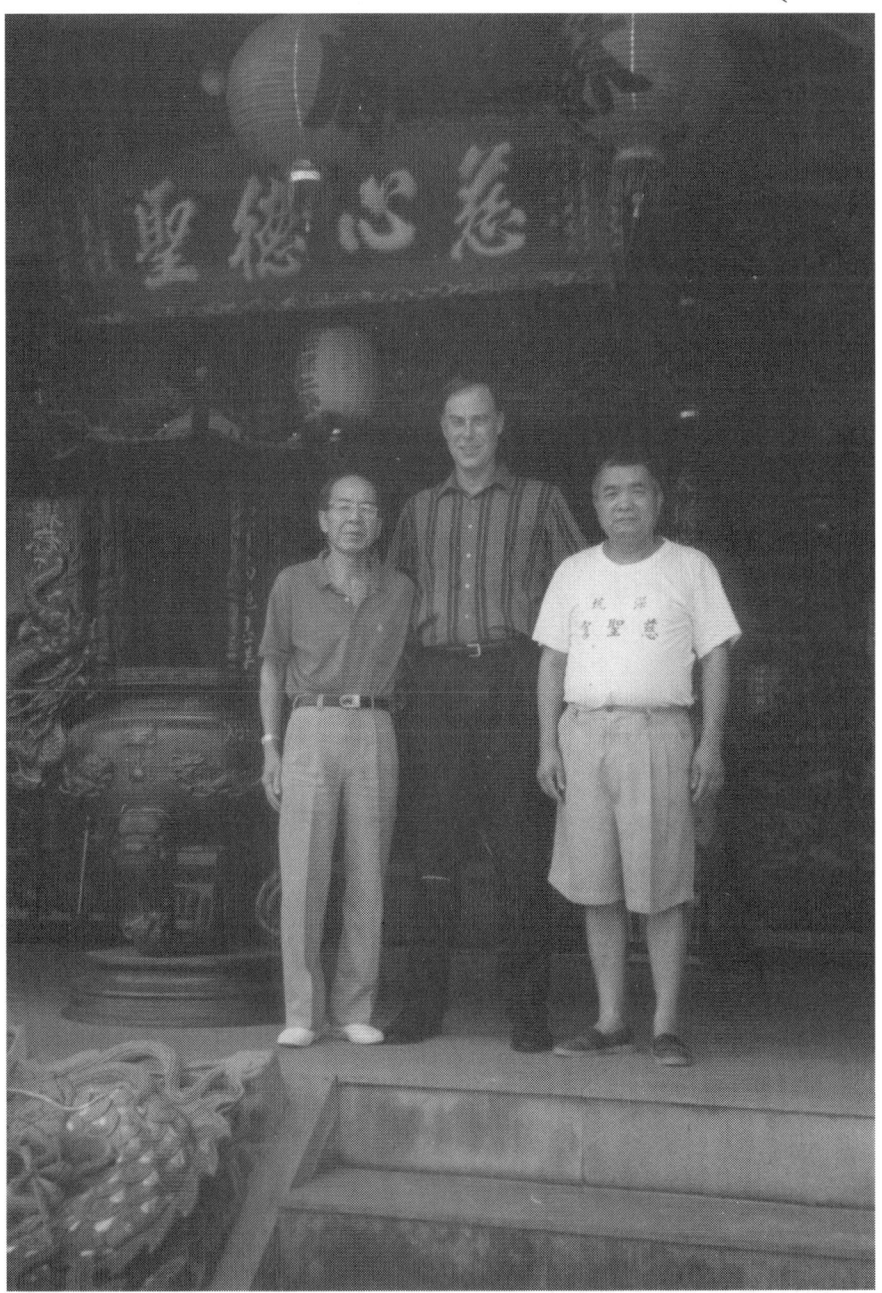

TOM SILVER DISCUSSES REINCARNATION WITH THE LOCAL RELIGIOUS FIGURES WHO HAVE WATCHED TOM CONDUCT A PAST LIFE REGRESSION ON TELEVISION

CHAPTER FOURTY-TWO

AN EXTRA GIFT FOR OUR CHINESE FRIENDS

BUDDHA'S "FLAME IN THE HEART" MEDITATION

We can think of nothing that we can give our Chinese friends of more meaningfulness than is this glorious meditation from the Buddha. We will begin by explaining a little about meditation.

The processes of meditation is not philosophical, it is existential. You cannot tackle such problems as your reality by just thinking about it, you have to live it through, go through it, allow yourself to be transformed by it. That is, to know love one will have to be in love. Then you will not remain the same. The experience will change you. The moment you enter love, you come out a different person; when you come out your will not be able to recognize your old face. It will no longer belong to you. A discontinuity will have happened and you come out a new being. Now there is a gap. The old person is gone and a new person has come. And the new person stands face to face with your inner SELF.

Meditation is Eastern the performance of which has swept into the Western. Hypnosis is Western, which is commencing to sweep into the Eastern. In Hypnomediation we have a blending and a combining of these two. It is like the forming of a developing union of a mental/spiritual bounding between people of the Orient with people of the Occident. Hypnomeditation will be found to be a remarkable process that are both scientific and operational -- objective and subjective -- it is functional. You don't have to believe in anything special to use the process. You don't have to have faith in anything. Really, you don't even have to understand the mental and spiritual levels upon which they operate, for they operate spontaneously for you. They are automatic because they are part of your very nature. And so this gift we give you is to become part of your very nature: The Buddha's beautiful "Flame In The Heart" Meditation.

Of this meditation, the sutra says, "Waking, dreaming, deeply sleeping, know yourself as light."

First start with waking. Your state of mind can be said to be mainly in three divisions. These are waking, sleeping and dreaming.

And consciousness is the fourth state, which is beyond mind. Consider the states of waking sleeping and dreaming as being like clouds in the sky (a waking cloud, a sleeping cloud, a dreaming cloud, and the sky in which they move is consciousness.

In the waking state you are not free, society is there, national boundaries are there, laws are there, moralities are there. Stress is there, for stress is innate to the waking state. One is in constant struggle with his, or her own desires; only in dreams are you free. Only in dreams are you authentically yourself.

You can do whatever you like in your dreams. No one is concerned. You are alone. Dreams are entirely your personal business, and belong exclusively to your private world. Because they are absolutely private and belong to no one beside yourself, you can be free. But still they are clouds -- private, freer, but still clouds, and you have to go beyond them also.

Appreciate that in your waking state you are one person; dreaming you become a different person, and while in deep sleep you are even more a different person. While in deep sleep you can't even remember your own name; you don't know whether you are or not; you have no identity; you have no image: you are boundless. Hence it can be said that in the waking state you exist with society. In the dreaming state, you exist with your own desires, and in the deepest sleep you exist with nature. Only beyond these three can you exist in the optima Whole. So these three must be passed beyond, transcended. The Buddha's Flame In the Heart Meditation is a transcendental technique, and you can do it by knowing yourself as light.

While awake -- moving, eating, working, whatever -- know yourself as light. Visualize the image as if your heart has become a flaming torch and is burning brightly, and your body is nothing but an aura around the flame. Allow this image to go deep within your mind and saturate your consciousness. Imbibe it! Let the image become an integral part of your very nature.

Go on imagining it and feel it. In this way, the image of yourself as a continuous flame will become part of your sense of yourself. While awake, always see yourself as a flame moving.

No one else will be aware of it in the beginning, but as you continue, others will also become aware. Never mention to others what you are doing -- just do the meditation and let others become aware of the change in yourself, through their own sensing. They will continue to sense to subtle light around you.

When you come near them they will feel a different warmth; if you touch them they will feel a "fiery" touch. Something beautiful is happening to you that is tangible.

Now, take this image of your flaming heart and your surrounding body as an aura of light into dreaming. Now it is no longer imagining, it has become a reality. Through visualization you have uncovered reality. It is reality because everything consists of light. You are light. Take this reality into your dreams.

When falling asleep, go on thinking of the flame, go on seeing it burning in your heart; feel it, feeling that you are light, condensed light. And so remembering fall asleep. In the beginning, you will start having some dreams in which you will feel you have a flame within and that you are light. By and by, in the dreams, also, you will move with the same feeling. And once this feeling enters your dreams your dreams will start disappearing -- there will be less and less dreaming and more and more deep sleep. When the dreams disappear, then you can carry this feeling into sleep. Now you are at the door. Now you can enter with the feeling. And once you enter sleep with the feeling that you are a flame, you will be aware of it, for this is a special kind of sleep that happiness only to your body, not to YOU.

This meditation -- this wondrous gift given you -- will help you go beyond these three states of mind if you can be aware that you are a flame and that sleep is not happening to you. You are consciousness, which is crystallized around that flame, you, yourself, are asleep but your SELF is not. This is transcendental sleep. While others are asleep YOU are awake. Your body sleeps, but only the body. The body needs rest because the body is a mechanism, but consciousness needs no rest because consciousness is not a mechanism. The way of the body is birth, youth, middle age old age and death. Consciousness is never born, never becomes old never dies.

If you can carry this image of flame and light through the door of sleep, your SELF will never sleep again, only your body will sleep. And when the body is sleeping you will know it. Once this happens, you become the fourth state -- consciousness. All the three states you have passed through are divisions of the mind's waking, dreaming, deep sleeping. As you become a "traveler," these states become "stations" along the way, so you can move from here to there and come back again. These "stations" are parts of the mind, and you have become the fourth -- one who goes through all of them and is none of them. You are the fourth, and that fourth is Divine.

"WORKING ON HYPNOSIS BOOKS AND HAVING FUN"

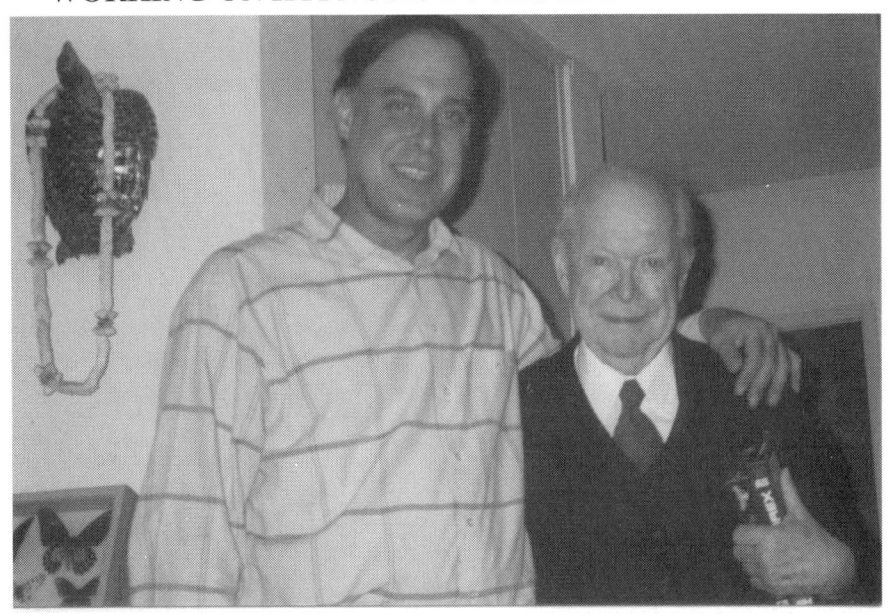

TOM SILVER SPENDING QUALITY TIME WITH ORMOND MCGILL AT ORMOND'S HOME IN NORHTERN CALIFORNIA *1995

THE "AURA" THAT SURROUNDS ORMOND MCGILL

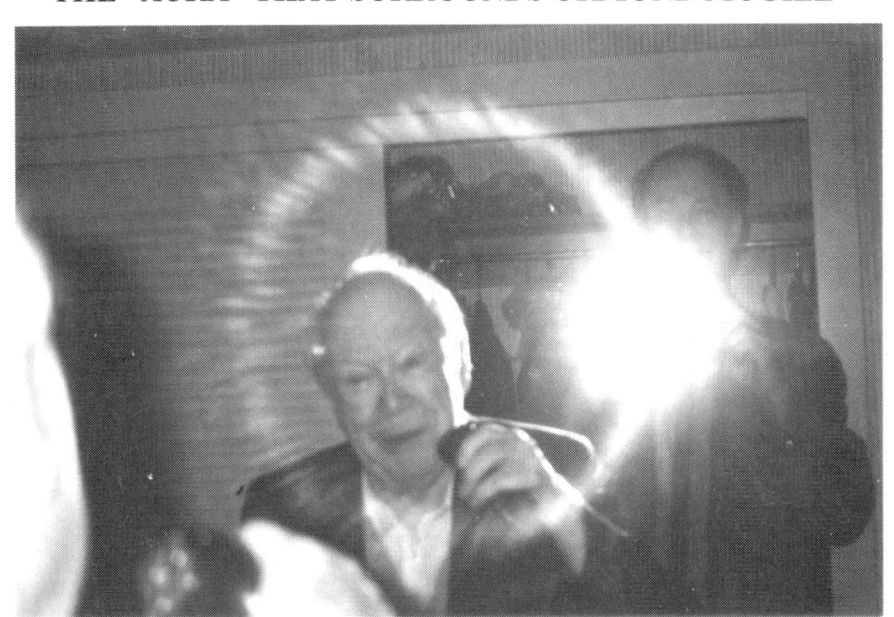

TOM SILVER PHOTOGRAPHS ORMOND MCGILL SHAVING IN THEIR HOTEL ROOM AND LOOK WHAT APPEARS ON THE PHOTOGRAPH
THE NATION GUILD OF HYPNOTISTS CONFERENCE IN LAS VEGAS NEVADA *1999

HAND LOCKING TOGETHER
RAPID HYPNOSIS INDUCTION

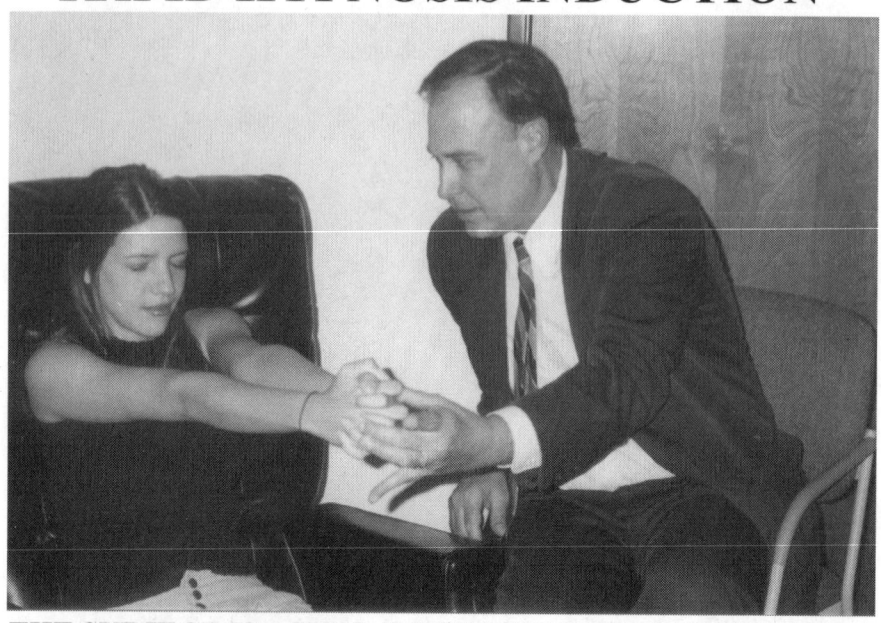

THE SUBJECT IS ASKED TO IMAGINE THAT HER HANDS ARE LOCKED AND STUCK TIGHTLY TOGETHER

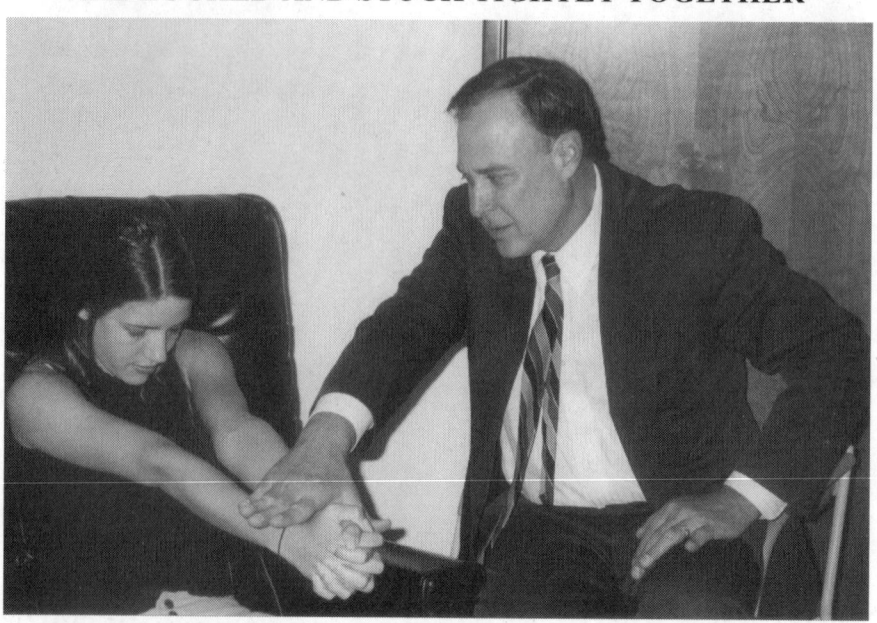

NEXT THE HYPNOTIST PUSHES THE SUBJECTS LOCKED HANDS DOWN AND SAYS THE WORD "SLEEP"

The Buddha's "Flame In the Heart" is one of the most remarkable meditative techniques in existence, but first try it in the waking state, and let others around you act as your guides, as to your stature in it. When others become aware of the change in yourself, as the flame burns brighter and brighter within you and your body radiates as an aura of light, then you can enter into the dream, then into deep sleep, and then you can awaken to that which YOU really are.

Make this meditation, this gift from The Buddha, become a part of yourself and implant it deeply in your subconscious. Place yourself in the Self-Hypnosis state, using the method that has been given you, and when you reach the point in the induction process where you are ready to receive the suggestions into your subconscious, place your hands over your ears and read aloud or to yourself this wonderful suggestion-formula. It will become your very own .

"I ACCEPT THE WHITE LIGHT OF PROTECTION INTO our INNER BEING AND "The Light Floods Me With Energy." I INSTINCTIVELY KNOW THAT our MIND HAS THREE DIVISIONS OF WAKEFULLNESS, DREAMING, AND SLEEPING. I KNOW THAT our REAL SELF IS A CONSCIOUSNESS BEYOND ANY OF THESE DIVISIONS. I KNOW KNOW THIS IS TRUE. AT ALL TIMES WHILE I AM AWAKE I WILL SENSE our SELF DEEP INSIDE our SELF AS BEING A FLAME. I AM A FLAME. I AM A FLAME. I AM LIGHT. our HEART HAS BECOME A FLAMING TORCH AND IS TURNING BRIGHTLY, AND our BODY IS AN AURA AROUND THE FLAME. I AM A FLAME. I AM LIGHT. our HEART IS A FLAMING TORCH OF FLAMING LOVE FOR ALL TO FEEL WHO COME NEAR ME. AND WHEN I SLEEP I WILL DREAM OF THIS FLAME WHICH BURNS WITHIN ME. IT IS BEAUTIFUL. IT IS GLORIOUS. IT IS LIGHT. I AM LIGHT! I AM LIGHT! I AM LIGHT! AND I STAND APART FROM our SELF AND RECOGNIZE our SELF AS THIS FLAME. I PASS BEYOND WAKING, BEYOND DREAMING, BEYOND SLEEPING, AND I RECOGNIZE our SELF as our SELF WHICH IS A FLAME. FOR I AM LIGHT!"

Sink down into the realm of Self-Hypnosis now. Go down deep into it. After a time, arouse your-self as you will. You will sense an inner warmth inside yourself, as the flame begins to burn in your heart. Brighter and brighter within you will burn the flame until its warmth is so great that others around you will sense it too.

Once the flame is kindled it is self-perpetuating. Others will feel your flame within for there is a difference in you now -- you have become a prince or princess.

Implant this meditation using Self-Hypnosis often. Meditation is pure gold, but this gift from Buddha adds to the gold a fragrance. All the great masters had "The Flame Within." Artists have shown it as a halo drawn about the heads of such as Christ, Buddha, Lao Tzu, Kirshna, and Shiva. This halo is not mere decoration, it is symbolic of the auric presence; a presence as a Being of Light: who brings hope and love to the world and all mankind. Use this gift often. Not only will it remove stress from yourself, but your very presence helps others as well. As the Masters have expressed it: Let your light so shine among mankind.

TRULY MAY YOUR ENLIGHTENMENT BE A BEACON THAT WILL SHINE SO BRIGHTLY THAT IT WILL LIGHT THE WAY FOR OTHERS IN FINDING THEIR OWN ENLIGHTENMENT

HAND LOCKING TOGETHER
RAPID HYPNOSIS INDUCTIONS BY TOM SILVER

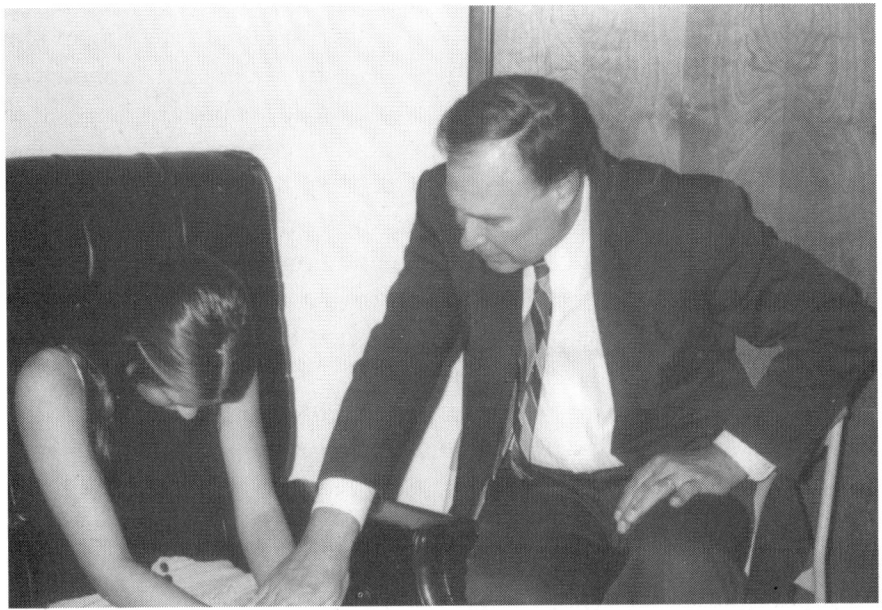

THE SUBJECT IS ASKED TO DROP HER HEAD DOWN HYPNOTIZED

HAND SLIPS OUT OF SUBJECT'S HAND

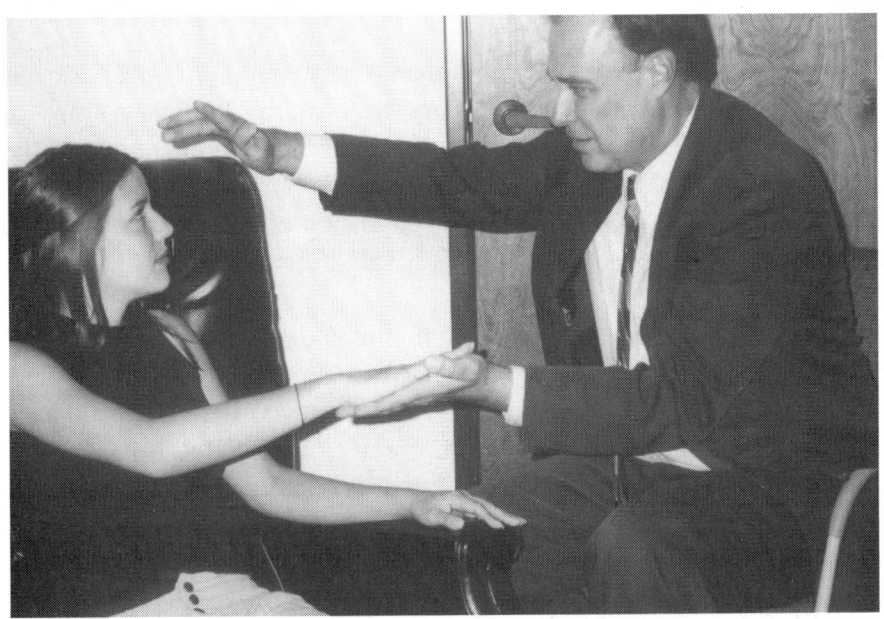

THE HYPNOTIST INSTANTLY SLIPS HIS HAND OUT OF SUBJECTS

ABOUT THE AUTHORS

Ormond McGill is a name with which to conjure to those who know mystery. He is known as the "Dean of American Hypnotists", and as a magician and hypnotist of international reputation has toured in many parts of the World with his exciting stage shows: "East Indian Miracles," "Mental-Magic", and the "Concert of Hypnotism". Ormond McGill is a member of the International Brotherhood of Magicians and the Society of American Magicians. In addition, he is also a naturalist of prominence, his contributions to entomology and conchology being well known. Among his previously published books are: *The How-To Book of Hypnotism (co-written by Tom Silver)*, *The Secret World of Witchcraft*, *Religious Mysteries of the Orient* (co-authored with Ron Ormond), *The Encyclopedia of Genuine Stage Hypnotism*, *The Art of Stage Hypnotism*, *How To Produce Miracles*, and *Entertaining With Magic* to name a few.

Tom Silver is a clinical hypnotherapist with a private practice in Southern California. He is the Founder and creator of The Silver Hypnosis Institute in Southern California. Tom Silver has been successful training students and currently teaches advanced courses in Hypnotherapy to hypnotherapists around the world. He is an expert in Group Hypnosis with over twenty years of experience. Tom Silver has toured the World conducting seminars, lectures, and demonstrations on hypnosis. Mr. Silver was one of the first clinical hypnotherapists in the world to create the method of Mass-Hypnosis through an interpreter in a foreign language. Tom Silver is the co-author along with Dr. Ormond McGill of the hypnosis book entitled "The How-To Book Of Hypnotism".

In February 1995, Tom Silver hypnotized over thirty-eight hundred people at the same time in Taiwan, R.O.C. setting the first "Interlingual Hypnosis World's Record". He hypnotized the entire audience in Mandarin Chinese through an interpreter. This method of hypnosis that Tom Silver created and authored is classified as "Interlingual Hypnotic Trance Induction" © 1995.

While in Taiwan, Tom Silver lectured about the positive therapeutic values of hypnosis on National Taiwan Television and to the Taiwan Police Academy, members of the Taiwan Olympic Committee, students, professors, doctors and businessmen. He also hypnotized famous celebrities weekly on the #1 most watched television show in Taiwan called "Super Sunday". Between 1997 and 1999, Tom Silver worked for The Taiwan Department Of Defense is helping to activate memories from some subjects that might have been involved in the biggest weapons procurement scandal and murder in Taiwan's history.

Tom Silver was awarded a "Gold Plate" of Honor from the Taiwan Minister Of Defense in July of 1997 for his work in using hypno-investigation to help retrieve memories of the crime and murder of Taiwan Navy Captain Yin Cheng-feng, which took place in Taiwan back in December of 1993.

Tom Silver has also lectured and performed for companies, universities, and corporations throughout the world, including Microsoft Corporation, Hughes Aircraft, Hitachi Corporation, the 3M Corporation, Costco Corporation, Atlantic Richfield, UCLA and Loyola Marymount University, just to name a few. Tom Silver has helped companies and their employees increase productivity in the workplace, creating a happy, motivated, stress-free environment. Students have also found Tom Silver's method of hypnotherapy and CYBERSUGGESTION™ to be very beneficial.

Tom Silver has appeared and performed live hypnosis demonstrations on such television shows as "The Sally Jesse Rafael Show", NBC "The Other Half" with Dick Clark, "WB" Beyond with "James Van Praagh" NBC "Life's Moments", TNN "Ultimate Revenge", FOX Television Special "Powers of The Paranormal", "Hypnotized", his own CBS television one hour special, Comedy Centrals "The Mans Show", the "Montel Williams Show" on UPN, the "Mike & Mattie Show" on ABC, and the "Home and Family Show" on the Family Channel. He has also been performing live on radio since 1990.

Tom Silver's hypnosis lectures and seminars are energizing, exciting, fun and inspiring. His abilities as a therapeutic technician and hypnotherapist have helped thousands of people around the world become happier, healthier, and more successful in their lives.

EEG BRAIN WAVE SCAN OF SUBJECT IN WAKING STATE
CONSCIOUS BRAIN WAVE FREQUENCY ACTIVITY OF "BETA" (30Hz)

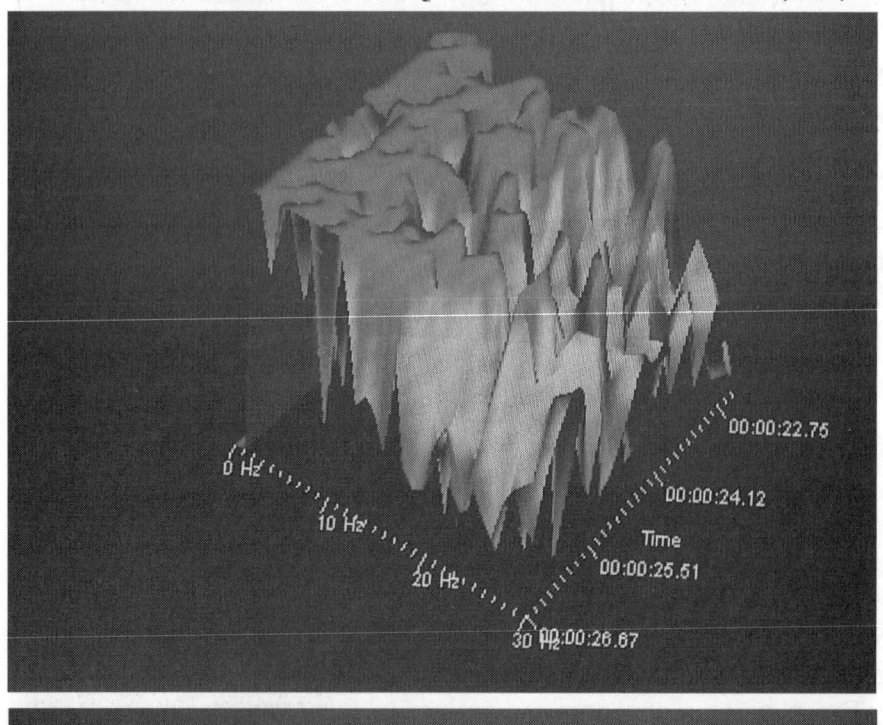

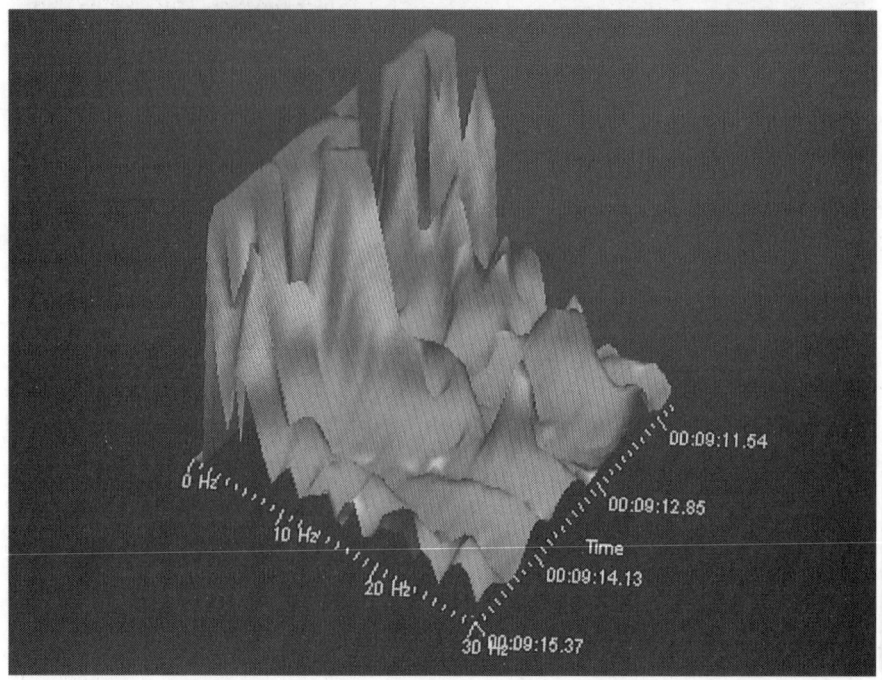

EEG BRAIN WAVE SCAN OF SUBJECT WHO HAS BEEN HYPNOTIZED
SUBCONSCIOUS BRAIN WAVE FREQUENCY "THETA" WITHIN 9 MINUTES!

THE SOUR LEMON TEST

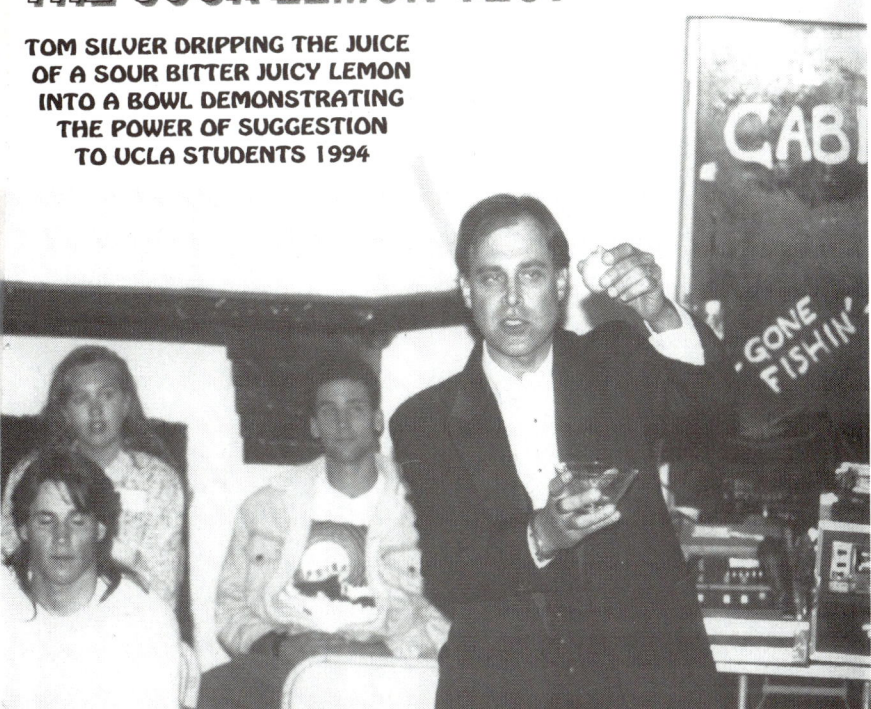

TOM SILVER DRIPPING THE JUICE OF A SOUR BITTER JUICY LEMON INTO A BOWL DEMONSTRATING THE POWER OF SUGGESTION TO UCLA STUDENTS 1994

TOM SILVER HYPNOTIZING UCLA STUDENTS USING THE HEAVY HAND LIGHT HAND INDUCTION TECHNIQUE

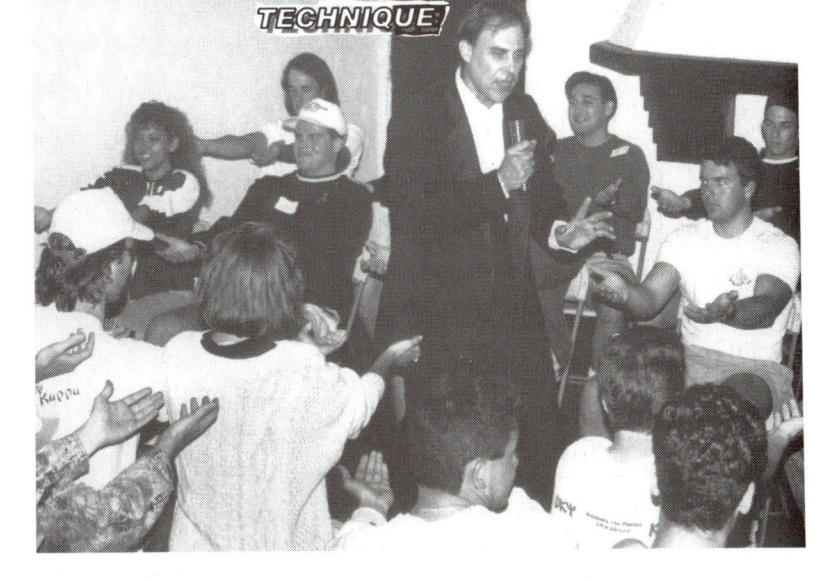

TOM SILVER'S HYPNOSIS VIDEO SEMINAR WORKSHOPS

Tom Silver

Hypnosis
Inductions That Work

TOM SILVER'S HYPNOSIS INDUCTIONS THAT WORK VIDEO SEMINAR WILL TEACH YOU HYPNOSIS INDUCTIONS THAT WILL CHANGE YOUR LIFE!

INSTANT HYPNOSIS INDUCTIONS!
RAPID HYPNOSIS INDUCTIONS!
INSTANT HYPNOSIS INDUCTIONS!
AND SHOCK INDUCTIONS!

THIS SEMINAR GIVES YOU STEP BY STEP INSTRUCTIONS AND ACTUAL LIVE HYPNOSIS INDUCTIONS AS TOM TEACHES HYPNOTHERAPY STUDENTS THE INDUCTION TECHNIQUES THAT HAVE MADE TOM TELEVISIONS FAVORITE HYPNOTIST!

TO ORDER THIS SEMINAR CALL TOLL FREE 1 888 646-3797 OR ON THE WEB AT www.tomsilver.com

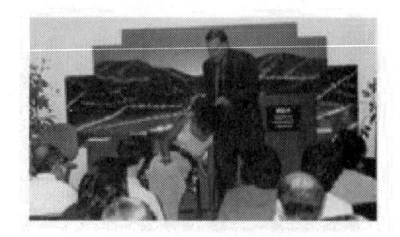

Instant Inductions
Rapid Inductions
Shock Inductions
and more!

VIDEO SEMINAR

HYPNOTHREAPIST
TOM SILVER
PRESENTS

FEARS & PHOBIAS

BECOME A FEARS AND PHOBIA EXPERT WITH THIS VIDEO SEMINAR AND WORKSHOP

THIS HYPNOSIS VIDEO SEMINAR WILL TEACH YOU EVERYTHING YOU NEED TO KNOW ABOUT FEARS AND PHOBIAS AND HOW TO USE HYPNOSIS TO REMOVE FEARS

RAPID * PHYSICAL * INSTANT AND SHOCK HYPNOSIS INDUCTION TECHNIQUES ARE DEMONSTRATED AND TAUGHT IN THIS VIDEO SEMINAR

CALL NOW TOLL FREE 1 888 MIND P.W.R.

Hypnotherapist
Tom Silver

FEARS & PHOBIAS
Emotion Replacement Therapy (E.R.T)
Subconscious Reconditioned Response

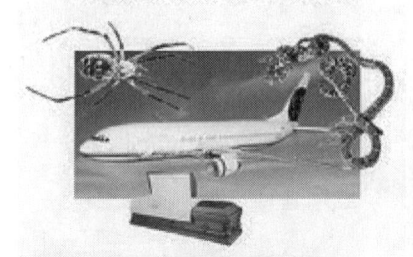

How To Remove Fears From The Subconscious Mind Through Hypnosis

Video Seminar

HYPNOTHERAPY STUDENTS PRACTICING SHOCK INDUCTION TECHNIQUES AT TOM SILVER'S HYPNOSIS INDUCTIONS SEMINAR AND WORKSHOP IN SOUTHERN CALIFORNIA (2000)

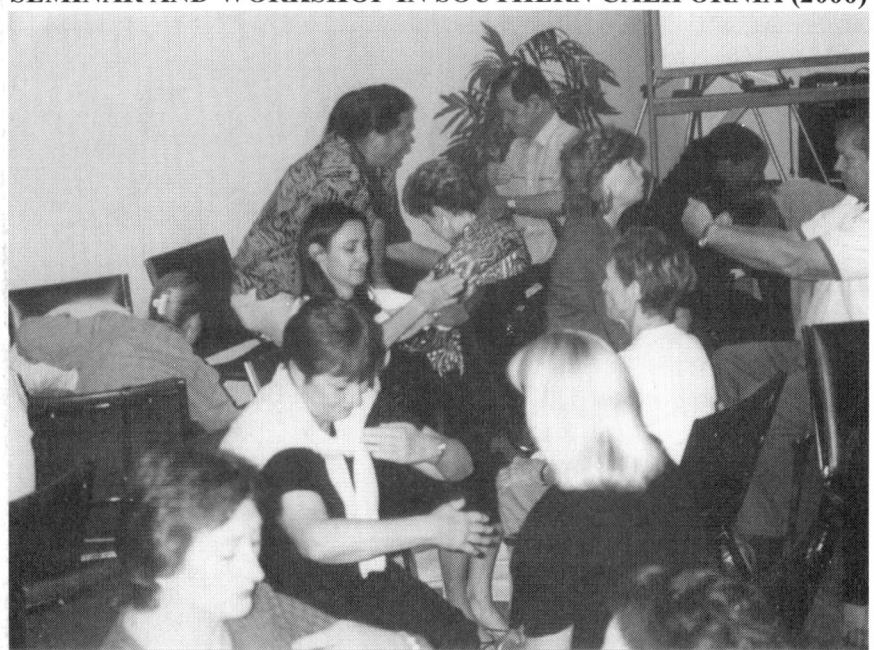

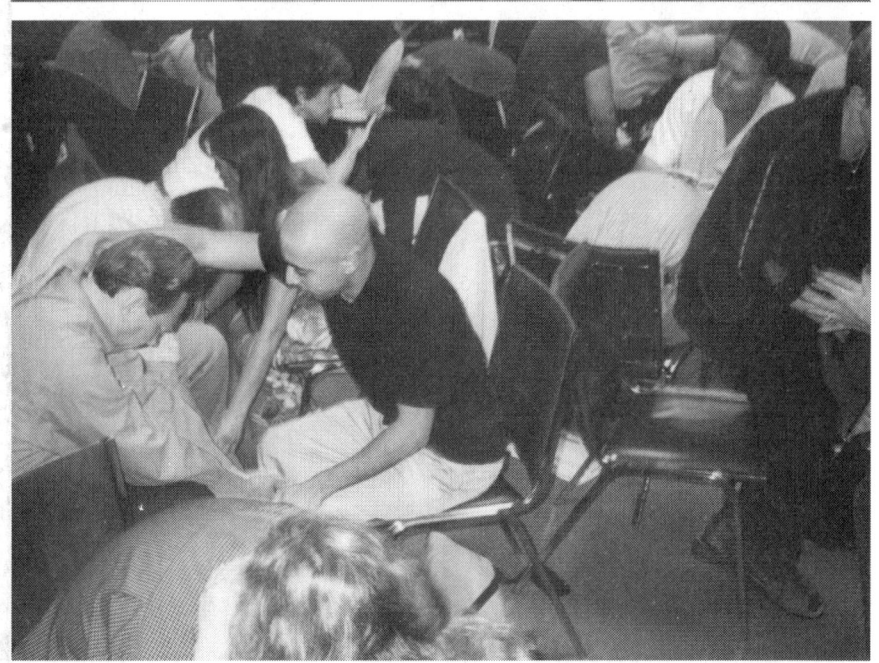

THESE HYPNOTHERAPY STUDENTS ARE BUILDING UP THEIR CONFIDENCE BY PRATICING SOME WONDERFUL HYPNOSIS INDUCTION TECHNIQUES THAT ARE FOUND IN THIS TRAINING AND TECHNIQUES MANUAL

READ THIS BOOK AND YOU CAN LEARN MORE ABOUT THE SCIENCE OF HYPNOSIS
THE ANCIENT ART OF MAGNETIC HEALING * TRANSLINGUAL HYPNOTISM *
STAGE HYPNOSIS ROUTINES FOR FUN ENTERTAINMENT* INSTANT INDUCTIONS

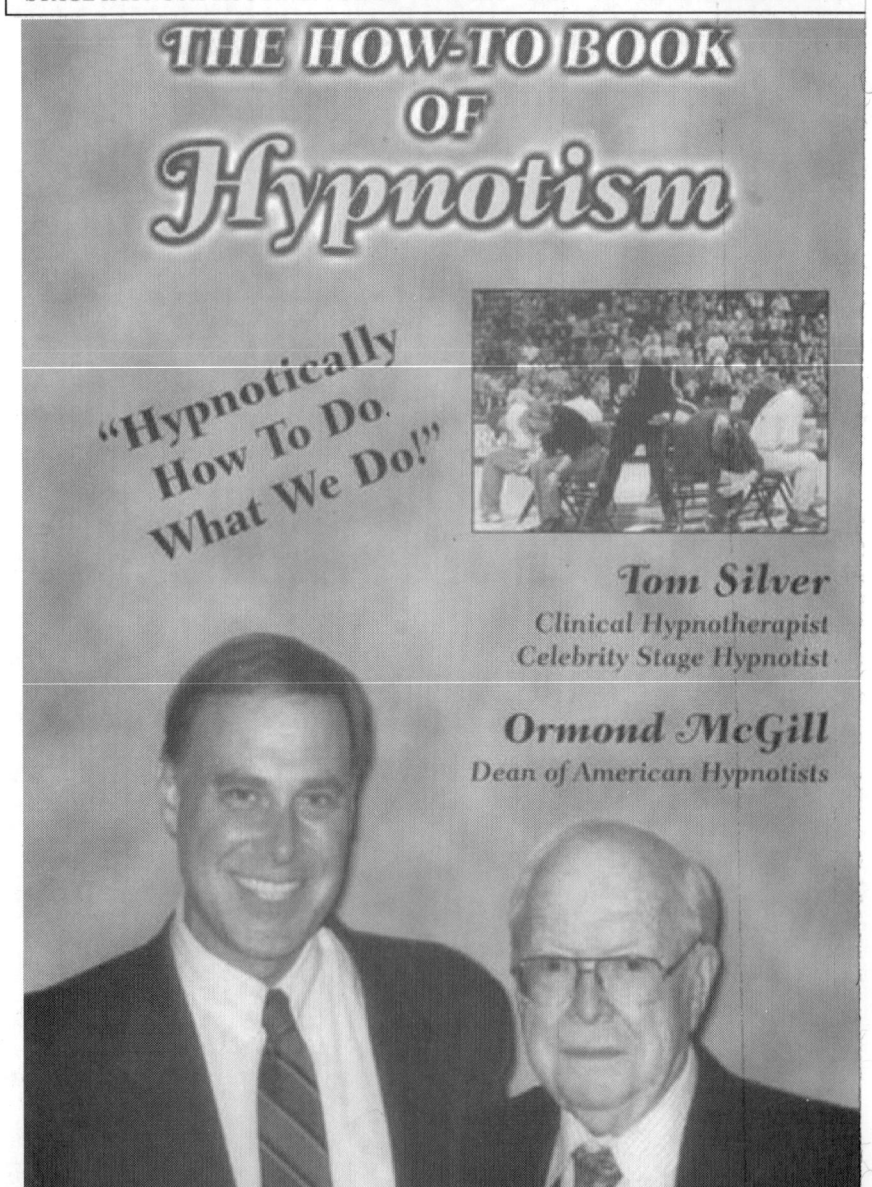

THE HOW-TO BOOK OF Hypnotism

"Hypnotically How To Do. What We Do!"

Tom Silver
Clinical Hypnotherapist
Celebrity Stage Hypnotist

Ormond McGill
Dean of American Hypnotists

Learn The Secrets of Hypnosis

TOM SILVER AND ORMOND MCGILL'S
THE HOW-TO BOOK OF HYPNOTISM